In: Health and Human Development Series

OBESITY AND ADOLESCENCE: A PUBLIC HEALTH CONCERN

HEALTH AND HUMAN DEVELOPMENT SERIES

Joav Merrick (editor)

Disability from a Humanistic Perspective: Towards a Better Quality of Life
Shunit Reiter
2008 ISBN 978-1-60456-412-9

Complementary Medicine Systems: Comparison and Integration
Karl W. Kratky
2008 ISBN 978-1-60456-475-4

Obesity and Adolescence: A Public Health Concern
Hatim A. Omar, Donald E. Greydanus,
Dilip R. Patel and Joav Merrick
2009 ISBN 978-1-60456-821-9

In: Health and Human Development Series

OBESITY AND ADOLESCENCE: A PUBLIC HEALTH CONCERN

HATIM A. OMAR,
DONALD E. GREYDANUS,
DILIP R. PATEL
AND
JOAV MERRICK
EDITORS

Nova Biomedical Books
New York

For permission to use material from this book please contact us:
Telephone 631-231-7269; Fax 631-231-8175
Web Site: http://www.novapublishers.com

Library of Congress Cataloging-in-Publication Data

Obesity and adolescence : a public health concern / editors, Hatim A. Omar, Donald E. Greydanus.
p. ; cm.
Includes bibliographical references and index.
ISBN 978-1-60692-821-9 (hardcover : alk. paper)
1. Obesity in adolescence. I. Omar, Hatim A. II. Greydanus, Donald E.
[DNLM: 1. Adolescent. 2. Obesity. 3. Public Health. WD 210 O112125 2009]
RJ399.C6O325 2009
616.3'9800835--dc22

2008050565

Published by Nova Science Publishers, Inc. ✦ New York

Contents

Preface

A mantra has developed in the late 20th century and early 21st century that has an underlying bias against overweight and obese individuals, who are blamed for their "disease" and told by society to lose weight or suffer the consequences. Art was used from 22,000 BC through the 19th century to glorify obesity, while art of the current era vilifies or mocks obesity. Considerable discrimination awaits the obese child, adolescent, or adult in current society, whether in the form of bullying in school, limited social life, or job refusal. Concern over obesity leads many youth to unhealthy diet practices that involve starvation and/or bulimic features. In this book, leading international experts discuss obesity in adolescence.

Indeed, what are the ethics of obesity management for the health care professionals of today? Perhaps proper obesity management begins with an examination of why obesity was desired for so many centuries, an acceptance that obesity is not the patient's fault, that many overweight/obese individuals are happy as well as healthy and that the economics of current obesity "treatment" must be reexamined and reconfigured.

This book has been created and edited by four leading physicians in child health and human development.

Chapter I - The link between obesity and hypertension is examined in this chapter. Underlying mechanisms include increase in sympathetic activity, sodium balance, renal tubular sodium reabsorption, glomerular filtration rate (GFR) and development of insulin resistance. The role of leptin is examined in the development of hypertension in obese adolescents. Also considered in this review are the definitions of hypertension and principles of management for obese youth with hypertension. Pharmacologic agents used for management of hypertension include diuretics, alpha blockers, beta blockers, angiotensin converting enzyme inhibitors (ACE inhibitors), angiotensin-2 receptor blockers (ARBs), and long acting calcium channel blockers. The importance of weight control, caloric restriction, and exercise in the management of obesity in youth is also stressed.

Chapter II - This chapter has a two-fold objective. One, it addresses the association of hyperandrogenism and obesity and the complex metabolic derangements that are part of the problem. Clinical management of these co-morbidities is challenging and complex. Second, this article will aid health care providers with the key features to an early diagnosis and intervention to decrease the morbidities in the short as well as long term. Method: Systematic review of articles and information on the topic of interest that were published in the last 15 years. Conclusion: Obesity and hyperandrogenism are integral parts of Metabolic Syndrome/Polycystic Ovarian Syndrome (PCOS)/Hyperandrogenism, Insulin resistance, and Acanthosis Nigricans (HAIR-AN). With the childhood obesity epidemic, the metabolic syndrome and the associated abnormalities are routinely seen in clinical practice and these have a tremendous economic burden on the society and the quality of life.

Chapter III - There has been a profound increase in the prevalence of obesity over the last 20 to 30 years causing the coining of the term "obesity epidemic" in children, adolescents and adults. It is believed to be due to a complex interaction of social and environmental factors in the overall lifestyle pattern. The increased rate of obesity is seen to be associated with increasing incidence of type 2 diabetes mellitus in adolescents, along with perturbations of the other endocrine axes, as well as, higher risk of long term complications. It is therefore of the utmost importance that concerns about overweight and obesity be addressed from early childhood and adolescence to avoid resultant significant morbidity and/or mortality.

Chapter IV - Obesity presents special challenges for skin care and is associated with several conditions that need careful attention. Conditions reviewed in this chapter will include acanthosis nigricans, papillomatosis of Gougerot and Carteaud, polycystic ovary syndrome, striae distensae, Cushing disease, and Cushing syndrome in relation to their dermatologic aspects. Various treatment modalities reviewed include bathing, soaps, cleansers, shampooing, emollients, topical corticosteroids, topical antibacterials, antifungals, and topical retinoids.

Chapter V - Although obesity is not classified as an eating disorder, there are associations between obesity and anorexia nervosa, bulimia nervosa, and binge eating disorder. This chapter reviews some of these associations. For example, a proportion of patients with anorexia nervosa eventually become bulimic and some of these patients eventually become overweight, while anorexia is often seen in a previously obese patient who loses weight successfully and then cannot stop losing weight or continues to try to lose weight even after reaching an otherwise normal weight range. There are possible genetic components for obesity as there are for anorexia nervosa and bulimia nervosa, but there are also associations with the family environment, particularly with family dietary habits. Obese patients should be screened for the presence of an eating disorder, especially bulimia nervosa and binge eating disorder. Obese patients who successfully lose weight should also be carefully observed for the possible development of anorexia nervosa. Principles of management are also reviewed.

Chapter VI - Adolescence is a critical period of growth and development in an individual's maturation from puberty to adulthood. A key component of normal adolescence is the process of healthy sexual development that is influenced by an inevitable passage through the stages of maturation from infancy to adulthood. Primary care clinicians should understand and appreciate the importance of sexuality in the lives of their adolescent patients. Obesity is one of the factors that influence sexuality in adolescents. The purpose of this chapter is to succinctly discuss the relationship between obesity and adolescent sexuality. In this regard, it is vital to examine whether obesity alone can derail healthy adolescent sexual development. Not all overweight adolescents experience severe negative outcomes because of their obesity. However, for those who do experience negative sexuality issues, the sensitive and caring clinician can help direct them to helpful resources to address these critical issues.

Chapter VII - All sexually active youth, whether obese or normal weight, should be offered counseling regarding contraception and appropriate contraceptive methods. However, obese youth who are sexually active may be less likely than their normal weight peers to use contraceptives correctly. Methods of contraception for obese adolescents are reviewed in this discussion. Combined oral contraceptives (COCs) and the contraceptive patch have higher failure rates in obese versus normal weight females, though failure rates are lower than noted with barrier contraceptives. The risk for venous thrombosis is higher in obese youth on COCs. Progestin-only pills and the levonorgestrel intrauterine system appear to be safe and effective methods in obese females. Depot-medroxyprogesterone acetate, intravaginal ring, and implants are also considered.

Chapter VIII - Obesity is increasingly prevalent in adolescents with significant lifelong medical complications. The exact prevalence of obesity among adolescent athletes is not known; however, there is research that suggests obesity prevalence varies by the type of sports. A few studies suggest that youth sport participation can be an effective tool in the management of obesity in children and youth. Regular physical activity and sport participation that is fun is strongly recommended. This discussion considers the role of sports in helping obese adolescents and also what physical activity is recommended. It is concluded that sports participation can be an important part of effective management of obese youth and setting the stage for a lifelong pursuit of physical activity to control and/or reduce obesity in the adolescent and adult population.

Chapter IX - Adolescents are becoming less physically active and are increasingly adopting a sedentary life-style in front of computers and television screens. In this chapter we look at self-related health, physical activity, sleeping habits, the prevalence of overweight and body complaints in two senior high schools with questions about weight and height, health, physical activity, type of physical activity/sport, intensity, sleeping habits and possible injuries or complaints during the last three months. Seventy seven percent % of the high school students participated in sports on a regular basis. In academic programs compared to vocational programs, more males and females in academic programs participated in sports (71% and 80% respectively). Males reported significantly better health than females, but 65% reported body complaints during the last three months. A higher number of females than males reported back and hip complaints. Good sleep was reported in 82.1% of the males (76.6% of the females). In males 44.3% were often sleepy in the daytime (females 56.6%). Underweight, physical activity and good sleep were found to be factors with significant positive effect on good health, whereas overweight was a negative factor. Proper sleep habits and higher physical activity levels should be promoted among high school students and TV viewing time and video game use restricted. Additionally, schools should provide opportunities for young people to participate in a wider range of physical activities that address their individual needs, while promoting the health benefits of engaging in regular exercise.

Chapter X - Lack of physical activity and overweight status continues to be a significant health problem in the United States. To assess the actual prevalence of these problems, we reviewed data from the School-based Health Promotion Centers in one middle school, and one high school in central Kentucky. A total of 232 6th graders and 607 9th graders were included. A total of 92% of 6th graders and 45% of 9th graders reported complete lack of regular exercise. 37% of 9th graders and 59% of 6th graders had inappropriate nutrition, 47% of 9th graders and 33% of 6th graders had Body Mass Index over the 85th percentile for age. Among overweight adolescents, only 16% of 9th graders and 1% of 6th graders thought they were overweight. Since the body mass index data is derived from actual objective measurement, we conclude that overweight status is a significant problem in Kentucky and that the actual numbers may be higher than those reported for the State based on surveys and estimates. Furthermore, many adolescents are not aware of their weight problem and most of them do not participate in regular exercise.

Chapter XI - Obesity has been deemed a public health epidemic, which carries with it high financial and psychological stakes, social consequences, and ethics of public, mental, and medical health care research pushing for all adolescents, who are "obese" to lose weight. This article reviews the psychological aspects of overweight in adolescents. No single factor has been shown to cause obesity; most researchers agree that the causes of obesity are multifaceted and complicated. Adolescents who are overweight may experience the deleterious effects of obesity on psychological functioning. Concepts of beauty, perceptions of body image and satisfaction all contribute to the psychological attitudes and beliefs about personal value, worthiness, self image, body satisfaction, and dieting. Not all adolescents who are at-risk-for-overweight or are overweight are unhealthy. Clinicians should consider that just as they warn the obese about the risks of obesity, they must expend as much energy evaluating the risks of successful weight loss. They must also remember that there are other standards of beauty and body size among ethnic groups and other cultures. The weight for height by body type tables that are used to calculate BMI should be changed to reflect the body types and fat distributions of Latino- and African-Americans.

Chapter XII - The global epidemic of childhood and adolescent overweight has become a major public health concern. Not only are these youth more likely to become obese as adults, and thus more prone to obesity-related diseases than their non overweight peers, they are also likely to suffer emotional and social effects associated with overweight. Overweight in youth has been linked to depression, low self-esteem, eating disorders, negative body image, and stigma. It appears to be bi-directional in nature, with overweight sometimes predicting certain psychological effects and psychosocial issues sometimes predicting overweight. Effective assessment and treatment of psychological and mental health issues in overweight youth will help overweight youth deal more effectively with their social and psychological milieus. Additionally, interventions for mental health concerns may have the added health benefit of increasing weight loss, thus decreasing obesity-related disease for which the overweight adolescent is prone.

Chapter XIII - This chapter in order to learn how female and male adolescents view their dissatisfaction body parts and to learn how gender-related body dissatisfaction parts of Thai adolescents differ from those studied in Western countries. We studies 400 Thai male and female adolescents in Bangkok, attending high school to freshmen level, and ranging from 16-19 years. Survey questionnaires containing questions related to the research objectives were distributed to every student. We also conducted in-depth follow-up interviews with 40 students to gain insightful data. We found that Thai female and male adolescents viewed their dissatisfaction body parts differently. While Thai female adolescents viewed their dissatisfied body parts individually and looked at their bodies in detail, Thai male adolescents tended to view their bodies as a whole and describe their dissatisfied body parts as problematic area(s). Moreover, some of the results in this study showed similarity with research conducted in the West. However, there were also differences that can be seen in detail that showed a variation on the gender-related dissatisfied body parts names, percentage to each body part/areas, and its beautified meanings. Like studies conducted in the West, female adolescents showed greater dissatisfaction with their bodies and felt more pressure to fix problematic parts than men.

Chapter XIV - This chapter will describe the self-perception of body weight and other weight-related factors among 2,665 Taipei high school students. A high percent of the girls (70.7%) and boys (42.2%) reported that they were too fat and these percentages were much higher than those reported by US students in a recent Youth Risk Behavior Survey. In addition, only 13.2% of girls and 22.0% of boys reported being completely satisfied with their weight and the level of dissatisfaction with weight appeared to be greater than among US students. Yet, in comparison to US students, the Taiwanese students were considerably less likely than their US counterparts to engage in weight management practices (e.g., dieting, eating less food, using diet pills). Taiwanese students with a self-perception of being too fat were more likely than those with perceptions of being just right or too thin to engage in weight management practices, to be dissatisfied with their weight, feel that they were unattractive, estimate that their same-sex peers were trying to loose weight, and have a higher body mass index. The findings from this study showed a relationship between self-perception of body size and engaging in weight control behaviors was consistent with other research. It suggested that self-perception of body weight, more so than objective weight status, was predictive of weight loss behavior and also negative psychological outcomes associated with poor body weight image. As a result, self-perception of weight may be an important point of focus for the design and implementation of clinical and public health initiatives targeted at this adolescent population as well as others.

Chapter XV - Weight perceptions and weight control behaviors have been documented with underweight and overweight adolescents, yet limited information is available on normal weight adolescents. This chapter investigates the prevalence of overweight misperceptions and weight control behaviors among normal weight adolescents in the United States by sociodemographic and geographic characteristics. We examined data from the 2003 Youth Risk Behavior Survey (YRBS). A total of 9,714 normal weight US high school students were included in this study. Outcome measures included self-reported height and weight measurements, overweight misperceptions, and weight control behaviors. Weighted prevalence estimates and odds ratios were computed. There were 16.2% of normal weight students who perceived themselves as overweight. Females (25.3%) were more likely to perceive themselves as overweight than males (6.7%) ($p < .05$). Misperceptions of overweight were highest among white (18.3%) and Hispanic students (15.2%) and lowest among black students (5.8%). Females (16.8%) outnumbered males (6.8%) in practicing at least one unhealthy weight control behavior (use of diet pills, laxatives, and fasting) in the past 30 days. The percentage of students who practiced at least one weight control behavior was similar by ethnicity. There were no significant differences in overweight misperception and weight control behaviors by grade level, geographic region or metropolitan status. A significant portion of normal weight adolescents misperceive themselves as overweight and are engaging in unhealthy weight control behaviors. These data suggest that obesity prevention programs should address weight misperceptions and the harmful effects of unhealthy weight control methods even among normal weight adolescents.

Chapter XVI - The prevalence of obesity has increased to epidemic proportions in the United States in recent years. Obesity in the Western world is a disease of poverty that is seen much more often in minority populations. Obesity-related illnesses, such as type II diabetes, are now seen frequently in adolescents and even in younger children. Caloric intake has increased in adolescents over the last two decades along with changes in dietary composition fueled by advertisements of unhealthy foods by various food producers. Nutritional modification is an essential part of any weight-loss program. This chapter discusses various diet changes that are important to reverse this current trend of increasing obesity in all populations and ages. Highly-restrictive diets should be reserved only for the morbidly obese child or for those with obesity-related problems such as sleep apnea.

Chapter XVII - Obesity rates among children around the world have reached an epidemic level. Having an option to walk or bike to school is important for mobility, health and equity purposes. However, fewer students are walking or biking to school today than a generation ago, and fewer students live within a walkable distance to schools. This chapter highlights the existing evidence from multiple disciplines on health and equity issues related to school transportation. It then assesses the literature dealing with the built environmental correlates of walking or biking to school. Travel distance and safety were found to be the strongest predictors of walking or biking to school. Studies suggested that about one-half to one mile (0.8-1.6 km) between home and school was generally considered walkable. Other factors such as roadway conditions, sidewalk continuity, bike lane availability, signals, lighting, and neighborhood design appeared important but with some inconsistencies in the findings. Many commonly reported environmental barriers were related to transportation infrastructure, such as high-volume and high-speed roadways, unsafe street crossings, and railroads. Compared with distance, safety and transportation infrastructure, neighborhood characteristics such as density, land use, and overall street patterns appeared less significantly associated with school transportation. Our review revealed evidence supporting the link between school transportation and the built environment. It also discovered many remaining questions for future research, such as interactions and causalities between personal and environmental factors, environmental influences from multiple spatial scales, and differences between objective and perceived measures.

Chapter XVIII - Obesity in childhood has particular concern, because if it continues into adulthood, the result will be increased morbidity and decreased life expectancy. An increase in obesity in the general population in the developed world has been documented in recent years. This trend is also seen in persons with intellectual disability and in particular in persons with Down syndrome (DS). Persons with DS are prone to obesity already at an early age and several studies have shown a high prevalence in this population compared to persons with intellectual disability without DS and the general population. Persons with DS have a low resting metabolic rate and low dietary intake of individual nutrients and therefore exercise and vitamin-mineral supplement diet must be instituted in this population to prevent or minimize obesity and its adverse consequences.

Chapter XIX - Adolescent obesity is a major public health problem in Australia, and in many other parts of the world. Recent data suggest that as many as one quarter of young people in Australia are either overweight or obese, and that the majority of obese young people have one or more risk factors for chronic disease. Efforts to reduce the health and economic burden of obesity must focus on both management of affected individuals and prevention of further cases. This chapter reviews some of the research currently underway in Australia, and includes recent data on both the prevalence of obesity and the associated complications, from large surveys and smaller cohorts. State and Federal governments have developed policies aimed at obesity prevention, but these are yet to be fully evaluated. Two large-scale community-based interventions are underway, one of which has reported positive preliminary findings. A number of smaller research programs are examining macro and individual level causation of obesity and include unique research examining the way adolescents perceive their environment. Other research includes the development and evaluation of service delivery models specifically targeting adolescents. A greater emphasis on environmental determinants and management of adolescent obesity is needed in future programs.

Chapter XX - Research has focused on adolescent's food choice with the hope of finding key factors preventing obesity. We aimed to specifically spot relevant key factors that influence Bangkok children, aged 9-11 years old, their food buying preferences and behaviors in schools. Nutritional anthropological research methodology namely, participant observation, in-depth interviews, and buying and eating behaviors-related observation questionnaires were carried out among 27 participating elementary schools in Central Bangkok. This research aimed to discover detailed factors associated with individuality, sociality, environmental, and external influence over children's food choices. First, individuality factors associated to children's food choices involved the amount of daily allowance, children's food preferences, students' perception towards food ability in correlation with the frequency of school breaks, and children's rationale of food prices (reasonable/affordable range). Second, sociality factors concerned how individual(s) have shaped children's knowledge of food, food-related beliefs, and individual(s) that accompany/are present at the moment when children are buying foods. Third, environmental factors discovered were the location, distance, and quality of where food is being sold, shelving/how food is being displayed, and the availability of food knowledge the school displayed/provided for their students. Last, external factors identified the variety of mass media channels, which triggered children to desire new food items, were tested and shown no influence over children's food choice on school days. In conclusion, the insights gained can enlighten ways in which in-depth understanding of children's food choice and behaviors can be obtained in order to create a more efficient and culturally suited future obesity prevention plan.

Chapter XXI - Childhood and adolescent obesity are risk factors for poor health later in life as well as decreased life expectancy. This short communication reviews literature on obesity in Israel and examines several recent studies, which have clearly demonstrated rising rates of childhood and adolescent obesity similar in magnitude to those trends observed in other Westernized nations. It is incumbent upon relevant authorities within Israel to reverse these trends so as to prevent the long-term adverse health consequences associated with childhood and adolescent obesity. We recommend initiating a national educational campaign to promote exercise and healthy eating. This campaign would target children and adolescents and would rely upon evidence based guidelines for diet and exercise.

Chapter XXII - This chapter describes the prevalence rate of overweight and thinness in a population of adolescents living in two different areas of Italy and explores the body self-image perception and unhealthy eating behaviours and strategies to lose weight. A questionnaire was administered to a sample of 2,121 teenage students (1,084 males, 1,037 females). We found that adolescent females and males build and perceive their body images in very different ways. Most of the overall sample perceived their weight as normal, while a relevant 31.6% defined themselves as overweight and another 4.4% as heavily overweight. Analysis based on BMI (calculated through self-referred weight and height) showed that only 9.2% of our sample could be considered overweight and 1.7% obese. Most of female students (485 out of 1,037) were trying to lose weight, demonstrating that strategies to lose weight were undertaken also by girls perceiving themsleves as normal in relation to body weight. 46.8% girls were using strategies to lose weight compared with 21.9% boys. These strategies included very problematic behaviours like self-induced vomiting (3.3% F vs 1.7% M) and dieting pills (2.8% F vs 1.5% M) undertaken along with more usual thinning strategies like dieting and exercising. Girls were more prone than boys to exercise as a way to lose weight (41% vs 31.7%). We found a deep gap between actual weight and perceived body-image and weight. We believe primary prevention and health education programs aimed at improving teen body-image should be adopted as a strategy to reduce the eating disorder epidemics spreading among young people.

Chapter XXIII - Obesity is the most prevalent metabolic disorder in the United States with adolescents and children being the fastest growing segment of the population affected by this disorder. The initial management of obesity entails modification of diet and exercise as well as a trial of medications. Unfortunately, this usually has unsatisfactory results; as a result, bariatric surgery has been used in the adult population and seems to offer improved long term results. Because the results have been quite favorable in the adult population, specialists are also looking at bariatric surgery for the adolescent population. This appears to be a safe approach in conjunction with diet and exercise and it offers improved long term results. This article discusses the use of bariatric surgery in obese adolescents.

Chapter XXIV - This chapter reviews various medications currently used and being studied for weight loss induction in adults and adolescents. The search for medication to induce weight loss was stimulated by the US FDA's 1959 approval of phentermine, a sympathomimetic amine, for short-term weight loss despite limited research supporting its claims of causing weight loss. In addition to noradrenergic products like phentermine, other reviewed medications include herbal products (such as Korean herbal formula based on Taeumjowi-tang), sibutramine (mixed noradrenergic-serotonergic chemical), orlistat (lipase inhibitor), metformin (biguanide), rimonabant (CB1-selective cannabinoid receptor antagonist), and others. Only two non-amphetamine-related medications are FDA-approved for adolescents: sibutramine for those 16 years of age and older, and orlistat for those 12 years of age and older. Pharmacotherapy for morbidly obese adolescents should only be used as part of a comprehensive weight loss program that involves diet, exercise, and behavioral modification. The side effects of these products should always be considered as well as the potential for serious adverse events.

In: Obesity and Adolescence: A Public Health Concern ISBN: 978-1-60692-821-9
Editors: H.A. Omar, D.E. Greydanus et al.

I. Introduction: Obesity as a Public Health Concern

Obesity is often linked to the development of so-called "thrifty" genes that allowed some humans to survive for millions of years in the face of the constant threat of starvation due to persistent lack of available food. This adaptive response was important to the survival of homo sapiens, because it allowed the development of heightened ability to store precious and limited calories in the form of fat deposits in the body. One of the earliest art figures of the human figure is the Venus of Willendorf, a small (4 and 3/8 inch or 11.1 cm) Paleolithic figure housed in the Naturhistorisches Museum in Vienna, Austria [1]. The Venus or Woman of Willendorf was discovered by the Jewish archeologist, Josef Szombathy (1853-1943), in 1908. It depicts a pregnant woman with no face (typical of the Paleolithic era), who is also obese and dates back to 22,000 to 24,000 BCE. This Nude Woman of Willendorf suggests that obesity was a normal, desirable, and even idealized feature of being human and/or being a female.

This idea of the desirability of obesity is repeated in society throughout the existence of homo sapiens for thousands of years, until the 20th century. Paintings, for example, by the Flemish artist, Peter Paul Rubens (1577-1640) are consistent with the positive notion of being overweight or obese [2]. The famous 1625 Rubens painting "Arrival of Marie de' Medici at Marseilles, France" at the Louve Museum in Paris clearly depicts the wealthy of the 17th century as being overweight. Likewise, his "Allegory of the outbreak of war" in 1638 depicts the theme of chronic war in Europe, which can be seen at the Pitti Gallory of Florence, Italy and reveals that healthy supernatural and human beings are obese.

Negative reactions to obesity are found in the 20th and now the 21st century after countless centuries of positive reactions to those who had enough food to be overweight or obese. Scientific literature of the past generation are repleat with articles bemoaning the high prevalence of obesity in the American and the world's population—including children, adolescents, and adults. Various methods are used to identify obesity, including body mass index (BMI), triceps skinfold thickness (TST), bioelectrical impedance analysis, dual x-ray absorptiometry and others. Many studies using these various methods suggest a prevalence of obesity of over 20% in the United States, Europe, Asia, China, India, and many other countries [3].

The result is that millions of obese children, adolescents, and adults are seeking to lose weight using methods that are often unsuccessful in the short or long run. In 2003, the US Surgeon General noted that "Obesity is the terror within… as real as weapons of mass destruction…." [4]. Governement, insurance, and medical officials complain about the high medical costs incurred in the United States because of obesity. The weight loss industry has become a multi-billion dollar endeavor that employs a large number of individual to help many unsuccessfully lose weight, sell costly "weight-loss" products, and support hospitals developing expensive bariatric programs. Weight loss programs have sprung up in the United States and elsewhere making millions of dollars despite no research evidence for significant weight loss in the long run.

A mantra has developed in the late 20th century and early 21st century that has an underlying bias against overweight and obese individuals, who are blamed for their "disease" and told by society to lose weight or suffer the consequences. Art was used from 22,000 BC through the 19th century to glorify obesity, while art of the current era vilifies or mocks obesity. Fernando Botero (1932-)[5] is a well-known artist born in Medellin, Columbia, South America, who has become famous for his drawings using obese and morbidly obese subjects as a way of providing satirical commentaries on contemporary life.

Considerable discrimination awaits the obese child, adolescent, or adult in current society, whether in the form of bullying in school, limited social life, or job refusal. Concern over obesity leads many youth to unhealthy diet practices that involve starvation and/or bulimic features. Some health care providers admit to being repulsed by dealing with obese patients, who may be shuffled between various primary care clinicians and specialists who may not want them in the first place [4]. Measures employed by clinicians willing to "help" their obese patients are often unproven, unhelpful, and potentially harmful to their patients.

Indeed, what are the ethics of obesity management for the health care professionals of today? [4]. Perhaps proper obesity management begins with an examination of why obesity was desired for so many centuries, an acceptance that obesity is not the patient's fault, that many overweight/obese individuals are happy as well as healthy, and that the economics of current obesity "treatment" must be reexamined and reconfigured [4,6]. As we debate various diets and the role of food intake in obesity management, the role of physical exercise for all homo sapiens must be remembered and emphasized [7-10].

Professor Donald E Greydanus, MD
Pediatrics and Human Development, Michigan State University College of Human Medicine, Kalamazoo, Michigan, United States. E-mail: Greydanus@kcms.msu.edu

Professor Dilip R Patel, MD
Pediatrics and Human Development, Michigan State University College of Human Medicine, Kalamazoo, Michigan, United States. E-mail: patel@kcms.msu.edu

Professor Hatim Omar, MD, FAAP
Adolescent Medicine and Young Parent programs, Department of Pediatrics, Kentucky Children's Hospital, University of Kentucky College of Medicine, Lexington, United States. E-mail: haomar2@uky.edu

Professor Joav Merrick, MD, MMedSci, DMSc
National Institute of Child Health and Human Development, Office of the Medical Director, Division for Mental Retardation, Ministry of Social Affairs, Jerusalem and Kentucky Children's Hospital, University of Kentucky, Lexington, United States. E-Mail: jmerrick@internet-zahav.net.

References

[1] McDermott L. Self-representation in upper Paleolithic female figurines. Curr Anthropol 1996;37(2):227-75.
[2] Belkin KL. Reubens: Art and ideas. New York: Phaidon,1998.
[3] Rowlett JR. Obesity in the adolescent. In: Greydanus DE, Patel DR, Pratt HD, eds Essential adolescent medicine. New York: McGraw-Hill Med Publ, 2006:651-65
[4] Fleck LM, Petersmarck KA. Ethical considerations related to obesity intervention" In: Fitzgerald HE, Mousouli V, eds. Obesity in childhood and adolescence. Westport, CT: Praeger, 2008:271-303.
[5] Sullivan EL, Tapest J. Fernando Botero: A monograph and catalog at Raisonne painting. Lausanne, Switzerland: Acatos Publ, 2000.
[6] Burgard D. Blinded by BMI. Health Every Size 2005;19:45-53.
[7] Phelan S. Diet: Obesity. In: Hillard PJA, ed. The 5-minute obstetrics and gynecology consult. Philadelphia, PA: Wolters Kluwer/Lippincott Williams Wilkins, 2008:274-5.
[8] Gardner CD. Comparison of the Atkins, Zone, Ornish, and LEaRN diets for change in weight and related risk factors among overweight premenopausal women. JAMA 2007;297:969-77.
[9] Greydanus DE, Bhave S. Obesity in the adolescent. Indian Pediatrics 2004;41(6):545-50.
[10] Greydanus DE, Bricker LA, Patel DR. The benefits of sports participation in childhood and adolescence to prevent obesity in adolescents and adults. Asian J Paediatr Pract 2006;9(4):1-7.

II. Medical Aspects

In: Obesity and Adolescence: A Public Health Concern
Editors: H.A. Omar, D.E. Greydanus et al.
ISBN: 978-1-60692-821-9

Chapter I

Hypertension and Obesity

Alfonso D. Torres*[*]*, and Colette A. Gushurst
Pediatric Nephrology, Pediatrics and Human Development Michigan State University/Kalamazoo Center for Medical Studies, Kalamazoo, Michigan, USA

Abstract

The link between obesity and hypertension is examined in this chapter. Underlying mechanisms include increase in sympathetic activity, sodium balance, renal tubular sodium reabsorption, glomerular filtration rate (GFR) and development of insulin resistance. The role of leptin is examined in the development of hypertension in obese adolescents. Also considered in this review are the definitions of hypertension and principles of management for obese youth with hypertension. Pharmacologic agents used for management of hypertension include diuretics, alpha blockers, beta blockers, angiotensin converting enzyme inhibitors (ACE inhibitors), angiotensin-2 receptor blockers (ARBs), and long acting calcium channel blockers. The importance of weight control, caloric restriction, and exercise in the management of obesity in youth is also stressed.

Introduction

World health organization (WHO) data indicates that one billion individual are overweight and over 300,000 obese. Epidemiologic data reveal that the prevalence rates of obesity are increasing not only in the industrialized nations but also in developing countries. The number of overweight and obese adults in the United States of America (USA) has dramatically increased in the last 20 years. Approximately 60 % of USA males and 51% of the USA

* Correspondence: Alfonso D Torres, MD, Pediatric Nephrology Director, Michigan State University/Kalamazoo Center for Medical Studies, 1000 Oakland Drive, Kalamazoo, MI 49008-1284 United States. Tel: 269-337-6450; Fax: 269-337-6474; E-mail: Torres@kcms.msu.edu

females are overweight or obese [1]. Of particular concern is the relatively new phenomenon of increasing prevalence in overweigh and obesity in children and adolescents. This is an alarming problem observed in industrialized as well as developing countries and in the urban centers more than in the rural areas. Overweight was reported in 40.9% of Mexican-American adolescents (12-19 years of age) 40.9% while obesity was noted in 22.9%; males had a higher prevalence of overweight and obesity than females [2]. In Pavia, northern Italy, the percent of overweight and obese boys were 20.9% and 4% while percentages of overweight and obese girls were 14.7% and 1.1% respectively [3].

In Pune, India the prevalence of overweight base on BMI was 27.5% in boys and 20.9 % in girls; hypertension was present in 12% of the overweight boys and in 9.75% of girls while the prevalence of hypertension increased with the increase in BMI [4]. In Lausanne Switzerland, of 2507 children studied with a mean standard deviation (SD) age 12.3 (0.5) years, 2.2 % were found to be hypertensive; of the hypertensive children, 16.1% of the boys and 12.4% of the girls were overweight or obese based on the CDC criteria of BMI > 85th percentile [5]. In a study in Poland (city of Lodz), involving 25,309 children and adolescents between 7-18 years of age, the mean prevalence of overweight was 15.1%; 13.2% of the girls and 17% of the boys were found to be overweight.6 Obesity was found in 4.4% of the boys and in 2.9 % of the girls [6]. Prehypertension was found in 11.1% and hypertension in 4.9 %; hypertension was more prevalent in the younger group ages 7-13 years than in the older group's age 14-19 years [6].

Similar observations have been made in Germany, China, and other countries. In the United States the prevalence of obesity increased from 5% to 13% in boys and from 5% to 9% in girls between 1996-1970 and 1988-1991 respectively [7]. In the United States, disparity exists in childhood and adolescent prevalence of obesity between regions and states of the Country [7]. South and central regions of the United States have an obesity prevalence of 18% while the mountain region has the lowest prevalence of 11.4% [7]. Children in West Virginia, Kentucky, Tennessee, Texas, and North Carolina all have an adjusted obesity prevalence >18.3%; this is over twice the odds of been obese than their Utah counterparts who have an adjusted prevalence of 10.4% [7]. Socioeconomic status, neighborhood, social capital, television viewing, recreational computer use, and physical activities account for 55% of the regional and states differences in the prevalence of obesity [7].

Substantial differences exist in the prevalence of overweight and obesity among different ethnic groups. African-American women and Mexican-American of both sexes have the highest prevalence of overweight in the United States today. However, the "epidemic" proportions of overweight and obesity can not be explained on the basis of familial or genetic factors alone. As a consequence of technologic advances over the past 30 years in agriculture, industry, communications, transport, commerce and medicine have brought changes in lifestyle all over the world, promoting a sedentary, self gratifying lifestyle in large number of children and adolescents. Education about appropriated nutrition and the importance of participation in physical activities has lagged behind [8].

Overweight and obesity are not variations of normal growth of children and adolescents, but that of illnesses requiring intervention. Excessive weight gain is an important risk for comorbidities involving multiple organ systems: endocrine, cardiovascular, gastrointestinal, pulmonary, orthopedic, neurologic, dermatologic, and psychosocial. Clinical manifestations of overweight and obesity are many, including those listed in table 1.

Based on the current prevalence of adolescent obesity in the United States, the prevalence of obesity in 35-years-olds will be in the range of 30% to 37% in men and 34% to 44% in women by the year 2020. A total increase in the number of patients with cardiovascular diseases is also expected to occur. Deaths secondary to coronary heart disease will increase in number and will occur in younger individuals as they approach middle age [9]. Recently a meta-analysis epidemiologic study involving 247 published papers indicated that there was a strong positive association between BMI and risk for kidney disease outcomes [10]. The authors concluded that 24.2% and 33.9% of kidney diseases among American men and women respectably (versus 13.8% in men and 24.9% in women in other industrialized countries) could be related to overweight and obesity [10]. Obesity by itself is clearly linked to glomerulomegaly and to a secondary form of focal segmental glomerulosclerosis, likely on the bassis of a hyperfiltration mechanism [11].

Obesity and Hypertension

The relationship between obesity and hypertension is well documented in children and adolescents, with blood pressure following an almost linear correlation though time; hypertension develops more often in those individuals that have been obese for over five years. Obesity is clearly related to type-2 diabetes mellitus and systemic arterial hypertension. Type 2 diabetes mellitus and hypertension are major risk complications of the development of coronary heart disease and chronic renal disease. Abundant clinical observations indicated that hypertension improves with reduction of body weight. Animal experimental observations that are highly reproducible demonstrate predictable elevation in blood pressure in association with high fat diets in dogs and rabbits as well as obese human beings [12].

Table 1. Complications of obesity

Hypertension
Type 2 Diabetes
Cardiovascular diseases
Cerebrovascular diseases
Sleep apnea
Back pain
Osteoarthritis
Non-alcohol-related fatty liver infiltration
Kidney diseases
Malignancies
Psychosocial disturbances

How Obesity Induces Hypertension?

Experimental data in obese animals and clinical observations in obese humans are associated with hemodynamic, neurohumoral, and renal changes that include increased arterial pressure, heart rate, and cardiac output. There is increase in sympathetic activity, sodium balance, renal tubular sodium reabsorption, glomerular filtration rate (GFR), and development of insulin resistance [13]. Endothelial dysfunction and carotid intimal thickening are also observed in children and adolescents with obesity and hypertension.

The increase in cardiac output observed in obese individuals is not necessarily directed to the increased adipose tissue. The change in blood flow is more likely due to general vasodilation induced by increase metabolic rate in many organs given the increase in organ size; this vasodilation is probably mediated by nitrous oxide (NO) produced by the endothelium and seems to occur early, before the development of vascular disease.

Increase heart rate early in obesity seems to be mediated by diminution of the parasympathetic tone in the heart, rather than change in sympathetic activity [14]. There are many studies however, linking obesity with hypertension and the role of the sympathetic nervous system activity in this relationship [15]. Ethnicity may be an important factor to consider given the fact that sympathetic nervous system activity as well as propensity to obesity and hypertension differ with different ethnic groups. In obesity, sympathetic nerve system activity is increased in skeletal muscle, as detected by microneurography that measures muscle sympathetic nerve activity; this technique has shown consistent elevation of such nerve activity in obesity [16]. One detrimental effect is to increase sympathetic activity to the peripheral vasculature resulting in vasoconstriction with time. Pharmacologic inhibition of the sympathetic nervous system(SNS) with alpha and beta blockers reduces blood pressure to a greater extent in obese than in lean individuals.

Examination of norepinephrine spillover in obesity has shown regional hyperactivity in the kidneys. Increase SNS activity in the kidneys cav lead to sodium retention and abnormal hemodynamics resulting in increased blood pressure. Patients with obesity-associated hypertension present with positive sodium balance and expanded extracellular volume. In normal subjects, expanded extracellular volume triggers mild increase in blood pressure, resulting in a significant sodium excretion by the kidney and restoration of normal volume. This phenomenon is known as "pressure natriuresis" and functions as a physiologic back-up system for preservation of the extracellular volume. In hypertensive obese individuals, pressure natriuresis is impaired, requiring higher blood pressure to excrete a sodium load. In experimental obese animals, sympathetic renal denervation attenuates renal sodium retention associated with high fat diet. Several other potential mechanism have been implicated in the activation of the SNS in obesity associated hypertension, including hyperinsulinemia, increase levels of free fatty acids, impaired baroreceptor reflexes, obstructive sleep apnea, and cytokines release from adipocytes. Visceral obesity is a high risk for obstructive sleep apnea that is often seen in association with hypertension. These patients have an increased peripheral chemoreflex response to hypoxia resulting in activation of the SNS.

Table 2. Interactions of adipose tissue

Central and Peripheral Nervous systems
Endocrine system
Cardiovascular system
Musculoskeletal system
Renal system
Immune system

There is also a clear link between visceral fat accumulation and SNS activity and hypertension is mediated through the visceral fat production of leptin. Leptin is a protein produced mainly by visceral adipose tissue that acts in the central nervous system. Leptin plasma concentration is elevated in obese humans [17]. One of the leptin pathways in the hypothalamus involves stimulation of the pro-opiomelacortin neurons in the arcuate nucleus that then send projections to the paraventricular nucleus and lateral hypothalamus releasing a-melanocyte-stimulating hormone (a-MSH) which is an agonist for acting on melanocortin receptors 3/4 (MC3/4-R). These neurons projections act on the nucleus of the solitary tract in the midbrain affecting changes in appetite, SNS activity, and blood pressure [18]. Currently leptin secreted by adipocytes is the main factor linking obesity with increased sympathetic nerve system activity and hypertension [19].

It is well known that the kidney contains all the elements for intrinsic activation of the renin-angiotensin-aldosterone system (RAAS). The intrarenal RAAS seems to be involved in hypertension associated with visceral obesity despite the fact that there is sodium retention and expansion of the extracellular volume. Possible explanations for the activation of renin secretion may involve activation of the sympathetic renal nerves and decrease sodium delivery to the macula densa due to increase sodium reabsorption early in the proximal tubule and the loop of Henle. In addition, increased renal pressure induced by visceral and intrarenal fat can stimulate renin secretion as seen in the peg kidney. Increase activity of RAAS causes efferent arteriole vasoconstriction and may result in hyperfiltration and nephrosclerosis. Aldosterone has direct mineralocorticoid receptor agonist effects resulting in increased sodium reabsorption in the cortical collecting duct and increasing blood pressure. Additionally, aldosterone is considered to promote fibrosis in organs such as the heart. Mineralocorticoid blockers are useful in the management of obese hypertensive patients.

The view that overweight and obesity represent simply a mater of caloric deposits is obsolete; we are learning that the adipose tissue is a very complex biologic system with surprising number of functions interacting with other organ systems including those listed in table 2. Adipose tissues are the source of numerous hormones, cytokines, growth factors, and complement factors that promote inflammation. Endothelial dysfunction eventually leads to promotion of vascular wall stiffness and is correlated with increase in carotid intimal-medial wall thickness [20].

A recently published epidemiologic meta-analysis involving 247 published papers from 1980 to 2006 demonstrated that compared with normal individuals, overweight and obese persons had significantly higher risk for kidney disease.21 The pooled relative risks (RRS) were 1.4 (1.30-1.50) for overweight and 1.83 (1.78-2.17) for obesity [21]. The association between obesity and kidney disease was stronger in women with RR=1.92 (1.78-2.07) than in men with RR=1.49 (1.36-1.63) [21]. This study indicated that there is a positive association between BMI and risk for kidney disease outcomes. The authors concluded that 24.2% and 33.9% of kidney diseases among men and women respectively in the United States versus 13.8% in men and 24.9% in women in other industrialized countries could be related to overweight and obesity [10].

Definitions of Hypertension in Children and Adolescents

The Fourth Report on the diagnosis, evaluation, and treatment of high blood pressure in children and adolescents uses blood pressure percentiles based upon demographic data from the National Health and Nutritional Examination Surveys (NHANES), taking in consideration information on gender, age, height, and blood pressure measurements on three separated occasions [21].

Table 3 lists hypertension definitions. Both systolic and diastolic blood pressures are of equal importance and the higher value determines the severity of the hypertension. The blood pressure should be measured in at least three different occasions to establish the diagnosis of hypertension. Stage 1 hypertension (see table 3) allows more time for evaluation. Treatment may be initiated with no pharmacologic approach that includes lifestyle modification such a weight loss, diet, and exercise. Stage-2 hypertension (se table 3) is more likely to be secondary hypertension and requires more rapid evaluation as well as initiation of pharmacologic intervention.

Table 3. Definitions of hypertension

1. Normal - systolic and diastolic blood pressure < 90 percentile
2. Prehypertension – Systolic and/or diastolic blood pressure >90th percentile but < 95th percentile, or if BP exceeds 120/80 mmHg even if <90th percentile
3. Stage 1 Hypertension – Systolic and/or diastolic BP between the 95th percentile and 5 mmHg above the 99th percentile.
4. Stage 2 Hypertension – Systolic and/or diastolic BP > 99% percentile + 5mmHg.

Treatment of Hypertension in Obese Adolescents

The treatment of the hypertensive obese adolescent is based on the same principles of treatment as used for management of other causes of hypertension. It is important to obtain a comprehensive history including a family history. The physical examination should be aimed to find possible secondary causes of hypertension that can be amenable to specific therapy, resulting in the cure or amelioration of the hypertension. Appropriate laboratory studies (see table 4) are helpful in investigating secondary forms of hypertension. Secondary forms of hypertension are more common in preadolescent children. Essential hypertension is more often seen in families with positive histories for hypertension and obesity.

Table 4. Selective list of key laboratory tests in hypertension evaluation

Urinalysis
Creatinine
Urea nitrogen
Electrolytes
Others

The cornerstone of management of hypertension secondary to obesity is body weight reduction and limiting caloric intake is necessary. Behavior modification is also very important. Better results are obtained by caloric restriction, behavior changes, and regular exercise [22]. The experience for weight reduction with pharmacologic agents is limited and in general not recommended in the United States for adolescents. There are reports of a few small series of morbidly obese adolescents with BMI > 40 Kg/ M^2 that have treated surgically for weight reduction [23]. However, lifestyle modification with behavior changes and exercise continues to be the best management option for most patients, particularly prehypertensive and stage 1 hypertensive adolescents. Adolescents with stage 1 hypertension should be monitored every few months. If the hypertension becomes more severe or symptomatic, stage 2 hypertension is diagnosed, and pharmacologic treatment is indicated.

Pharmacologic Therapy for Obese Hypertensive Adolescents

Several classes of medication are able to successfully control elevated blood pressure in adolescents as listed in table 5. The decision to utilize a specific medication however, requires consideration of the potential undesirable side effects, including metabolic consequences. It is well known that diuretics decrease blood pressure and offer cardiovascular protection in many hypertensive patients and are recommended as the fist line therapy for hypertensive adults. However in obese patients, there is an increase in the fasting blood glucose (FBG) levels in patients that were started on treatment with thiazides for hypertension. The magnitude of change in FBG and the development of new onset diabetes mellitus after thiazide initiation have been associated with increase in BMI and base line FBG [24]. Additionally, diuretic use is associated with electrolyte disturbances, particularly hypokalemia, hyponatremia, and abnormalities in uric acid metabolism.

Table 5. Medications for treatment of hypertension in adolescents

Diuretics
Alpha blockers
Beta blockers
Angiotensin converting enzyme inhibitors (ACE inhibitors)
Angiotensin-2 receptor blockers (ARBs)
Long acting calcium channel blockers

The experience with beta blockers for the treatment of hypertension in pediatrics is extensive. In the older adult population, beta blockers are particularly beneficial after myocardial infarction. However, beta blockers make glucose control more difficult; they are also associated with increased lipid levels and make it more difficult for the individual to loss weight. In younger obese individuals, other metabolically more neutral alternatives for treatment of hypertension are available.

Increasing experience in the use of angiotensin converting enzyme (ACE) inhibitors and angiotensin-2 receptor blockers (ARBs) is accumulating in the treatment of hypertensive adolescents and in children. In general, these medications are well tolerated by adolescents. Precautions are necessary in those adolescents with decrease renal function because for the risk of aggravating the decreased glomerular filtration rate and the development of hyperkalemia. These drugs are effective in controlling the elevated blood pressure, and because most are long acting medications, compliance is better. One drawback with these medications is the possibility of development of angioedema, a rare but serious complication. Another important consideration is their use in the adolescent female at risk of becoming pregnant given the teratogenic effects of ACEs and ARBs in the fetus.

Long acting calcium channel blockers are used for different forms of hypertension and are well tolerated in adolescents. They are associated with less metabolic abnormalities than diuretic or beta blockers [25]. The dihydropyridine calcium channel blocker, amlodipine, induces tachycardia and ankle edema that are of no clinic consequence; gum hypertrophy is also noted. Recent publications seem to indicate that that long term thiazide diuretics can increase fasting blood glucose and BMI levels and predispose to development of diabetes mellitus in hypertensive patients [24,25]. These studies indicate that the selection of antihypertensive medications is important to prevent or diminish the undesirables metabolic consequences that may be induced in susceptible individuals by certain medications.

Conclusions

Overweight and obesity in adolescents is now a global problem affecting developed and developing societies around the world. It is predictable that childhood and adolescent obesity will translate into adulthood obesity and its consequent morbidities including hypertension, hyperlipidemia, as well as type 2 diabetes mellitus and cardiovascular diseases. The causes of overweight and obesity in children and adolescents are the result of excessive caloric intake and concomitant decline in levels of physical activity in association with various socioeconomic, cultural, and genetic factors. There are populations that are at higher risk than others to be affected by these factors, including Asian Pacific Islanders, Australian Aborigine, African American Hispanics, and Native Americans; however no populations are exempt.

Adolescent hypertension is one of the co-morbidities of obesity that can be detected, prevented, and treated. The diagnosis of hypertension in adolescents in the United States is based on the recently published guidelines [21]. The cornerstone in the treatment of obesity-associated hypertension in adolescents is weight reduction by decreased caloric intake, behavior modification, and exercise. Organized physical activities and sport programs at schools and/or in the community in important in this regard. When pharmacologic therapy becomes necessary the prescribing physician needs to become familiar with the different antihypertensive medications as well as their side effects noted in obese diabetic patients, in those with cardiovascular diseases, and in patients with diminished kidney function. The best approach to the management of the obese "epidemic" is prevention and in this regard, health education of the population at large is critical.

References

[1] Jensen MD. Obesity. In: Goldman L, Ausiello D, eds. Cecil medicine, 23rd ed. Philadelphia, PA: Saunders Elsevier, 2008:1643-52.
[2] Forrest KY, Leeds MJ. Prevalence and associated factors of overweight among Mexican-American adolescents. J Am Diet Assoc 2007;107(10):797-800.
[3] Turconi G, Guarcello M, Maccarini L, Bazzano R, Zacardo A, Roggi C. BMI values and other anthropometric and functional measurements as predictors of obesity in selected group of adolescents. Eur J Nutr 2006;45(3):136-43.
[4] Rao S, Kanade A, Kelkar R. Blood Pressure among overweight adolescents from urban school children in Pune, India. Eur J Clin Nutr, 2007;61(5):633-41.
[5] Chiolero A, Cachat F, Burnier M, Paccaud F, Bovet P. Prevalence of hypertension in schoolchildren based in repeated measurements and association with overweight. J Hypertension 2007;25(11):2209-17.
[6] Ostroswska-Nawarycz L, Nawaricz T. Prevalence of excessive body weight and high blood pressure in children and adolescents in the city of Lodz. Kardiol Pol 2007;65(9):1079- 87.
[7] Singh GK. Kogan MD, VanDick PC. Multilevel analysis of state and regional disparities of children and adolescents obesity in the United States. J Community Health 2007;34:222-5.
[8] Pazmino P A, Pazmino A K, Diabetic renal failure in Texas: Influence of ethnicity and household income. Tex Med 2003;99:57-65.
[9] Bibbins-Domingo K, Coxon P, Pletcher MJ, Lightwood J, Goldman L. Adolescent overweight and future adult coronary heart disease. N Engl J Med 2007;357:2371-9.
[10] Wang Y, Chen X, Song Y, Caballero B, Cheskin LJ. Association between obesity and kidney disease: A systemic review and meta-analysis: Kidney Int 2008;73:19-33.
[11] Kambham N, Markowitz GS, Valeri AM, et al. Obesity and related glomerulopathy: An emerging epidemic. Kidney Int 2001;59:1498-1509.
[12] Hall JE Brands MW, Dixon WN, et al Obesity induced-hypertension: Renal function and systemic hemodynamics. Hypertension 1993;22:292-9.
[13] Messereli FH, Christie B, DeCarvalho JG, Obesity and essential hypertension: Hemodynamics, intravascular volume, sodium excretion, and plasma renain activity. Arch Intern Med 1981; 141:81-5.
[14] Vaz M, Jennings G, Turner A, et al. Regional sympathetic nervous activity and oxygen consumption in obese normotensive human subjects: Circulation 1997;96:3423-9.

[15] Lambert E, Staznicky M, Esler M, Dawood T, Hotchkin E, Lambert G. Differing patterns of sympathoexitation in normal-weight and obesity related hypertension. Hypertension 2007;50(50):862-8.

[16] Corry DB, Tuck ML. Obesity, hypertension and sympathetic nerve system activity. Curr Hypertens Rep 1999;1(2):119-26.

[17] Haynes WG, Interaction between leptin and sympathetic system activity in hypertension. Curr Hypertens Rep 2000;2(3):311-8.

[18] John E. Hall, Alexander A da Silva, Elizabeth Brandon, et al. Pathophysiology of obesity induced hypertension and target organ damage. In: Lip GYH, Hall JE, eds. Comprehensive hypertension. Philadelphia, PA: Mosby Elsevier, 2007:441-68.

[19] Francischetti EA, Genelhu VA. Obesity-hypertension: An ongoing pandemic. Int J Clin Pract. 2007;61(2):269-80.

[20] Sorof JM, Turner J, Martin DS, et al. Cardiovascular risks factors and sequelae in hypertensive children identified by referral versus school base screening. Hypertension 2004;43:214-8.

[21] The Fourth Report on diagnosis, evaluation and treatment of high blood pressure in children and adolescents. Bethesda, MD: Nat Heart Lung Blood Inst Health. Pediatrics 2004;114:555-76.

[22] Rocchini AP, Cutch V, Anderson J, Becker D, Martin M, Mark C. Blood pressure in obese adolescents, effect of weight loss. Pediatrics 1998;82(1):16-23.

[23] Widhalm K, Dietrich S, Prager G, Silberhummer G, et al. Bariatric surgery in morbidly obese adolescents: A 4-year follow-up of ten patients. Int J Pediatr Obes 2008;3(suppl 1):78-82.

[24] Siegel D, Meier J, Maas C, Lopez J. Swislocki AL. The effect of body mass index on fasting blood glucose after initiation of thiazide therapy in hypertensive patients. Am J Hypertension. 2008; [Epub ahead of print]

[25] Gupta AK, Dahlof B, Dobson j, Sever PS, Wedel H, Poulter NR; on behalf of ASCOT Investigators. Determinants of new-onset diabetes Among 19,251 hypertensive patients randomized in the ASCOT-BPLA Trial and relative influence of antihypertensive medication. Diabetes Care 2008; [Epub ahead of print].

In: Obesity and Adolescence: A Public Health Concern ISBN: 978-1-60692-821-9
Editors: H.A. Omar, D.E. Greydanus et al.

Chapter II

Obesity and Hyperandrogenism

Amit M. Deokar, Shawn J. Smith, Amanda J. Goodwin and Hatim A. Omar*

Division of Adolescent Medicine, Department of Pediatrics, University of Kentucky, Lexington, Kentucky, United States of America

Abstract

This chapter has a two-fold objective. One, it addresses the association of hyperandrogenism and obesity and the complex metabolic derangements that are part of the problem. Clinical management of these co-morbidities is challenging and complex. Second, this article will aid health care providers with the key features to an early diagnosis and intervention to decrease the morbidities in the short as well as long term. Method: Systematic review of articles and information on the topic of interest that were published in the last 15 years. Conclusion: Obesity and hyperandrogenism are integral parts of Metabolic Syndrome/Polycystic Ovarian Syndrome (PCOS)/Hyperandrogenism, Insulin resistance, and Acanthosis Nigricans (HAIR-AN). With the childhood obesity epidemic, the metabolic syndrome and the associated abnormalities are routinely seen in clinical practice and these have a tremendous economic burden on the society and the quality of life.

Introduction

Obesity in children and adolescents has increased at an alarming rate in the last two decades. Over the years, researchers have acquired a better understanding about the strong association of obesity in metabolic syndrome (MS, previously known as metabolic syndrome X) [1].

* Correspondence: Hatim A Omar, MD, FAAP, Professor of Pediatrics and Obstetrics/Gynecology, Chief, Adolescent Medicine and Young Parent programs, J422, Kentucky Clinic, University of Kentucky, Lexington, KY 40536 United States. Tel: 859-323-6426 ext. 311; Fax: 859-257-7706; E-mail: haomar2@uky.edu

Patients with MS have various metabolic abnormalities that can include abnormal glucose and insulin ratio, insulin resistance, high blood pressure, altered lipid profile, pro-thrombotic and pro-inflammatory state. Teenagers with MS are predisposed to long term morbidities, such as early coronary artery disease, hepatic steatosis, type 2 diabetes, and stroke [1]. Evidence suggests that an overweight teenager has an 80 percent chance of continuing to be overweight in the adult life [2].

Approximately 17 percent of children aged 2-19 years are considered overweight based on a survey by National Health and Nutrition Examination Survey of 2003-2004 [3]. As noted earlier, the rate of obesity has doubled in adolescents, who are in the 12-19 year age group [4]. The prevalence of obese and overweight children may be different depending on the gender and ethnicity. For example, the obesity rates are higher in African Americans, Hispanic Americans, males, and those living in the southern states [2]. The definition of obesity varies in adolescents when compared to adults due to different proportion of body fat in boys and girls at different ages [5]. Body Mass Index (BMI) is a reliable tool to assess obesity, because it is easy to obtain and correlates well with the body fat [6]. Any adolescent with a BMI of 30 kg/m^2 or 95th percentile for gender and age falls in the overweight category. They are considered at risk of being overweight if their BMI is between 85th and = 95th percentile. In the US, the economic burden of direct and indirect healthcare cost due to obesity and co-morbidities is estimated to be well over $ 117 billion annually. As the obesity rates have doubled and tripled respectively in children and adolescents, so have the health care costs [7]. This impacts the healthcare burden directly.

Obesity and hyperandrogenism (HA) are strongly associated in patients who have been diagnosed to have polycystic ovarian syndrome (PCOS)/HA/MS. This article addresses their relationship with one another and specific management options. A subset of (PCOS) includes hyperandrogenism, insulin resistance and acanthosis nigricans, abbreviated as HAIR-AN [8,9]. Historically PCOS was described based on findings of multiple cysts in the ovaries, irregular or no menstrual periods, and hirsuitism. However, absence of ovarian cysts does not rule out this syndrome [10]. Women with high androgen levels have associated HAIR-AN features in about 5-10 percent of cases [11]. The onset of PCOS/HAIR-AN may occurs in adolescent years and the diagnosis is likely to be delayed until early adulthood [8,9].

Pathophysiology

As PCOS/HAIR-AN is being studied more over the last two decades, different theories have been proposed to explain the features of the syndrome, including obesity. The primary problem in HA appears to be due to an altered hypothalamo-pituatary-ovarian axis. The anovulation and thus abnormal or absence of menstrual periods is from a persistent leutenizing hormone (LH) surge and its high concentration in the blood. There is also an increased GnRH surge as the negative feedback from estrogen and progesterone is ineffective due to relative hypothalamic insensitivity. The LH surge results in increased production of androgens. The level of follicle stimulating hormone (FSH) is less when compared to the LH resulting in decreased enzymatic (aromatase) conversion of androgen to estrogen and thus anovulation.

Another key association of HA is hyperinsulinsm. This is due to peripheral insulin resistance, which can result in a hyperglycemic state. The level of sex hormone binding globulin (SHBG) is decreased due to the high insulin levels and consequently there is a rise in the free testosterone level [8]. Insulin also increases the androgen production by directly stimulating the theca cells [12]. Both hyperinsulinism and HA predispose an individual to have an athrogenic lipid profile. Total cholesterol, triglycerides (TG) levels are also elevated. Increased activity of the enzyme lipase affects the cholesterol metabolism and could result in a decreased level of the high density lipoprotein-cholesterol (HDL-C) [13]. Another postulated mechanism for HAIR-AN is a genetic mutation of the insulin receptor (tyrosine kinase domain) [9].

Effects of HA can be multi-fold. Even though increased androgen production in women is associated with obesity, one study in 2002 by Gapstur et al [14] in obese men have found to have lower testosterone and dehydroepiandroterone sulfate (DHEAS) levels. High androgen levels in children and adolescents are linked to precocious puberty, accelerated bone growth, height, features of PCOS, and are more commonly seen in obese subjects compared to non-obese. In pre-pubertal obese children the level of DHEAS is often elevated [14].

Recently, researchers have looked at the effects of proteins like adiponectin, resistin, leptin, and TNF-a on the fat metabolism, peripheral insulin resistance, and energy expenditure [15]. Resistin is produced by the mature visceral and subcutaneous adipocytes and influences insulin sensitivity. Adiponectin and leptin, also secreted from the adipocytes, have similar roles [16]. A recently published study by Shin et al [17] suggested obesity as an inflammatory process due to findings of increased levels of C-reactive protein (CRP) and TNF found in obese children. The adiponectin level was found to be much lower concentration in these children. Retinol Biding Protein 4 (RBP4) is present in omental and subcutaneous fat and is expressed more in women with PCOS [18]. The high levels of androgen and features of metabolic syndrome have shown to normalize in post-menarche obese adolescents after weight reduction [19].

Diagnostic Criteria

A standard list of the diagnostic criteria for MS in children and adolescents is still lacking. However, a modified diagnostic criteria for children using the NCEP criteria and data from the National Health and Nutrition Examination Survey (NHANES, 1988-94) is widely used. The National Cholesterol Education Program (NCEP) and the Adult Treatment Panel III (ATP III) include at least 3 of 5 of the following criteria for the diagnosis of MS in adults [1,2,20,21].

- Abnormal lipid panel: Hypertriglyceridemia (>150 mg/dl) and low HDL-C (<40mg/dl in males and <50 in females).
- High fasting glucose level. Hyperglycemic state is defined as fasting glucose level of 100 mg/dl or more.

- Elevated blood pressure, systolic, diastolic, or both using reference ranges. From example, blood pressure of >135/85 mmHg is considered abnormal.
- Increased waist circumference/abdominal girth. BMI is fairly reliable in assessing obesity in children.
- High insulin resistance (criterion in children).
- The World Health Organization (WHO) criteria required elevated insulin or glucose level (>110mg/dl) in addition to at least two of the following:[2]
- Abdominal obesity
- Waist size >94 cm or waist to hip ratio of >0.9
- Triglycerides > 150 mg/dl or HDL <35 mg/dl
- Blood pressure >140/90 mmHg.

HAIR-AN is a clinical diagnosis and includes the following, in addition to criteria mentioned above [9]:

a) Acne, hirsuitism, temporal balding, clitoromegaly, and deepening of voice (suggestive of high androgen level).
b) Acrochordons (skin tags), acanthosis nigricans (usually found on the neck, axillae, and back). These are suggestive of insulin resistance and altered hormonal levels.

Suggested Workup

Anthropometric measurement, vital signs, with a complete history and physical exam (including genital) is recommended. A detailed family, past medical, and medication history should also be documented. Laboratory data that may be useful includes, fasting levels of insulin, glucose (complete metabolic panel to assess liver and renal function), lipid panel, glucose/insulin ratio, HgA1c, and AM cortisol level. Oral glucose tolerance test (2 hour) is also recommended to document hyperglycemic state. One test that has high sensitivity and specificity is the euglycemic hyperinsulinemic clamp. This may be impractical in a clinical setting due to the time consuming and complex nature of the test [9]. A thorough endocrine evaluation should include thyroid function tests, serum prolactin, DHEA-S, am 17-hydroxyprogesterone (17-OHP), SHBG level, and free and total testosterone. IGF-1 level may be helpful in a suspected growth hormone producing tumor [22].

In order to establish the diagnosis of PCOS, the presence of multiple ovarian cysts is not necessary. Likewise, an abdominal/pelvic ultrasound detection of multiple ovarian cysts does not confirm that diagnosis either. Occasionally a computed tomography (CT) or an MRI of the abdomen/pelvis may be necessary in situations where there are progressive signs of hyperandrogenism [22].

Outcome

Metabolic syndrome (PCOS and HAIR-AN subset) in children can lead to potentially complicated short and long term medical problems. This exhaustive list includes but is not limited to the following [6]:

- Distorted body image and perception
- Low self-esteem and depression
- Acne
- Obesity associated problems like snoring, obstructive sleep apnea, disordered sleep, gastro esophageal reflux disease (GERD), gall stones, joint pain, exercise intolerance, features of diabetes, coronary artery disease, and skin changes, etc.
- Amenorrhea (predisposing to subsequent inadequate bone mineralization) and possibly infertility.

Treatment Options

The timeframe for the diagnosis of metabolic syndrome/HAIR-AN to the outcome of the treatment varies from patient to patient and can be often protracted. A multidisciplinary approach is often required to address the metabolic as well as the psychological stressors associated with this syndrome. reatment should be geared toward specific metabolic abnormalities as well [6,9,23]. It is important for the healthcare provider to be aware of the concerns that teenagers may have when it relates to cosmetic appearance. At a psychological developmental stage where bodily appearance plays an important role in a teenager's life, skin related problems such as acanthosis nigricans, acne, and hirsuitism may be quite troubling [22]. This can affect their self-esteem directly. Health care providers should have a low threshold for referring these teenagers to counseling services.

Lifestyle Modification

Although compliance can play a big role with this approach, it is considered one of the most favored and successful mode of treatment in obese patients, who also have HA [22]. Weight loss can dramatically improve the ovarian function and decrease the levels of androgens [24]. Different dietary changes such as caloric restriction of carbohydrates or fat with increased protein intake have been previously studied. There is no sufficient data available if restriction of carbohydrates is better than that of fat intake. It is therefore prudent to use the expertise of a dietician or nutritionist who can work with obese/overweight individuals.

Medication Management

Typically, in addition to the lifestyle modification, medical treatment may include a combination of one or more of these therapies such as anti androgens, insulin-sensitizing agents, combined hormonal contraceptives, bariatric surgery, and complementary and alternative medicine treatment options. As part of a multidisciplinary approach, psychological counseling is very crucial.

Insulin-Sensitizing Agents

Biguanide: Metformin (trade names such as Glugophage®, Rhiomet®), a pregnancy category B drug, has traditionally been used in type 2 diabetes mellitus (DM). From a glycemic stand point, Metformin interferes with the hepatocyte mitochondrial respiratory oxidative process and decreases gluconeogenesis. This however, is not a complete blockade of gluconeogenesis. It also facilitates the glucose transport in tissues such as the skeletal muscles, by activating the enzyme tyrosine kinase (TK) on the insulin receptors and enhancing the glucose transporter system. Some of this action is also on the adipocytes. It also acts against the gluconeogenic effects of glucagon. Metformin is particularly useful in obesity associated with HA. Due to its insulin lowering effect, there is a consequent decrease in the free and total testosterone and an increase in the estradiol level [25]. This has a beneficial effect on ovulation, hirsuitism and acne.

As obesity is strongly associated with cardiovascular morbidity and mortality, metformin has an added benefit of being cardioprotective. It has shown to decrease the free fatty oxidation, which helps improve the insulin sensitivity as well. It may also help lower the total cholesterol (TC), very low density lipopoprotein cholesterol (VLDL-C), low density lipoprotein cholesterol (LDL-C), and increase the high density lipoprotein cholesterol (HDL-C). It also lowers the platelet aggregation and adhesion, and decreases the levels of tissue plasminogen inhibitor 1 and von Willebrand factor. This has a positive effect on homeostasis [26]. It can induce vascular relaxation and reduce the oxidative stress [25,26]. A combination of flutamide (an androgen receptor blocker) and metformin with an addition of drosperinone (a 4th generation progesterone) has shown to decrease abdominal fat [27].

Usual side effects from metformin may include gastrointestinal symptoms such as nausea, flatulence and diarrhea. These may be reduced by taking it with food. Treatment may be started with a single daily dose, preferably at a lowest possible dose. It may then be increased to a twice daily dose. It is not recommended to go over the maximum dosage of 2.25 grams/day [25]. One must be aware of the potential toxicity from metfromin that includes lactic acidosis in rare situations. Metformin is fairly safe for the mother and baby during pregnancy and lactation [28].

Thiazolidinediones: Rosiglitazone is an insulin sensitizing agent, whose action on the peroxisome proliferator-activated receptor (PPAR) on the adipocytes improves glucose transport into the cell by increasing the adiponectin secretion [29]. In studies done earlier on overweight women with PCOS, there was a decrease in the insulin resistance and return of ovulation as indicated by regular menses. The SHBG level also shows an increase that helps with the ovulation. Some of the side effects include weight gain and cardiac failure in susceptible individuals [30].

Regulation of the Hormonal/Androgen Imbalance and Use of Oral Contraceptives

Combination birth control pills (BCP's) are the cornerstone in the treatment of HA. Their mechanism of action includes the following:

- Increase the SHBG production and level: This allows a reduction of free testosterone.
- Suppress LH: Decreases androgen production from the ovaries.
- Anti-minerelocorticoid activity: Certain progestins such as Drosperinone have low androgenic activity and are generally preferred in HA. The brand name contraceptives Yasmin® and Ortho-Tri-Cyclen® contain Drosperinone.

The effects of combination BCP's include normalization of menses and a decrease in acne and hirsuitism [22]. In addition to the above, other pharmacologic agents have been tried in HA states are cyproterone acetate, finastreride, glucocorticoid, such as prednisone (patients with late onset congential adrenal hyperplasia (CAH) having PCOS features), and spironolactone.

Surgical Options

Bariatric Surgery: A decrease in obesity-related morbidity has been well documented in individuals that have undergone Roux-en-Y gastric bypass surgery. Although this is an optional procedure that has been evaluated mostly in morbidly obese adults, the guidelines are quite conservative for the adolescent population. Morbidly obese teenagers, who have failed the non-surgical approach may be considered for a gastric bypass surgery. Other justifications in addition to the above includes a BMI of 40 kg/m^2 or more, physical and psychosocial co morbidities from obesity [31]. Bariatric surgery intended to result in weight loss can positively impact obesity, PCOS, and reverse anovulation. The risks from obesity during pregnancy in morbidly obese teens is also decreased by the procedure [31]. A 1 to 2 year wait post operatively for becoming pregnant is usually recommended. As there can be potential complications from this surgical procedure, careful multidisciplinary evaluation for the need for surgery is needed.

Complementary and Alternative Medicine

Alternative approaches in the treatment of PCOS have been recently gaining popularity. In view of side effects from the traditional medical and surgical treatment, researchers have looked at the benefits of acupuncture, a traditional form of Chinese medicine. Acupuncture has been shown to modulate neuro-endocrine systems that results in lowering of the increased sympathetic tone in individuals with PCOS. By releasing ß-endorphins the technique of acupuncture can directly influence the HPA axis and lower the cortisol and LH levels [32]. As a result, its beneficial effects on metabolic, ovulation, and other neuro-endocrinal endogenous systems can positively influence the features of PCOS/HA. Other forms of alternative medicine such as homeopathy, Ayurveda, diet supplements, and hypnotherapy have been tried to treat obesity in adults with some encouraging results even though some are not very convincing [33].

Federal/State Program

The CDC (Center for Disease Control and Prevention), the Division of Nutrition and Physical Activity (DNPA) and the health departments of 28 states have established the Nutrition and Physical Activity Program to Prevent Obesity and Other Chronic Diseases (NPAO) since 1999 using the social ecological model [34]. Healthcare providers are encouraged to contact their individual health departments to learn more about the program, where available.

Conclusions

Metabolic syndrome, hyperandrogenism, and PCOS are integral part of complex metabolic abnormalities that have a great impact on the health and general well-being of an individual. The diagnosis is often late and this adds to the economic burden from obesity related problems. The following key points will aid the healthcare provider with the timely diagnosis of HA/MS/PCOS and appropriate interventions.

- Healthcare provider awareness of obesity in childhood and adolescence.
- Utilizing diagnostic criteria and/or clinical diagnosis of PCOS/HA/MS. One may refer to the NCEP, NHANES, ATP III, WHO diagnostic criteria.
- A complete history, including that of the individual, family, past, and medications.
- Complete physical exam. As noted earlier, the diagnosis of HAIR-AN is clinical.
- Laboratory and radiological work up. The list includes fasting insulin, glucose (complete metabolic panel to assess liver and renal function), lipid panel, glucose/insulin ratio, HgA1c, and AM cortisol level. Oral glucose tolerance test (2 hour), thyroid function tests, serum prolactin, DHEA-S, am 17-hydroxyprogesterone (17-OHP), SHBG level, free and total testosterone, IGF-1 level are also recommended.
- Management that includes medical, surgical, lifestyle modification techniques, and appropriate referrals to other sub-specialty providers for addressing associated co morbidities. Keeping in mind that some patients may desire to utilize alternative and complimentary medicine options as well.

- Multidisciplinary approach that includes, the primary care provider, sub-specialist, social worker, nutritionist, and counselor/psychologist.

References

[1] Kranz S, Mahood LJ, Wagstaff DA. Diagnostic criteria patterns of US children with metabolic syndrome: NHANES 1999-2002. Nutrition J 2007;6:38.

[2] Strasburger VC, Braverman PK, Rogers PD, Holland-Hall CM. Adolescent medicine: A handbook for primary care, 1st ed. Philadelphia, PA: Lippincott Williams Wilkins, 2005.

[3] CDC. Prevalence of overweight among children and adolescents: United States, 2003-2004. 2007 [cited 2008 05/16/2008]; Health E-Stat. National Center for Health Statistics. Centers for Disease Control.]. Available from: http://www.cdc.gov/nchs/products/pubs/pubd/hestats/overweight/overwght_child_03.htm

[4] National Association of Children's Hospitals and Related Institutions (NACHRI). Childhood Obesity Statistics and Facts. 2007 [cited 2008 05/16/2008]; Available from: http://www.childrenshospitals.net/AM/Template.cfm?Section=Homepage&TEMPLATE=/CM/ContentDisplay.cfm&CONTENTID=34357

[5] CDC. Defining overweight and obesity, 2007 [cited 2008 05/14/2008]; Definition for children and teens]. Available from: http://www.cdc.gov/nccdphp/dnpa/obesity/defining.htm

[6] Krebs NF, Himes JH, Jacobson D, Nicklas TA, Guilday P, Styne D. Assessment of child and adolescent overweight and obesity. Pediatrics 2007;120(Suppl 4):S193-228.

[7] Stein CJ, Colditz GA. The epidemic of obesity. J Clin Endocrinol Metab 2004;89(6):2522-5.

[8] McCartney CR, Prendergast KA, Chhabra S, Eagleson CA, Yoo R, Chang RJ, et al. The association of obesity and hyperandrogenemia during the pubertal transition in girls: obesity as a potential factor in the genesis of postpubertal hyperandrogenism. J Clin Endocrinol Metab 2006;91(5):1714-22.

[9] Rager KM, Omar HA. Androgen excess disorders in women: the severe insulin-resistant hyperandrogenic syndrome, HAIR-AN. ScientificWorldJournal 2006;6:116-21.

[10] Mukhtar I Khan DMK. Polycystic ovarian syndrome. 2006 [cited 2008 05/14/2008]; Available from: http://www.emedicine.com/med/topic2173.htm

[11] Barbieri RL, Hornstein MD. Hyperinsulinemia and ovarian hyperandrogenism. Cause and effect. Endocrinol Metab Clin North Am 1988;17(4):685-703.

[12] McCartney CR, Blank SK, Prendergast KA, Chhabra S, Eagleson CA, Helm KD, et al. Obesity and sex steroid changes across puberty: evidence for marked hyperandrogenemia in pre- and early pubertal obese girls. J Clin Endocrinol Metab 2007;92(2):430-6.

[13] Valkenburg O, Steegers-Theunissen RP, Smedts HP, Dallinga-Thie GM, Fauser BC, Westerveld EH, et al. A more atherogenic serum lipoprotein profile is present in

women with polycystic ovary syndrome: a case-control study. J Clin Endocrinol Metab 2008;93(2):470-6.

[14] Gapstur SM, Gann PH, Kopp P, Colangelo L, Longcope C, Liu K. Serum androgen concentrations in young men: a longitudinal analysis of associations with age, obesity, and race. The CARDIA male hormone study. Cancer Epidemiol Biomarkers Prev 2002;11(10 Pt 1):1041-7.

[15] Zou CC, Liang L, Hong F. Relationship between insulin resistance and serum levels of adiponectin and resistin with childhood obesity. Indian Pediatrics 2007;44(4):275-9.

[16] Hendler I, Blackwell SC, Mehta SH, Whitty JE, Russell E, Sorokin Y, et al. The levels of leptin, adiponectin, and resistin in normal weight, overweight, and obese pregnant women with and without preeclampsia. Am J Obstet Gynecol 2005;193(3 Pt 2):979-83.

[17] Shin JY, Kim SY, Jeung MJ, Eun SH, Woo CW, Yoon SY, et al. Serum adiponectin, C-reactive protein and TNF-alpha levels in obese Korean children. J Pediatr Endocrinol Metab 2008;21(1):23-9.

[18] Stanley T, Misra M. Polycystic ovary syndrome in obese adolescents. Curr Opin Endocrinol Diabetes Obes 2008;15(1):30-6.

[19] Wabitsch M, Hauner H, Heinze E, Bockmann A, Benz R, Mayer H, et al. Body fat distribution and steroid hormone concentrations in obese adolescent girls before and after weight reduction. J Clin Endocrinol Metab 1995;80(12):3469-75.

[20] de Ferranti SD, Gauvreau K, Ludwig DS, Neufeld EJ, Newburger JW, Rifai N. Prevalence of the metabolic syndrome in American adolescents: Findings from the Third National Health and Nutrition Examination Survey. Circulation 2004; 110(16):2494-7.

[21] Cook S, Weitzman M, Auinger P, Nguyen M, Dietz WH. Prevalence of a metabolic syndrome phenotype in adolescents: Findings from the third National Health and Nutrition Examination Survey, 1988-1994. Arch Pediatr Adolesc Med 2003; 157(8):821-7.

[22] Harwood K, Vuguin P, DiMartino-Nardi J. Current approaches to the diagnosis and treatment of polycystic ovarian syndrome in youth. Horm Res 2007;68(5):209-17.

[23] McClanahan KK, Omar HA. Navigating adolescence with a chronic health condition: a perspective on the psychological effects of HAIR-AN syndrome on adolescent girls. ScientificWorldJournal 2006;6:1350-8.

[24] Huber-Buchholz MM, Carey DG, Norman RJ. Restoration of reproductive potential by lifestyle modification in obese polycystic ovary syndrome: role of insulin sensitivity and luteinizing hormone. J Clin Endocrinol Metab 1999;84(4):1470-4.

[25] Kirpichnikov D, McFarlane SI, Sowers JR. Metformin: an update. Ann Intern Med 2002;137(1):25-33.

[26] Bailey CJ. Metformin--an update. Gen Pharmacol 1993;24(6):1299-309.

[27] Ibanez L, De Zegher F. Flutamide-metformin plus an oral contraceptive (OC) for young women with polycystic ovary syndrome: switch from third- to fourth-generation OC reduces body adiposity. Hum Reprod 2004;19(8):1725-7.

[28] Goldenberg N, Glueck C. Medical therapy in women with polycystic ovarian syndrome before and during pregnancy and lactation. Minerva Ginecol 2008;60(1):63-75.

[29] Majuri A, Santaniemi M, Rautio K, Kunnari A, Vartiainen J, Ruokonen A, et al. Rosiglitazone treatment increases plasma levels of adiponectin and decreases levels of resistin in overweight women with PCOS: a randomized placebo-controlled study. Eur J Endocrinol 2007;156(2):263-9.

[30] Lago RM, Singh PP, Nesto RW. Congestive heart failure and cardiovascular death in patients with prediabetes and type 2 diabetes given thiazolidinediones: a meta-analysis of randomised clinical trials. Lancet 2007;370(9593):1129-36.

[31] Miller RJ, Xanthakos SA, Hillard PJ, Inge TH. Bariatric surgery and adolescent gynecology. Curr Opin Obstet Gynecol 2007;19(5):427-33.

[32] Stener-Victorin E, Jedel E, Manneras L. Acupuncture in polycystic ovary syndrome: current experimental and clinical evidence. J Neuroendocrinol 2008;20(3):290-8.

[33] Pittler MH, Ernst E. Complementary therapies for reducing body weight: a systematic review. Int Journal Obes 2005;29(9):1030-8.

[34] Hamre R, et al. CDC's state-based nutrition and physical activity program to prevent obesity and other chronic diseases. July 2006 January 17, 2008 [cited 2008 06/24/08]; Available from: http://www.cdc.gov/nccdphp/dnpa/obesity/state_programs/pdf/NPAO_Performance_Report_2005.pdf

In: Obesity and Adolescence: A Public Health Concern ISBN: 978-1-60692-821-9
Editors: H.A. Omar, D.E. Greydanus et al.

Chapter III

Obesity and Endocrinology

Manmohan Kamboj*

Pediatrics and Human Development, Michigan State University College of Human Medicine, Division of Pediatric Endocrinology, Pediatrics Program, Michigan State University/Kalamazoo Center for Medical Studies, Kalamazoo, Michigan, United States of America

Abstract

There has been a profound increase in the prevalence of obesity over the last 20 to 30 years causing the coining of the term "obesity epidemic" in children, adolescents and adults. It is believed to be due to a complex interaction of social and environmental factors in the overall lifestyle pattern. The increased rate of obesity is seen to be associated with increasing incidence of type 2 diabetes mellitus in adolescents, along with perturbations of the other endocrine axes, as well as, higher risk of long term complications. It is therefore of the utmost importance that concerns about overweight and obesity be addressed from early childhood and adolescence to avoid resultant significant morbidity and/or mortality.

Introduction

Obesity has become a significant health problem worldwide over the last few years. The prevalence of obesity has reached epidemic proportions both in the pediatric as well as adult populations. Obesity in children and adolescents correlates directly to obesity in adulthood. This high prevalence of obesity is leading not only to an increased incidence of a multitude of

* Correspondence: Manmohan Kamboj, MD, Associate Professor, Pediatrics and Human Development, Michigan State University College of Human Medicine, Division of Pediatric Endocrinology, Pediatrics Program, Michigan State University, Kalamazoo Center for Medical Studies, Kalamazoo, MI 49008-1284 United States. Tel: 269-337-6450; Fax: 269-337-6474; E-mail: Kamboj@kcms.msu.edu

medical problems, but also increasing the financial burden on the health systems all over the world.

Definition

Obesity and overweight have been defined in a variety of ways by different institutions. For the purposes of the following discussion, the definitions considered in this article are a Body Mass Index (BMI) of 25-29.9 kg/m2 is considered overweight and BMI > 30 kg/m2 is labeled obese in adults.1 For children and adolescents definitions of the Institute of Medicine label BMI between 85th to 95th percentile for age and sex as overweight and BMI values >95th percentile are classified as obesity. The Centers for Disease Control and Prevention (CDC) labels both these categories as 'risk for overweight' and 'overweight' respectively [1-3].

Incidence and Prevalence

Approximately 17.1 % of children and adolescents in the US were overweight while 33.6% were overweight or at risk for overweight in 2003-2004 [4]. The prevalence of overweight/obesity increased from 5% to 17.1% in adolescents (12-19 years of age) between 1976-1980 and 2003-2004 [4]. Prevalence of obesity is more common among Native Americans, non-Hispanic blacks, and Mexican Americans than in whites [4]. The risk of obesity increases if one of the parents is obese.

Medical Conditions Associated with Obesity

Obesity in childhood and adolescence is associated with morbidity involving multiple body systems. These include abnormalities of the endocrine, cardiovascular, gastrointestinal, dermatological, pulmonary, neurologic, and psychosocial systems. Many of these effects are primarily caused by metabolic dysfunction while others may be due more to the physical impairment caused by obesity. Although the medical dysfunction is multi-systemic with function of each system closely linked to the other, only the endocrine dysfunction is discussed in this chapter.

Endocrine Dysfunction in Obesity

Obesity can cause alteration in functioning of most endocrine axes leading to disturbances of growth and pubertal development, thyroid, adrenal, gonadal as well as parathyroid function. Metabolic function in context of insulin and glucose metabolism is a major concomitant of obesity. These disturbances predispose the individual to develop hyperinsulinemia, insulin resistance, impaired glucose tolerance, and ultimately type 2 diabetes mellitus. The coexistence of insulin resistance and dyslipidemias with obesity is referred to as the dysmetabolic syndrome (or Syndrome X). Obesity together with hyperandrogenemia may predispose to the development of the polycystic ovarian syndrome (PCOS). Hyperandrogenism and PCOS are discussed elsewhere in this edition.

Disturbances of the Insulin and Glucose Metabolism

The spectrum of disturbances seen in the glucose and insulin metabolism include insulin resistance and hyperinsulinemia with normal glucose tolerance, insulin resistance and hyperinsulinemia with impaired glucose tolerance (IGT), and type 2 diabetes mellitus (type 2 DM). The relationship of obesity, BMI, IGT and type 2 DM has been well illustrated in a study where 25% of children and 21% of adolescents with BMI >95th percentile for sex and age were found to have IGT, while 4% of these adolescents had type 2 DM [5].

Insulin resistance (IR) is defined as a subnormal glucose response to a given concentration of insulin. IR is found to be an easy and good predictor of IGT. Various methods have been devised to study IR including the fasting glucose to insulin ratio (FGIR), the homeostasis model assessment of insulin resistance (HOMA), and the quantitative insulin sensitivity check index (QUICKI) [6-8]. In routine clinical practice fasting glucose and insulin levels are commonly done. However, it is also important to evaluate the post-prandial response with a two hour oral glucose tolerance test (OGTT) with fasting and two hour post-prandial glucose as well as insulin level determinations. The diagnostic criteria for normoglycemia, IGT and frank diabetes mellitus are outlined in table 1 by the American Diabetes Association (ADA) [9].

Table 1. Diagnostic criteria for diabetes mellitus

Criterion	Fasting plasma glucose (mg/dl)	2 hr postprandial glucose (mg/dL)
Normoglycemia	<100	<140
Impaired fasting glucose	≥100 but <126	___
Impaired glucose tolerance but	<200	≥140
Diabetes	≥126	≥200
Symptoms of diabetes and random blood glucose ≥200 (repeated on two separate occasions)		

Adapted from American Diabetes Association. Screening for Diabetes (Position Statement). Diabetes Care 2004;27(Suppl1):S11-14.

An important clinical marker of IR in children and adolescents is acanthosis nigricans (AN) which is a velvety dark pigmentation seen at the nape of the neck and flexural folds of the body. Nevertheless, there is an ongoing controversy about whether or not AN should be considered a reliable clinical marker for hyperinsulinemia in overweight children [10,11]. With the increasing prevalence of type 2 DM in children and adolescents, it becomes increasingly important to be able to differentiate between the two major types of diabetes mellitus, namely type I DM and type 2 DM; this is an issue that may not be as straight forward as previously believed. The important differentiating features are listed in table 2. The increasing prevalence of type 2 DM children and adolescents is noted to closely parallel the obesity curve. Varying incidences of new onset, non-autoimmune diabetes mellitus (with a majority of patients having type 2 DM) in children and adolescents have been reported to be between 8-45 % [12].

Management

Early diagnosis of IGT and type 2 DM is very important for early initiation of interventional strategies resulting in early and improved glycemic control. This would lower the incidence of chronic complications. Recommendations have been made by the American Diabetes Association for testing guidelines in high risk individuals as outlined in table 3 [13].

The spectrum of obesity – IR – IGT – type 2 DM is a clear example of prevention being the cornerstone of intervention strategies. The key to prevention of type 2 DM remains addressing the root concern of obesity by early introduction of life-style modifications. These include reduced caloric intake coupled with initiation of structured exercise/activity programs. Exercise regimens improve insulin sensitivity, metabolic profile, and cardiovascular functioning independent of weight loss [14]. Daily caloric intake is lowered by making quantitative and qualitative modifications in daily food intake by decreasing portion sizes and making healthy food choices. Moderate intensity exercise as 30 minutes/day for seven days a week has been recommended for everyone while 60 minutes have been advised for weight loss [14,15].

Table 2. Common factors differentiating between Type 1 and Type 2 diabetes mellitus

Parameters	Type 1 DM	Type 2 DM
Age	Usually younger age groups	Usually older Increasing in adolescents
Ethnicity	More common in Caucasian	More common in African American, Hispanics, Native Americans
Obesity	Less common	More common
Family history	Less often associated	More often associated
DKA	Relatively common	Relatively uncommon
Insulin levels	Absent/low	High
C-peptide	Low	High
Antibodies • Anti-Insulin • Anti-Islet cell • Antiglutamic acid decarboxylase 65 (GAD-65)	Usually positive	Usually negative
Treatment	Insulin	Oral Hypoglycemic agents Insulin may be needed

Table 3. Testing for type 2 diabetes mellitus in children and adolescents

Weight-BMI >85th percentile for reference standards

Risk factors-Presence of two risk factors:

- Presence of signs of insulin resistance – acanthosis nigricans, PCOS, hypertension, dyslipidemias
- Race and ethnicity: with high incidence of type 2 DM – African-American, Latin American, Hispanic, Pacific Islander, Asian American
- Family history of type 2 DM in first or second degree relative

Testing Recommendations

- Should be started at 10 years or at pubertal onset
- Repeated every 2 years
- Testing with fasting plasma glucose should be done

Adapted from: American Diabetes Association: Standards of medical care in diabetes (Position Statement). Diabetes Care 2004;26 (Suppl 1): S15-35.

Pharmacologic agents are being extensively investigated for prevention and treatment of obesity. Medications available include orlistat and sibutramine but lack long term study information regarding benefits and side effects in children and adolescents. Metformin has increasingly been used in this group of patients to improve insulin sensitivity. A small, randomized study in adolescents reported metabolic improvement and a small decrease in BMI, while lifestyle modifications were noted to be more effective than metformin in preventing progression from IGT to type 2 DM [16,17]. Newer options being investigated include topiramate, Peptide YY, rimonabant, and magnesium. Unfortunately not enough long term studies have been done to justify their use in children and adolescents [18]. Once obese patients develop type 2 DM, pharmacologic therapeutic agents need to be added to the lifestyle modifications which should be continued. Metformin remains the most common oral hypoglycemic agent used in adolescents. Other oral hypoglycemic agents available and used extensively in adults are not used in children and adolescents very commonly. Insulin may also have to be added to the treatment regimen if adequate glycemic control is not achieved with oral medications. A list of the commonly available hypoglycemic agents is available in table 4 [19].

Effect of Obesity on other Endocrine Axes

Effect of Obesity on Growth Axis

Although obesity is associated with accelerated growth, obese patients are noted to have low growth hormone (GH) levels [20]. Both the spontaneous growth hormone levels as well as stimulated GH levels are low [21-23]. Interestingly the IGF-1 levels are normal or even elevated inspite of low growth hormone levels. The mechanism for this complex interaction is not clear. Multiple mechanisms have been proposed for low growth hormone levels including decreased synthesis and increased clearance of growth hormone; others include an increase in the somatostatinergic tone causing inhibition of GH secretion, or a compromised response to growth hormone releasing hormone (GHRH)[24,25]. Possible explanations for normal IGF-1 levels offered include increased hepatic IGF-1 production by high insulin levels, adipose tissue being a source of IGF-1 production, and the effect of some obesity related factors possibly leptin [26].

Effect of Obesity on Thyroid Axis

Hypothyroidism may cause obesity and an important point to remember in this regard is that exogenous obesity is associated with accelerated growth while obesity due to hypothyroidism is associated with poor growth.21 There is controversy regarding the effect of obesity on thyroid function. Overall, it is believed that the hypothalamic-pituitary-thyroid axis is generally intact and normal in obesity. A retrospective study noted a 20% incidence of TSH elevation in obese patients versus an incidence of 0.3% in non-obese patients, in the face of normal free T4 levels and negative antithyroid antibodies [27]. At present there is no consensus on role of thyroid hormone replacement in this subgroup of patients with apparent subclinical or compensated hypothyroidism [21].

Table 4. Oral medications for the treatment of type 2 diabetes mellitus

Medications	Usual daily dose in mg
Sulfonylureas: (act at the β cell; increase insulin secretion)	
Glimepiride (Amaryl)	1-4
Glipizide (Glucotrol)	10-20
Glyburide (Glynase)	5-20
Micronised glyburide (Micronase)	3-12
Glipizide extended release (Glucotrol XL)	5
α-glucosidase Inhibitors (act at the small intestine; increase insulin sensitivity)	
Acarbose (Precose)	50-100
Miglitol	50-100
Thiazolidinediones (act at the muscle and fat; increase insulin sensitivity*)	
Rosiglitazone	4-8
Pioglitazone	15-45
Biguanides (act at the liver and muscle; increase insulin sensitivity)	
Metformin (Glucophage)	1000-2500
Other (act at the β cell; augment supply of insulin)	
Repaglinide (Prandin)	1-4

* Probably via PPARγ. With permission: Kamboj MK, Diabetes on college campus. Pediatr Clin N Am (2005) 279-305.

Effect of Obesity on Puberty and Reproductive Function

Obesity can interfere with the hypothalamic-pituitary-gonadal (HPG) axis function causing disruption of pubertal development. Obesity in boys may be associated with delay of pubertal development and maturation [28-30]. On the other hand, obesity in girls may be associated with early puberty and early menarche [29,30]. Interference with the HPG axis may cause low FSH, high LH, and high LH:FSH ratios with elevated estrogen levels, presenting clinically with disturbances and irregularity of menstrual function [20,31]. There may be early adrenarche, PCOS, hirsutism, and infertility [32,33]. Free testosterone levels are generally normal, although total testosterone and SHBG levels are low.

Effect of Obesity on Adrenal Axis

In the face of the ongoing obesity epidemic, complex interactions of obesity including the hypothalamic-pituitary-adrenal axis (HPA axis) and the central complex mechanisms of appetite control, are areas of active research work. Over activity of the components of the HPA axis result in hypercortisolemia and cause Cushing's syndrome. These patients exhibit central obesity and increased cortisol levels with disruption of the normal diurnal rhythm. The majority of adolescents with simple, exogenous obesity are believed not to have significant perturbations of the HPA axis. There is increased cortisol secretion rate with normal diurnal rhythm, normal dexamethasone suppression and normal 24 hour free urine cortisol (for body surface area) levels. Recent studies however highlight the role of adreno-cortical dysregulation as a major player in causing insulin resistance and obesity [34]. The enzyme 11βHSD1 present in the liver and adipose tissue regenerates active cortisol from inactive cortisone. Multiple studies have explored the role of dysregulation of 11βHSD1 in adipose tissue in the pathogenesis of insulin resistance and obesity [35,36].

Effect of Obesity on Parathyroid/vitamin D Axis

Abnormalities of the mineral metabolism in calcium, parathyroid, and vitamin D homeostasis are seen in obesity [37]. These changes have suggestions of secondary hyperparathyroidism with elevated parathyroid hormone levels, normal calcium levels, and increased urine calcium levels [31]. A recent study looked at vitamin D and parathyroid hormone level status in obese children before and after weight loss. PTH levels were positively, and 25 hydroxy vitamin D levels were negatively related to the weight status; these changes were believed to be consequences rather than the cause of overweight [38].

Conclusions

The incidence of obesity is rapidly increasing at epidemic proportions in the adolescent age group. Obesity is associated with multi-systemic pathophysiologic alterations leading to a wide array of complications. The endocrine system is one of the systems which is extensively involved with changes in its multiple axes as mentioned in this discussion. It is therefore essential that clinicians recognize and manage obesity early emphasizing life-style modifications to prevent long-term morbidity and mortality.

Acknowledgments

The author thanks Dr Martin Draznin for his critical review of the manuscript and Ms Amy Esman for her expert administrative assistance.

References

[1] Department of Health and Human Services, Centers for Disease Control and Prevention. Atlanta, GA: Centers for Disease Control and Prevention; updated 2007 November 17; cited 2008 February 13. Available from: http://www.cdc.gov/nccdphp/dnpa/obesity/

[2] Institute of Medicine of the National Academies. Washington DC: National Academy of Sciences; 2008; updated 2006 April 7; cited 2008 February 13. Available from: www.iom.edu/cms/22593.aspx

[3] Ogden CL, Flegal KM, Carroll MD, Johnson CL. Prevalence and trends in overweight among US children and adolescents, 1999-2000. JAMA 2002;288:1728-32.

[4] Ogden CL, Carroll MD, Curtin LR, McDowell MA, Tabak CJ, Flegal KM. Prevalence of overweight and obesity in the United States, 1999-2004. JAMA 2006;295:1549-55.

[5] Sinha R, Fisch G, Teague B, Tamborlane WV, Banyas B, Allen K et al. Prevalence of impaired glucose tolerance among children and adolescents with marked obesity. N Engl J Med 2002;346:802-10.

[6] Matthews DR, Hosker JP, Rudenski AS, Naylor BA, Treacher DF, Turner RC. Homeostasis model assessment: insulin resistance and beta-cell function from fasting plasma glucose and insulin concentrations in man. Diabetologia 1985;28:412-9.

[7] Keskin M, Kurtoglu S, Kendirci M, Atabek ME, Yazici C. Homeostasis model assessment is more reliable than the fasting glucose/insulin ratio and quantitative insulin sensitivity check index for assessing insulin resistance among obese children and adolescents. Pediatrics 2005;115:500-3.

[8] Katz A, Nambi SS, Mather K, Baron AD, Follmann DA, Sullivan G et al. Quantitative insulin sensitivity check index: a simple, accurate method for assessing insulin sensitivity in humans. J Clin Endocrinol Metab 2000;85:2402-10.

[9] American Diabetes Association. Screening for type 2 diabetes. Diabetes Care 2004; 27(Suppl 1):S11-4.

[10] Nguyen TT, Keil MF, Russell DL, Pathomvanich A, Uwaifo GI, Sebring NG. Relation of acanthosis nigricans to hyperinsulinemia and insulin sensitivity in overweight African American and white children. J Pediatr 2001;138:474-80.

[11] Stuart CA, Gilkison CR, Smith MM, Bosma AM, Keenan BS, Nagamani M. Acanthosis Nigricans as a risk factor for non-insulin dependent diabetes mellitus. Clin Pediatr (Phila) 1998;37:73-9.

[12] American Diabetes Association. Type 2 diabetes in children and adolescents. Diabetes Care 2000;23:381-9.

[13] American Diabetes Association. Standards of medical care in diabetes. Diabetes Care 2004;27 Suppl 1: S15-35.

[14] Jakicic JM. Exercise in the treatment of obesity. Endocrinol Metab Clin North Am 2003;32:967-80.

[15] Cummings S, Parham ES, Strain GW; American Dietetic Association. Postion of the American Dietetic Association: weight management. J Am Diet Assoc 2002;102:1145-55.

[16] Knowler WC, Barrett-Connor E, Fowler SE, Hamman RF, Lachin JM, Walker EA, et al. Diabetes Prevention Program Research Group. Reduction in the incidence of type 2 diabetes with lifestyle intervention or metformin. N Engl J Med 2002;346:393-403.

[17] Freemark M, Bursey D. The effects of metformin on body mass index and glucose tolerance in obese adolescents with fasting hyperinsulinemia and a family history of type 2 diabetes. Pediatrics 2001;107:E55.

[18] Thearle M, Aronne LJ. Obesity and pharmacologic therapy. Endocrinol Metab Clin North Am 2003;32:1005-24.

[19] Kamboj MK. Diabetes on the college campus. Pediatr Clin North Am 2005;52:279-305.

[20] Gungor N, Arsalanian S. Nutritional disorders. Integration of energy metabolism and its disorders in childhood. In: Sperling M, ed. Pediatric endocrinology, 2nd ed. Philadelphia, PA: Saunders Elsevier, 2002:689-724.

[21] Boston BA. Obesity. In: Kappy MS, Allen DB, Geffner ME, eds. Principles and practice of pediatric endocrinology. Springfield, IL: Charles C Thomas, 2005:577-606.

[22] Vanderschueren-Lodeweyckx M. The effect of simple obesity on growth and growth hormone. Horm Res 1993;40:23-30.

[23] Bowers CY. A new dimension on the induced release of growth hormone in obese subjects. J Clin Endocrinol Metab 1993;76:817-8.

[24] Maccario M, Grottoli S, Procopio M, Oleandri SE, Rossetto R, Gauna C, et al. The GH/IGF-I axis in obesity: Influence of neuro-endocrine and metabolic factors. Int J Obes Relat Metab Disord 2000;24(Suppl 2):S96-9.

[25] Veldhuis JD, Iranmanesh A, Ho KK, Waters MJ, Johnson ML, Lizarralde G. Dual defects in pulsatile growth hormone secretion and clearance subserve the hyposomatotropism of obesity in man. J Clin Endocrinol Metab 1991;72:51-9.

[26] Woelfle JF, Harz K, Roth C. Modulation of circulating IGF-I and IGFBP-3 levels by hormonal regulators of energy homeostasis in obese children. Exp Clin Endocrinol Diabetes 2007;115:17-23 .

[27] Stichel H, L'Allemand D, Grüters A. Thyroid function and obesity in children and adolescents. Horm Res 2000;54:14-9.

[28] Wang Y. Is obesity associated with early sexual maturation? A comparison of the association in American boys versus girls. Pediatrics 2002;110:903-10.

[29] Laron Z. Is obesity associated with early sexual maturation? Pediatrics 2004;113:171-2.

[30] Kaplowitz PB, Slora EJ, Wasserman RC, Pedlow SE, Herman-Giddens ME. Earlier onset of puberty in girls: relation to increased body mass index and race. Pediatrics 2001;108:347-53.

[31] Kokkoris P, Pi-Sunyer FX. Obesity and endocrine disease. Endocrinol Metab Clin North Am 2003;32:895-914.

[32] L'Allemand D, Schmidt S, Rousson V, Brabant G, Gasser T, Grüters A. Associations between body mass, leptin, IGF-I and circulating adrenal androgens in children with obesity and premature adrenarche. Eur J Endocrinol 2002;146:537-43.

[33] Ibañez L, Potau N, Virdis R, Zampolli M, Terzi C, Gussinyé M et al. Postpubertal outcome in girls diagnosed of premature pubarche during childhood: increased frequency of functional ovarian hyperandrogenism. J Clin Endocrinol Metab 1993;76:1599-603.

[34] Roberge C, Carpentier AC, Langlois MF, Baillargeon JP, Ardilouze JL, Maheux P. Adrenocortical dysregulation as a major player in insulin resistance and onset of obesity. Am J Physiol Endocrinol Metab 2007;293:1465-78.

[35] Stewart PM, Boutlon A, Kumar S, Clark PM, Shackleton CH. Cortisol metabolism in human obesity: impaired cortisone – cortisol conversion in subjects with central adiposity. J Clin Endocrinol Metab 1999;84:1022-7.

[36] Weigand S, Richardt A, Remer T, Wudy SA, Tomlinson JW, Hughes B, et al. Reduced 11beta-hydroxysteroid dehydrogenase type 1 activity in obese boys. Eur J Endocrinol 2007;157:319-24.

[37] Glass AR. Endocrine aspects of obesity. Med Clin North Am 1989;73:139-60.

[38] Reinehr T, de Sousa G, Alexy U, Kersting M, Andler W. Vitamin D status and parathyroid hormone in obese children before and after weight loss. Eur J Endocrinol 2007;157:225-32.

In: Obesity and Adolescence: A Public Health Concern
Editors: H.A. Omar, D.E. Greydanus et al.
ISBN: 978-1-60692-821-9

Chapter IV

Obesity and Dermatologic Issues

Donald Hare*

Department of Pediatrics and Human Development, Michigan State University College of Human Medicine, MSU/Kalamazoo Center for Medical Studies, Kalamazoo Michigan, United States of America

Abstract

Obesity presents special challenges for skin care and is associated with several conditions that need careful attention. Conditions reviewed in this chapter will include acanthosis nigricans, papillomatosis of Gougerot and Carteaud, polycystic ovary syndrome, striae distensae, Cushing disease, and Cushing syndrome in relation to their dermatologic aspects. Various treatment modalities reviewed include bathing, soaps, cleansers, shampooing, emollients, topical corticosteroids, topical antibacterials, antifungals, and topical retinoids.

Introduction

Obesity in adolescents presents special challenges for skin care and is associated with several conditions that need careful attention. First, this article considers basic dermatologic anatomy and physiology followed by mention of some basic research perspectives regarding clinical dermatologic conditions. Then the discussion reviews dermatologic conditions including acanthosis nigricans, papillomatosis of Gougerot and Carteaud, polycystic ovary syndrome, striae distensae, Cushing disease, and Cushing syndrome in relation to their dermatologic aspects. Various treatment modalities reviewed include bathing, soaps, cleansers,

* Correspondence: Donald Hare, MD, Associate Professor, Department of Pediatrics and Human Development, Michigan State University College of Human Medicine, MSU/Kalamazoo Center for Medical Studies, 1000 Oakland Drive, Kalamazoo MI 49008-1284 United States. Tel: 269-337-6450; Fax: 269-337-6474; E-mail: hare@kcms.msu.edu

shampooing, emollients, topical corticosteroids, topical antibacterials, antifungals, and topical retinoids.

Anatomy and Physiologogy

The skin has the largest surface area of the body and in the obese individual, the area gradually increases with body size. When obesity starts in childhood as it usually does, the skin increases in growth at a normal pace; however, if weight gain is rapid, at some point stretching may occur resulting in striae or stretch marks which may leave atrophic lines. These may be permanent or may heal and disappear.

The skin is a dynamic organ. The epidermis provides mechanical, physical (e.g. U-V), chemical, and immunological protection from the external environment maintaining a homeostatic internal environment for the body. The subcutaneous fat layer provided protection from cold and heat. The inner layer of the epidermis is the stratum spinosum. The basal layer is a factory of metabolism providing Vitamin D and antibody production. Oil glands provide lubrication and sweat glands help with heat regulation. The dermis which meshes with the epidermis through the rete peges consist of fibroblasts and collagen and is a tough protective layer.

The subcutaneous layer underneath is a vascular layer that contain the fat cells that dynamically produce the endocrine leptin which when called upon along with gastric grehlin controls appetite to maintain a balanced intake of fuel. The color of the skin depends on many factors. Melanocytes in the stratum spinosum are increased in numbers in dark skinned people but are also stimulated to increase in numbers in areas around the neck, axillae, and other areas in obesity and are a marker for insulin resistance and type 2 diabetes mellitus.

Current Researh Perspectives

The agouti gene defect causes obesity and yellow coat color in mice. In these mice, the agouti-signaling protein α133 amino acid peptide is over abundant in many tissues. This protein inhibits the binding of melanocyte stimulating hormone (MSH) to its receptor in the skin (melanocortin-1 receptor) and therefore, reduces melanin pigmentation in the stratum spinosum [1]. The agouti gene defect then could explain the increase in melanocyte stimulating hormone and increase in melanin pigmentation as seen in acanthosis nigricans. When transgenic mice are developed deleting the melanocortin-4 receptor, the mice become hyerphagic and obese [2]. When melanocortin-3 receptors are deleted mice also become obese.

Leptin is actively produced in fat cells and it signals the brain to reduce food intake. Defects in leptin receptors have been shown in the mouse model to increase fat mass. These hormones and their receptors in the skin and subcutaneous tissue as well as other parts of the body are part of the complex metabolic disorder that is responsible for obesity and insulin resistance. Leptin deficient mice (OB or LEP gene) have hyperphagia, insulin resistance, and hyperinsulinemia. The study of the human genome has advanced rapidly and may identify many gene defects responsible for obesity and may lead to new therapies to identify and treat these gene disorders.

Children born with an absence of leptin have been identified. They gain rapidly after birth with a voracious appetite [3,4]. People with leptin mutation defects have been identified and have been treated successfully with recombinant leptin. It has been suggested that obese children and youth should have leptin levels to compare with the normal. One child with leptin deficiency was treated with recombinant leptin and lost 16.4 kg of adipose tissue over a 12-month period [5]. Leptin used for obese adults with normal leptin levels has resulted in some weight loss. Issues regarding such medication as sibutramine, octreotide and metformin therapy are discussed elsewhere. Selected specific dermatologic disorders are now considered.

Acanthosis Nigricans (AN)

AN is a cutaneous disorder characterized by light brown to black veruccous or papillomatous lesions that may appear in any part of the body, but characteristically in the neck, axillae, and in the groin. It may be seen on the knuckles, the perineum, and the breasts. It may appear in childhood or adolescence as a marker for insulin resistance and it is found in various ethnic groups as noted in table 1. AN may be rarely associated with malignancy.

Therapy for AN is not very successful. It seems to be related to circulating peptides, C-peptide or other unknown factors associated with insulin resistance. Good management of the metabolic syndrome or type 2 diabetes seems to improve the AN in patients with these problems [6,7].

Confluent and Reticulate Papillomatosis of Gougerot and Carteaud

This condition can be confused with AN. There is black papillomatosis but no true hyperpigmentation. It appears around the neck and chest. It will not wash off with soap and water but will come off with alcohol. It responds to the tetracycline class of antibiotics.

Table 1. Percentage appearance of acanthosis nigricans in ethnic groups

Adolescents of European origin – 0.5%
Adolescents of Hispanic origin – 6.0%
Adolescents of African American origin – 13.0%
Adolescents of Native American origin – 40%

Polycystic Ovary Syndrome (PCOS)

This is another disorder of insulin resistance with obesity that must be recognized in the adolescent female. It is associated with ovulatory dysfunction and hyperandrogenism. There are increased testosterone and adrenocorticosteroid levels and it is the most common cause of sterility in women PCOS has life long implications for increased risk of infertility, metabolic syndrome, type 2 diabetes mellitus, and possible cardiovascular disease. It is a syndrome and not a disease and must be considered in adolescent females with hirsuitism, acne vulgaris, menstrual irregularities, and obesity. Many cases are atypical and a diagnosis may be challenging because some features will be present and others will not [8].

Striae (Striae Distensae)

Stretch marks are linear depressions of the skin that are initially pink and later become white, shiny, and atrophic. They are seen in areas subject to stretching such as the lower back, buttocks, thighs, breast, abdomen, inguinal areas, and shoulder. They develop in 35% of girls and 15% of boys between 9 and 16 years at a time when the adrenal gland is producing an increased amount of glucocorticoids. They appear at times of rapid growth, obesity, adolescence, and pregnancy. They seem to be due to stress induced rupture of connective tissue damage to collagen as well as elastin and healing is slowed by glucocorticoid activity. Cushing's disease and prolonged use of potent topical steroids aggravate the healing, although in time the striae become less noticeable. In one report, retinoic acid 0.1% cream once per day for eight weeks improved and even faded pink striae [9]. Breast and hip striae showed the best results. Pulsed dye laser treatment has produced good results in the inflammatory (rubra) stage, and this treatment should be limited to experienced dermatologists because some skin types result in hyperpigmentation [9].

Cushing's Disease and Cushing's Syndrome

Cushing's disease is a disorder of overproduction of adrenal cortical hormones from pituitary and hypothalamic overstimulation. Cushing's syndrome is most commonly due to the iatrogenic use of steroid drugs usually systemic but rarely topical. All causes of Cushing's syndrome, except due to exogenously administered corticosteroids, produce signs of combined adrenocortical and androgen excess. A study of 36 children and adolescents with pituitary Cushing's disease had features as noted in table 2 [10].

New onset acne (steroid acne) and/or hirsuitism may be the presenting complaint. Hyperpigmentation of the striae is associated with the generalized hyperpigmentation due to adrenocorticotrophic hormone (ACTH) excess and the melanocyte stimulating hormone (MSH) excess as in Addison's disease. The glucocorticoids also cause a change in the distribution of fat to the cheeks (moon faces), the buffalo hump, the abdomen, and buttocks while sparing the extremities. This is an example of the influence of the endocrine system on the distribution of body fat. Glucocorticoids cause fine downy hair on the sides of the face but the androgens cause true sexual hair excess in pubic and face as well as the mid-chest and abdominal areas.

Other cutaneous features of glucocorticoid excess are due to superinfection with organisms that normally colonize the skin. Tinea versicolor may appear; oral and vaginal candida may also be seen. Fungal infections of the nails may present early. Perleche at the corners of the mouth and intertrigo with candida may appear at the neck, axillae, under the breasts, and in the groin. Glucocorticoids cause distinct perifollicular pustules on the back, upper arms, chest, and face. They are all at the same stage of development and present like a folliculitis; this is called "steroid acne." These dermatologic problems require usual management but may be difficult to treat until endocrinologic management is also started [10].

Table 2. Features of pituitary Cushing's disease in 36 children and adolescents [10]

Striae	77.7%
Acne	58.3%
Hirsutism	63.7% of 22 girls
Acanthosis nigricans	27.7%
Ecchymosis	27.7%
Hyperpigmentation	16.6%
Fungal infections	11.1%

Treatment

Bathing, Soaps and Cleansers

Principles of bathing and skin cleansing do not differ for the obese patient and daily bathing and shampooing is not necessary because the skin is self cleansing. However, daily bathing and shampooing is not harmful and is a ritual in American life. Soap should be mild with a low alkaline pH for sensitive skin but for normal skin any soap that pleases the patient should be acceptable. Soapless cleansers such as Aquanil or Cetaphil are useful as moisturizers for sensitive skin such as eczema. This should be put on the skin before towel drying. After the bath topical steroids should be put on the skin before the emollient for eczema. Retinoids and other potent medications for acne vulgaris should be applied only after the skin is dry because of the rapid absorption of wet skin. Eczema and xerosis present with itching problems that start the scratch-itch cycle in itchy and dry skin. Pramoxine topical and Pramosone have been helpful but not as helpful as topical corticosteroids. Benadryl has been used at bedtime but is not as effective as the newer non-sedating antihistamines. Loratadine is approved to age 3 and Cetirizine to age two years.

Shampooing

Daily shampooing may not be necessary but is not harmful. Medicated shampoos used for dermatitis should be applied before the bath and left on for 15-20 minutes after the bath before rinsing.

Emollients

The best skin emollient is petrolatum or mineral oil. These may not be comfortable in hot weather and may aggravate acne vulgaris when creams and lotions are used. They are important for dry skin especially in cold weather. Lanolin and vegetable oils may be more sensitizing.

Soaks and Bathing

Intertrigo and Staphylococcal pyoderma may require wet compresses for cleansing using dilute chlorhexidine, 2% acetic acid or a 1:40 aluminum acetate (Domeboro) solution. Betadine is not recommended because of iodine absorption from damaged skin. The wet skin after a soothing soak will absorb medications such as Bactroban, Lotrimin, and corticosteroids better when indicated. Poison ivy contact dermatitis responds well to astringent soaks followed by steroid creams or ointments. Intertriginous dermatitis found in the folds of the skin in the neck, groin, axillae, and beneath the folds of the breasts respond well to this plan.

Topical Corticosteroids

Topical cortiocosteroids have been used since 1952 for the treatment of atopic dermatitis and soon after for other inflammatory dermatoses in children and adolescents. They have an immediate and delayed effect on cytokines and immune mediated as well as inflammatory skin conditions. Hydrocortisone was first used as a low potency medication. Its potency has been increased by fluorination, methylation, and acetylation with more potent products being developed as a result. The lowest strength that will clear the eruption in the shortest time should be used. For lesions on the face, skin folds, and diaper areas, use a low potency cream or ointment such as hydrocortisone 1%. For problems that are moderately severe or for thickened dry lesions, use a mid or high potency cream or ointment for a short time and follow with a moisturizing cream or lotion. Continuous use for longer than 4-6 weeks is not recommended because tachyphylaxis can develop. For chronic eczema, intermittent use is much more effective and patients can be given pulsed on and off treatment with a calcineurin inhibitor or moisturizing cream. Prolonged use will cause dermal atrophy, striae, and petechiae. These skin changes will resolve if discontinued after 4 weeks. Striae will not disappear. Prolonged use of medium to high potency steroids will affect the adrenal-pituitary axis and Cushing's syndrome will develop though this is rare with topical steroids. Peri-oral dermatitis is made worse by steroid preparations. The treatment of scabies or tinea with corticosteroids will improve initially only to return with vigor.

Antibacterials and Antifungals

The skin of the obese person is subject to an increased risk for intertrigo with the problem of moist skin folds, increased friction, increased sweating, and rubbing from tight clothing. The female has an increased risk for vulvo-vaginitis and leucorrhea. There is an increased risk for the metabolic syndrome and type 2 diabetes mellitus which leads to monilial infections. The skin may be colonized and infected with Staphylococcal aureus while Pseudomonas may be contracted from hot tubs. Folliculitis in the bearded area as well as areas on the legs from shaving may develop. Skin cultures are indicated to identify resistant organisms and plan appropriate systemic treatment if needed. Topical 1% Clotrimizole or 2% Miconazole cream or vaginal tablets can be used. They are effective for dermatophytes and yeasts. Staphylococcal or streptococcal impetigo of the face may be treated with mupirocin three times daily for 7-10 days. Nasal carrier for streptococcus is common and can be eliminated in 2-4 days with mupirocin ointment but recurrences are expected in 2-4 months. Trimethoprim/sulfamethoxazole is effective, but there is a risk of Stevens-Johnson's Syndrome or hemolytic reaction with G-6-PD deficiency. Nizoral 2% (ketoconazole) cream or shampoo is useful for problems with topical fungal or candida infections; its use systemically is fraught with risks of prolonged QT and sudden death from ventricular tachycardia.

Onychomycosis is common in the older adolescent and is easier to prevent than to treat. Good foot care, frequent bathing, careful drying beneath the toes, the use of foot powder such a Tinactin and appropriate nail care is essential. If fungal nail infection develops, topical nail treatment with ciclopirox or fluconazole is safer but less effective than systemic Sporonox.

Tinea corporis, tinea cruris, tinea pedis, and tinea versicolor are common problems in which fungal cultures and KOH preps confirm the correct diagnosis. Patients with tinea corporis do not need to be excluded from school but wrestlers can spread it. Keeping the area dry and application of antifungal powder or cream such as Nystatin is usually effective. Rarely a systemic antifungal may be needed in which griseofulvin is safer and preferred over ketaconazole. A dermatophytid reaction may occur as an immune reaction in the hands, arms, legs, and trunk, while skin testing shows a positive reaction to dermatophytes.

Tinea versicolor responds to topical Selenium sulphide shampoo or Ketaconozole shampoo. If persistent, fluconazole (Diflucan) 400 mg is given in one dose that may be repeated if necessary. Candidal infections should be looked for as mycelial forms or budding yeasts on KOH preparation or cultures on Sabouraud's media. It is seen as vulvovaginitis or oral candida infection, including moist areas at the corner of the mouth. Treat with Nystatin, clotrimozole, or if persistent, Diflucan 150 mg (one dose) in the older child or adolescent. If these infections persist, check for underlying HIV infection.

Retinoids

There is no published evidence that obesity is related to more or less trouble with acne vulgaris than the average patient; however, when acne occurs, retinoids may be clinically useful. The biologic action of this medication is targeted to intracellular receptors with stimulation of cellular growth, apoptosis, and control of skin cytokines. The newer synthetic retinoids, adapalene and tazarotene, have more selective retinoid receptor interactions than Retin-A (retinoic acid). Retinoids have a comedolytic action and are effective with benzoyl peroxide topical management. Pomade acne consists of multiple closed comedones on the forehead of patients using various hair oils. Topical azelaic acid is effective for inflammatory acne vulgaris but may cause hypopigmentation in dark skinned patients.

Systemic antibiotics may be needed for more severe cases of acne and these include tetracycline, erythromycin, minocycline, and doxycycline. Tetracycline is probably the safest for long term use if effective for the selected patient. Topical preparations of benzoyl peroxide and either erythromycin or clindamycin are often helpful. The estrogenic role of oral contraceptive medications may suppress androgens and may be helpful, although depo-medroxyprogesterone acetate may aggravate acne.

Genetic Disorders Associated with Obesity

Families often enquire regarding a genetic cause for the obesity problem. Obesity as a genetic disorder is rare but frequently seen in conditions listed in table 3 [12]. Many dermatologic features may be present in these syndromes. Skin fibroblasts are affected with streaks of hyperpigmentation in KTN Syndrome. If suspected a genetic referral is indicated [11]

Table 3. Genetic disorders associated with obesity [11-13]

Albright Hereditary osteodystrophy (Intracutaneous ossification from infancy or childhood) Bardet-Biedl Syndrome (Laurence-Moon Biedl's Syndrome) [12]
Borjeson-Forsman Lehman Syndrome
Carpenter Syndrome
Cohen Syndrome
Grebe Syndrome
45 X0 Syndrome
Prader Willi S. (acanthosis nigricans)
Killian Teschler-Nicola S. (Tetrosomy 12p) (streaks of hyperpigmentation)

Conclusions

Dermatologic conditions in children and adolescents with obesity can be challenging conditions for patients and clinicians alike. This discussion considers a variety of skin conditions, including acanthosis nigricans, papillomatosis of Gougerot and Carteaud, polycystic ovary syndrome, striae distensae, Cushing disease, and Cushing syndrome in relation to their dermatologic aspects. Various treatment modalities are also reviewed include bathing, soaps, cleansers, shampooing, emollients, topical corticosteroids, topical antibacterials, antifungals, and topical retinoids. Complex and resistant cases should be referred to dermatologic colleagues.

References

[1] Lu D, Willard D, Patel IR, et al. Agouti protein is an antagonist of the melanocyte stimulating hormone receptor. Nature 1994; 371:799-802.

[2] Vaisse C, Clement K, Duzant E, et al. Melanocyte-4 receptor mutations are frequent and heterogeneous cause of morbid obesity. J Clin Invest 2000;106(2):253-62

[3] Montague CT, Farouki IS, Whitehead JP, et al. Congenital leptin deficiency is associated with early onset obesity in humans. Nature 1997; 387:903-8.

[4] Farouki IS, Yeo GS, Keogh JM, et al. Dominant and recessive inheritance of morbid obesity associated with melanocortin-4 deficiency. J Clin Invest 2000;106(2):185-7

[5] Farouki IS, Jebb, SA , Langmack G, et al. Effects of recombinant leptin therapy in a child with congested leptin deficiency. New Eng J Med 1999;341(12):879-84

[6] Kahn CR, Flier JS, Bar RS, et al. The syndromes of insulin resistance and acanthosis nigricans. N Engl J Med 1976;294:739.

[7] Stuart CA, Gilkison CR, Smith M. Acanthosis nigricans as a risk factor for non-insulin dependent diabetes mellitus. Clin Pediatrics 1998;37:73-80.

[8] Rosenfield RL. Current concepts of polycystic ovary syndrome. Bailliere's Clin Obstet Gynecol 1997;11:307.

[9] Marcus J, Horan, DB, Robinson JK. Tissue expansion, past, present and future. J Am Acad Dermatol 1990;23:813-25.

[10] Stratakis C, Mastorakos G, Mitsiades NS, et al. Skin manifestations of Cushing's disease in children and adolescents before and after the resolution of hypercortisolemia. Ped Dermatol 1998;15(4):253-8.

[11] Schachner LA, Hansen RC. Pediatric dermatology. New York: Mosby 2003.

[12] Slarotinek, AM, Stone EM, Mykytyn K, et al. Mutations in MKKS cause Bardet-Biedle syndrome. Nat Genet 2000;26:15-6.

[13] Greydanus DE, Feinberg AN, Patel DR, Homnick DN. The pediatric diagnostic examination. New York: McGraw-Hill Med Publ, 2008.

In: Obesity and Adolescence: A Public Health Concern
Editors: H.A. Omar, D.E. Greydanus et al.
ISBN: 978-1-60692-821-9

Chapter V

Obesity and Eating Disorders

Vinay N. Reddy [*]
Pediatrics and Human Development, Michigan State University College of Human Medicine, Pediatrics Program, MSU/Kalamazoo Center for Medical Studies, Kalamazoo, Michigan, United States of America

Abstract

Although obesity is not classified as an eating disorder, there are associations between obesity and anorexia nervosa, bulimia nervosa, and binge eating disorder. This chapter reviews some of these associations. For example, a proportion of patients with anorexia nervosa eventually become bulimic and some of these patients eventually become overweight, while anorexia is often seen in a previously obese patient who loses weight successfully and then cannot stop losing weight or continues to try to lose weight even after reaching an otherwise normal weight range. There are possible genetic components for obesity as there are for anorexia nervosa and bulimia nervosa, but there are also associations with the family environment, particularly with family dietary habits. Obese patients should be screened for the presence of an eating disorder, especially bulimia nervosa and binge eating disorder. Obese patients who successfully lose weight should also be carefully observed for the possible development of anorexia nervosa. Principles of management are also reviewed.

* Correspondence: Vinay N. Reddy, MD, Assistant Professor, Pediatrics and Human Development, Michigan State University College of Human Medicine, Pediatrics Program, MSU/Kalamazoo Center for Medical Studies, 1000 Oakland Drive, Kalamazoo, Michigan 49008-1284 United States. Tel: 269-337-6450; Fax: 269-337-6474; E-mail: Reddy@kcms.msu.edu

Introduction

Anorexia nervosa, bulimia nervosa, and binge eating disorder are all classified as eating disorders by the American Psychiatric Association Manual of Mental Disorders (DSM-IV TR)[1]. Obesity is often not regarded as an eating disorder per se and differs from the DSM-IV eating disorders in that distortion of body image, a hallmark of and a diagnostic criterion for anorexia nervosa and for bulimia nervosa, is not common in obese patients. However, there are many connections between obesity and the eating disorders, and especially close associations between obesity and bulimia nervosa as well as between obesity and binge eating disorder.

The term anorexia nervosa (Greek: "nervous loss of appetite") is used to describe patients with self-restriction of food intake, increased physical activity, psychological disturbance including distorted self-perception of appearance, severe weight loss, and, in females [2,3]. In contrast, bulimia nervosa (Greek: "nervous ravenous hunger") is "an irresistible urge to overeat, followed by self-induced vomiting or purging" [4], which may or may not be associated with weight loss; in fact, many adolescents with bulimia nervosa are not underweight, and some are obese or morbidly obese.

Anorexia nervosa and bulimia nervosa were described in DSM-III and -III-R [5,6], while the diagnostic criteria were made more specific in DSM-IV [1] with subtyping of anorexia nervosa patients into "restrictors" and "binge/purgers;" in addition, more stringent criteria was applied for "binge eating" in the definition of bulimia. DSM-IV also includes a category of "eating disorders not otherwise specified" (acronym: EDNOS). This category includes patients with "binge eating disorder", a term used to describe marked binge eating or overeating with significant associated distress, but not followed by purging or other compensation for excessive food intake. Excessive weight is not a required criterion for the diagnosis of binge eating disorder, or of bulimia nervosa, but many patients with binge eating disorder are overweight, as are a smaller but still significant proportion of patients with bulimia nervosa.

Epidemiology

About 0.5-2% of females will meet all of the criteria for diagnosis of anorexia nervosa during their lifetimes. Some patients have only some of the clinical features of anorexia but are still sufficiently ill to require medical treatment for its complications. Bulimia nervosa is much more common with a lifetime prevalence of bulimia of 1-3% [7-9].

Both anorexia nervosa and bulimia nervosa predominantly affect females. Males are also seen with both disorders, but the ratio of affected females to affected males is about 10-20:1 for anorexia and about 10:1 for bulimia. The higher incidence of eating disorders in females may be related to societal and cultural pressures regarding appearance, as considered later in this discussion.

Risk Factors

Eating disorders are by their nature biological, psychological, social, and developmental. They are diseases of affluence, in that they occur in societies where food is plentiful and yet in which "thinness" is valued over "fatness". In such societies people, especially the young, constantly receive both overt and covert messages that fat is bad and "the thinner is the winner" (a phrase that appears on many so-called "pro-ana" or pro-anorexic Web sites). Many eating disorder patients start wanting to lose weight because of specific stimuli of this type; often a patient starts to lose weight after critical remarks about her weight or appearance from family, teachers (especially physical education or health teachers), peers, or romantic interests, or after disorders related to excess weight are diagnosed in family or friends. This can also occur in the previously obese. A small but non-negligible percentage of obese people who try to lose weight by dietary restriction and increased exercise, and who reach a normal weight and BMI, "overshoot" and continue to lose weight until they meet the diagnostic criteria for anorexia. Conversely, a proportion of patients with anorexia nervosa "recover" from their anorexia but then meet the diagnostic criteria for bulimia nervosa; many of these patients are overweight or obese.

As with anorexia nervosa and bulimia nervosa, there is evidence for a genetic component to obesity. Candidate genes have been identified, including genes coding for leptin receptors. Leptin is produced by fatty tissue and appears to be the transmitter involved in feedback regulation of weight [10] and obesity has been induced in experimental animals deficient in these candidate genes. As with anorexia and bulimia, the familial component is most likely environmental as well as genetic, and the environmental component includes the immediate family's dietary habits and is quite significant in itself.

Clinical Features

Bulimia and anorexia have many risk factors in common, as do bulimia and binge eating disorder. Abnormally low body weight excludes the diagnosis of bulimia, and many bulimic patients are also obese; however, excess concern with body image and weight is a diagnostic criterion for bulimia. As many as 30% of those with bulimia have a prior history of anorexia; bulimia, like anorexia, tends to run in families [11]. Childhood and parental obesity are more common in those with bulimia than in the general population or in patients with non-eating-disorder-related psychiatric problems, in contrast to those with anorexia nervosa; also, criticism by family and friends regarding diet and habitus are more common in patients with bulimia [12,13].

Anxiety, mood disorders, personality disorders, and substance abuse are also more common in those with bulimia than in other groups [11]; in particular, up to 75% of patients with bulimia also have or have had an affective disorder [14] and as many as 37% of those with bulimia meet DSM-IV criteria for the diagnosis of borderline personality disorder [15]. A history of abuse, particularly sexual abuse, in childhood is associated with the later development of eating disorders, particularly bulimia. Many theories have been advanced as to the mechanisms, including development of a disassociative coping style, poor self-esteem and self-hatred, and attempts to reexert control over the patient's own life [16,17]. Adolescents with bulimia also seem to have a higher incidence of novelty-seeking behavior and impulsivity, and an increased incidence of self-injurious behavior including self-mutilation, substance abuse, and suicidal behavior [18], which is consistent with the association between bulimia and borderline personality disorder.

Bulimia usually develops in early adulthood or late adolescence, in contrast to the association with puberty seen in anorexia. Disordered eating in bulimia typically begins during or after a period of dieting, when a patient comes to believe that it is possible to cut caloric and nutritional absorption by purging after eating; however, many patients begin bingeing before making other diet changes [19]. Emetics such as ipecac are sometimes used to purge, but more often patients learn to induce vomiting with their fingers or with objects such as toothbrush handles, and with practice patients learn to vomit voluntarily without adjuncts. Others use laxatives or enemas in an attempt to increase stool output, reduce weight, and hopefully decrease absorption of nutrients, or take diuretics to lose weight acutely; they do not understand that these measures simply redistribute fluid. Bulimic (and anorexic) diabetics have been known to stop their own insulin to cause hyperglycemia leading to hyperglucosuria and osmotic diuresis, while some with bulimia and anorexia have resorted to stimulants or thyroid hormone to induce weight loss.

As bulimia develops, the initial feeling of control over weight and the satisfaction of eating large amounts of food without gaining weight decreases. Hunger after purging leads to "compensatory" bingeing, and a vicious cycle develops, made worse by other provocations to binge such as anxiety, depressed mood, boredom, and use of alcohol and other substances that reduce inhibition. Certain "forbidden" foods may also trigger binges. Binges tend to occur while alone, and patients may hoard food for later bingeing in privacy. As with anorexia, bulimic patients will go to great lengths to conceal their disordered eating behavior from family and friends. The amount of food ingested may be massive (i.e., >10,000 kcal in a single binge), but may also be no larger than a normal meal and distinguished from normal eating only by the patient's perceived loss of control during the meal.

Assessment

The high prevalence of eating disorders in adolescents makes screening patients for signs and symptoms imperative; such screenings should involve obese adolescents as well. An obese patient may be even more at risk for development of an eating disorder, and may already have bulimia nervosa or binge eating disorder. The reported mortality rates for those with anorexia exceeds that for bulimia, but a bulimic patient may appear relatively normal physically with no outward signs of potentially lethal metabolic derangements. Patients in the early stages of anorexia, especially if they are or have recently been overweight, may not yet show the stigmata of chronic malnutrition.

Table 1. Screening questions for patients with disordered eating (adapted from Sigman) [20]

For the patient:

- Are you dieting now?
- Do you diet often?
- Are you comfortable with your weight and appearance? Do you want it to change?
- Do you think about food and food choices often? Do you wish you could think about it less?
- Do you do things to control your weight that you wish you didn't have to do as often?
- Do you feel in control of the way you eat?

For the parents:

- Has the way your child has been eating changed?
- Is your child overly concerned about weight or food choices?
- Have you noticed any compulsive weight control behaviors, such as dieting, excessive exercise, or frequent weighing?
- • Has your child been eating fewer meals with the family than in the past?

When taking a history, initial screening questions for disordered eating are noted in table 1 [20]. Diagnosis of an eating disorder in an obese patient may be complicated by the patient's and physician's desire to maintain or reduce her current weight and diet. When working with an obese patient, it is important to watch for and avoid "undershoot" of weight; similarly it is important to avoid "overshoot" of weight in treating an anorexic patient, both to maintain a good therapeutic relationship and to avoid the possible development of frank obesity.

The physician's own attitude toward obesity is a potential pitfall in caring for the obese patient, and may itself contribute to the development of an eating disorder. The negative reaction to obese people seen in their peers is, consciously or not, shared by many of clinicians, and to treat these patients effectively the physician must set these reactions aside. Also, as with the eating disorders, treatment of obesity may be lengthy and drawn-out, complicated by socioeconomic factors affecting both patients and their families; these issues may make it difficult for these adolescents to improve their diet and exercise. Simply helping the adolescent patient to maintain a stable weight may be more feasible than trying to achieve actual weight loss.

Treatment

There are many aspects in common in the management of patients with anorexia nervosa or with bulimia nervosa. The psychological aspects of treatment are especially similar. The treatment of obesity, which inevitably involves recommended or imposed dietary restriction, may in fact trigger anorexia or bulimia. For example, in the World War II-era study by Keys [21,22] volunteer subjects who were subjected to severe dietary restriction for several months continued to restrict their own intake for some time after the imposed restriction was lifted; also, a similar phenomenon is seen in some -- but not all -- obese persons who develop clinical features of anorexia after losing an appropriate amount of weight.

The patient with an eating disorder is treated most effectively by a team approach whether the youth is in an outpatient or as an inpatient setting [23,24]. The multifactorial nature of eating disorders makes it unlikely that any one person will have all the therapeutic and medical skills an eating disorders patient needs to be treated effectively. The core of a typical treatment team includes a physician, a psychotherapist, and a dietitian. The physician is responsible for the patient's medical supervision, including overall regulation of nutrition and medication, monitoring of symptoms, physical findings as well as laboratory studies, and management of such complications as malnutrition, refeeding, and purging. Often a pediatrician or internist works in partnership with a psychiatrist, since the latter is more familiar with psychotropic agents including their uses and side effects. Subspecialists in adolescent medicine and pediatric hospitalists are often well-versed in eating-disorder management.

The therapist concerns herself with the psychological and social aspects of the patient's eating disorder, as well as concurrent and contributing problems such as obsessive-compulsive disorder or prior abuse. A clinical psychologist or a psychiatric social worker experienced in working with adolescents with eating disorders and their families is recommended. Family therapy and parent coaching are also important in treating adolescents with eating disorders, since these adolescents live in the context of their families. Some therapists can provide both individual and family therapy, or collateral therapy in which the patient is seen separately from the parents by the same provider; however, in other situations, separate individual and family therapists may be required.

Cognitive-behavioral therapy (CBT) has been shown in randomized controlled trials to be effective in the treatment of bulimia nervosa, and is felt by some to be the psychotherapy of choice in those patients, whether conducted on an individual or a group basis [25-28]. Dialectical-behavioral therapy, which combines CBT with principles derived from Zen Buddhism, is a frequently-used modality for patients with borderline personality disorder (BPD) and has been found effective in treating patients with BPD and bulimia nervosa or binge eating disorder [29,30].

Table 2. Hospital admission indications for eating disorder patients

- Body weight that is dangerously low or has dropped rapidly
- Electrolyte disturbances, including hypokalemia and hypophosphatemia
- Symptomatic bradycardia or orthostatic hypotension, or signs of heart failure
- Risk of self-injury (suicide, or ED behaviors that have potential for physical injury)
- Concomitant medical or psychiatric conditions requiring hospitalization
- Failure of outpatient treatment to arrest the progress of the disease

Although the medical aspects of refeeding need close medical supervision, a dietitian is also an essential part of the team. Her role includes not only helping to determine patients' nutritional needs, but educating patients and their families on the role of specific nutrients, assisting in planning menus, and addressing the adolescent patient's beliefs, attitudes, and misconceptions about various foods. As with other members of the team, a dietitian who has experience working with adolescents with eating disorders is desirable, but dietitians without such experience can be helpful in communication with other, more experienced professionals on the patient's team.

A social worker can contribute to treatment in ways other than providing direct therapy to the patient and family. She or he can assist in resolving conflicts between the patient and family, and can help identify patient/family needs and locate other management resources. A recreational therapist or child-life specialist can be very valuable in helping patients improve their social interactions and with learning relaxation techniques.

The majority of eating disorder patients, and in particular most bulimic patients, can be managed as outpatients. Anorexic patients are hospitalized more often than bulimic patients in part because of physiologic changes that accompany chronic malnutrition. Table 2 provides indications for admission.

Medical Management

Eating disorder patients and those who treat them have a common goal, that is, they all want the patient to "eat healthy". The difference between patients and therapists is in the definition of "healthy eating." One feature of eating disorders is distortion of the patient's view of what healthy eating really involves. The modern Western world values thinness, and society is continuously bombarded with messages extolling thinness and denigrating fatness. The effects of societal pursuit of thinness are magnified in obese patients, for whom frequent weight-based criticism may trigger an eating disorder. As a result, many ED patients learn to fear fat and to avoid fat intake at all costs, not realizing that fatty acids are essential to many physiological functions, from hormone production to nerve-fiber myelination. Providing nutrition to an ED patient is a matter of helping the adolescent patient maintain a healthy weight range and to do so with as little food-related anxiety as is possible. In an obese patient this may require initial weight reduction, while simultaneously helping the patient avoid "undershoot".

The ultimate goal is for the patient to reach and maintain good health in a healthy weight range. The concept of a range must be emphasized, since the patient will focus on a particular number as a goal and feel that she has failed if her weight is above or below that number. The healthy range, or goal range, is that in which she has normal physical, endocrine, metabolic, and reproductive functioning. The latter is one factor used in choosing a healthy weight range for a patient. It is common to choose a goal weight range corresponding to 10-15 percentiles below the anorexic patient's height percentile, based on National Center for Health Statistics standard growth charts. This may be appropriate for a formerly obese patient who is now anorexic. For an adolescent patient who presents with obesity, an appropriate goal range may be at or above the mean for age and/or height, especially since weight loss of 10-15 pounds is associated with improvement in other physiologic markers such as blood pressure and glucose regulation.

Even before admission, cardiac dysrhythmias due to electrolyte imbalance are the most concerning complication of anorexia and bulimia nervosa. Electrolyte imbalances are most often due to purging, whether by vomiting (which results in both potassium loss and hypochloremic metabolic alkalosis), laxative abuse (leading to metabolic acidosis because of bicarbonate loss in stools), or excessive use of diuretics (also leading to metabolic alkalosis). Prolonged QT intervals are also often seen in ED patients; the mechanism for this is unclear but may be related to deficiency of magnesium and/or potassium. Prolonged QT intervals may also be a contraindication to many medications that might otherwise be useful in these patients. Abuse of ipecac for purging may result in skeletal and cardiac myopathy due to toxic effects of emetine. Excessive vomiting, regardless of how it is induced, may cause upper gastrointestinal trauma ranging from a Mallory-Weiss tear to rupture of the esophagus or stomach.

Counseling and Therapy

Since eating disorders are biopsychosocial in nature, individual therapy and family therapy are essential to recovery and to preventing relapse. This is true for inpatients and outpatients, and therapy for these two groups is largely similar. Psychotherapy, including individual, family, and group therapy, should begin as soon as possible after diagnosis, and is generally started or restarted almost immediately after inpatient medical admission; it is, of course, the mainstay of residential therapy for eating disorder patients. Initial therapy for patients hospitalized for severe malnutrition may consist of little more than supportive counseling, coupled with basic explanations of the disease and its effect on the patient that can be repeated and varied as necessary.

Psychotropic Medications

Psychotropic medications have also been used to treat patients with eating disorders, especially in bulimia nervosa where the use of selective serotonin reuptake inhibitor (SSRI) antidepressants such as fluoxetine is supported by randomized controlled trials. However, the salutary effect of SSRIs in these patients is not as great, or as long-lasting, as that of CBT, and it appears that the most effective treatment for bulimia is the combined use of CBT and an SSRI [26,31].

Conclusions

Although obesity is not classified as an eating disorder, there are associations between obesity and the DSM-IV-defined eating disorders. Many patients with binge eating disorder are overweight, as are a smaller but still significant proportion of patients with bulimia nervosa. Anorexia nervosa, for which abnormally low body mass is a diagnostic criterion, is not immediately associated with obesity. However, a proportion of patients with anorexia nervosa eventually become bulimic and some of these patients eventually become overweight, while anorexia is often seen in a previously obese patient who loses weight successfully and then cannot stop losing weight or continues to try to lose weight even after reaching an otherwise normal weight range.

There are possible genetic components for obesity as there are for anorexia nervosa and bulimia nervosa, but there are also associations with the family environment, particularly with family dietary habits. Bulimia runs in families, and both childhood and parental obesity are more common in patients with bulimia compared with the general population. Bulimia often begins after a period of dieting when a patient starts thinking that purging after eating will result in weight loss, then worsens when post-purging hunger leads to "compensatory" bingeing which is then followed by further purging. Obese patients should be screened for the presence of an eating disorder, especially bulimia nervosa and binge eating disorder. Obese patients who successfully lose weight should also be watched for the possible development of anorexia nervosa.

References

[1] American Psychiatric Association. Diagnostic and statistical manual of mental disorders, 4th ed, text revision. Washington, DC: APA, 2000.

[2] Gill W. Anorexia nervosa (apepsia hysterica, anorexia hysterica). Trans Clin Soc London 1874;7:22-28.

[3] Silverman J. Sir William Gill (1819-1890). Limner of anorexia nervosa and myxoedema. An historical essay and encomium. Eat Weight Disord 1997;2(3):111-6.

[4] Russell G. Bulimia nervosa: an ominous variant of anorexia nervosa. Psychol Med 1979;9(3):429-48.

[5] American Psychiatric Association. Diagnostic and statistical manual of mental disorders, 3rd ed. Washington, DC: APA, 1980.

[6] American Psychiatric Association. Diagnostic and statistical manual of mental disorders, 3rd revised ed. Washington, DC: APA, 1987.

[7] Quintero-Parraga E, Perez-Montiel A, Montiel-Nava C, Pirela D, Acosta M, Pineda N. Eating behavior disorders. Prevalence and clinical features in adolescents in the city of Maracaibo, Zulia State, Venezuela. Invest Clin 2003;44:179-93.

[8] Kendler K, MacLean C, Neale M, Kessler R, Heath A, Eaves L. The genetic epidemiology of bulimia nervosa. Am J Psychiatry 1991;148:1627-37.

[9] Garfinkel P, Lin E, Goering P, Spegg C, Goldbloom D, Kennedy S, et al. Bulimia nervosa in a Canadian community sample: prevalence and comparison of subgroups. Am J Psychiatry 1995;152:1052-8.
[10] Zhang Y, Proenca R, Maffei M, Barone M, Leopold L, Friedman JM. Positional cloning of the mouse obese gene and its human homologue. Nature 1994;372 (6505):425-32.
[11] Klump K, Kaye W, Strober M. The evolving genetic foundations of eating disorders. Psychiatr Clin North Am 2001;24(2):215-25.
[12] Fairburn C, Doll H, Welch S, Hay P, Davies B, O'Connor M. Risk factors for binge-eating disorder: A community-based case-control study. Arch Gen Psychiatry 1998;55:425-32.
[13] Fairburn C, Welch S, Doll H, Davies B, O'Connor M. Risk factors for bulimia nervosa: A community-based case-control study. Arch Gen Psychiatry 1997;54:509-17.
[14] Brewerton TD, Lydiard RB, Herzog DB, Brotman AW, O'Neil PM, Ballenger JC. Comorbidity of axis I psychiatric disorders in bulimia nervosa. J Clin Psychiatry 1995;56:77-80.
[15] Sansone RA, Levitt JL, Sansone LA. The prevalence of personality disorders among those with eating disorders. Eat Disord 2004;13(1):7-21.
[16] Smolak L, Murnen S. Meta-Analytic Examination of the relationship between child sexual abuse and eating disorders. Int J Eat Disord 2002;31:136-50.
[17] Rayworth B, Wise L, Harlow B. Childhood abuse and risk of eating disorders in women. Epidemiology 2004;15:271-8.
[18] Paul T, Schroeter K, Dahme B, Nutzinger D. Self-injurious behavior in women with eating disorders. Am J Psychiatry 2002;159:408-11.
[19] Haiman C, Devlin M. Binge Eating before the onset of dieting: A distinct subgroup of bulimia nervosa? J Eat Disord 1999;25:151-7.
[20] Sigman G. Eating disorders in children and adolescents. Ped Clin North Am 2003;50:1139-77.
[21] Keys A. The residues of malnutrition and starvation. Science 1950;112(2909):371-3.
[22] Taylor HL, Keys A. Adaptation to caloric restriction. Science 1950;2904(2899):215-8.
[23] Rome E, Ammerman S, Rosen D, Keller R, Lock J, Mammel K, et al. Children and adolescents with eating disorders: The state of the art. Pediatrics 2003;111:e98-e108.
[24] Joy E, Wilson C, Varechok S. The multidisciplinary team approach to the outpatient treatment of disordered eating. Curr Sports Med Rep 2003;2(6):331-6.
[25] Walsh B, Wilson G, Loeb K, Devlin M, Pike K, Roose S, et al. Medication and psychotherapy in the treatment of bulimia nervosa. Am J Psychiatry 1997;154(4):523-31.
[26] Fairburn C, Harrison P. Eating disorders. Lancet 2003;361:407-16.
[27] Lundgren J, Danoff-Burg S, DA. A cognitive-behavioral therapy for bulimia nervosa: An empirical analysis of clinical significance. Int J Eat Disord 2004;35(3):262-74.
[28] Mitchell J, Pyle R, Pomeroy C, Zollman M, Crosby R, Seim H, et al. Cognitive-behavioral group psychotherapy of bulimia nervosa: importance of logistical variables. Int J Eat Disord 1993;14(3):277-87.

[29] Safer D, Telch C, Agras W. Dialectical behaviou therapy for bulimia nervosa. Am J Psychiatry 2001;158(4):632-4.

[30] Telch C, Agras W, Linehan M. Dialectical behavior therapy for binge eating disorder. J Consult Clin Psychol 2001;69(6):1061-5.

[31] Greydanus DE, Calles J, Patel DR: Pediatric and adolescent psychopharmacology: A primer for the pediatrician. Cambridge: Cambridge Univ Press, 2008.

III. Sexuality

In: Obesity and Adolescence: A Public Health Concern
Editors: H.A. Omar, D.E. Greydanus et al.
ISBN: 978-1-60692-821-9

Chapter VI

Obesity and Sexuality

Helen D. Pratt*, Donald E. Greydanus, and Kazue Ishitsuka

Division of Behavioral and Developmental Pediatrics, Pediatrics Program, Michigan State University/Kalamazoo Center for Medical Studies, Kalamazoo, Michigan, United States of America and Division of Child and Adolescent Psychiatry, Tokyo Metropolitan Umegaoka Hospital, Setagaya-Ku, Tokyo, Japan

Abstract

Adolescence is a critical period of growth and development in an individual's maturation from puberty to adulthood. A key component of normal adolescence is the process of healthy sexual development that is influenced by an inevitable passage through the stages of maturation from infancy to adulthood. Primary care clinicians should understand and appreciate the importance of sexuality in the lives of their adolescent patients. Obesity is one of the factors that influences sexuality in adolescents. The purpose of this chapter is to succinctly discuss the relationship between obesity and adolescent sexuality. In this regard, it is vital to examine whether obesity alone can derail healthy adolescent sexual development. Not all overweight adolescents experience severe negative outcomes because of their obesity. However, for those who do experience negative sexuality issues, the sensitive and caring clinician can help direct them to helpful resources to address these critical issues.

Introduction

Adolescence is a critical period of growth and development in an individual's maturation from puberty to adulthood [1,2]. The hallmark of adolescence is the process of puberty, a profound neurobiological/psychological event in the life of each child that prepares the way

* Correspondence: Helen D Pratt, PhD, Pediatrics Program, MSU/KCMS, 1000 Oakland Dr, Kalamazoo, MI 49008 United States. Tel: 269 337-6450; Fax 269-337-6474; E-mail: pratt@kcms.msu.edu

for eventual adulthood. The onset of puberty is often accompanied by acts of daydreaming, fantasizing, feelings of confusion, fears about the future, peer rejection, strong emotions, and strong physiological reactions to a variety of stimuli. These accompaniments are a part of the continued process of human sexual development (see table 1) [3]. A key component of healthy sexual development involves how the adolescent moves through the stages of maturation from infancy to adulthood (see table 2) [4-12]. As adolescents matriculate through puberty into adulthood they generally will come to terms with their own sexuality.

Table 1. Components of sexuality biologic sex (XX or XY)

Gender identity
Gender role behavior
Behaviors associated with masculinity or femininity and androgyny

Sexual orientation:
- Physical and emotional attractions to individuals
- Heterosexual, gay lesbian or bisexual

Cultural environment
Family inter- and intra- personal intimacy
Peer inter- and intra- personal relationships and intimacy
Personal
Physical health

Mental health
- Emotional
- Intellectual

Psychosocial Health
Exposure to interpersonal violence or abuse
Perceptions of attractiveness to others
Body image (positive negative view of physical attributes)
Self esteem (negative/positive views of value/worthiness)
Body satisfaction/dissatisfaction

Sexual activity
- Masturbation
- Mutual masturbation

Petting/kissing
Sexual intercourse

Table 2. Factors that may impede development of healthy sexuality in adolescents

Cognitive factors

- Poor self esteem
- Negative body image
- Body dissatisfaction
- Negative perceptions of physical characteristics
- Poor intimate peer relationships
- Feeling overweight or fat

Physical factors

- Delayed physical or mental development
- Being overweight
- Being physically different from peers

Exposure to violence or trauma

- Sexual molestation
- Sexual assault
- Rape
- Being harassed physically or sexually
- Dating violence
- Constant exposure to sexual media content.

Unwanted pregnancy

Sexually transmitted diseases

Physical disabilities or chronic illness

Growing up during adolescence brings with it a number of inevitable stresses and obstacles without the potential burden of additional issues, such as obesity. It is important to examine whether obesity alone can derail healthy adolescent sexual development. Research shows that not all obese adolescents grow up to be maladjusted. Obese adolescents are sexual individuals as can be readily observed by simply watching and counting the number of pregnant young women in any area of the United States. Many of the psychosocial outcomes of obesity are also common psychosocial outcomes of adolescence itself. Additionally, physiological and biological processes of adolescence may promote or predispose to the condition of being overweight or obese in females.13 Since obesity is one of the factors that influences sexuality in adolescents, the purpose of this discussion is to consider the relationship between obesity and the development of sexuality in adolescents.

Defining Sexuality

Sexuality begins at conception and the physiologic components to sexuality are evident at an early age (see table 1)[4-12]. Sexuality is comprised of the interactions between a complex set of individual, family, environmental, peer, and community variables as well as processes. Sexuality is affected by various family, legal, ethical, moral, and religious issues. An individual's personal history of exposure to violence (i.e., rape, abuse, molestation) can have a significant impact on that adolescent's sexuality. Factors such as hormonal problems, body dissatisfaction, poor self image, and interest in sexual activity also impact an individual's sexuality [13].

A person's sexuality is based on his or her body image. Body image, a vital component of sexuality, is influenced by factors that include: a) attitudes about intimacy, b) perceptions about attractiveness, c) views about peer reactions to his or her physical characteristics, d) mental depiction of his or her personal body size and e) the feelings concerning those characteristics [2,13].

Defining Obesity

The term "at risk for overweight" is defined by the Centers for Disease Control and Prevention (CDC), when an adolescent's age- and sex specific body mass index (BMI) is over the 85th percentile, but below the 95th percentile [14]. "Overweight" has been defined by the CDC as a sex- and age-specific BMI at or above the 95th percentile based on revised CDC growth charts. The classic formula for calculating BMI is weight in kilogram devided by height in meter squared ($BMI=kg/m^2$).

Sexuality Development

Beginning in infancy, youth discover their bodies first through internal and external sensations. Next, they learn how their specific actions/reactions cause changes in their environments. A combination of their ability to process these sensations and the resulting cause and effect relationships in their environments help to shape aspects of their sexuality. Early experiences with sexuality include the activities of daily living (i.e., feeding, changing diapers, bathing, nurturing, and soothing). How an infant is held, how gentle the care giver is when the child is bathed, how the genitalia are handled when a diaper is changed are all events that help the child and youth develop body image and feelings of value. The infant who has caregivers who can interpret her needs, and responds to those needs in a manner that nurtures or soothes, is learning about her self and how to get her needs met. The infant who sees the caregiver smile and talk in a soothing nature is learning to see themselves as able to make others happy.

The child that grows with these same levels of care begins to develop self-confidence, enjoys others, and behaves in a way that encourages others to see them as lovable and valuable. For example, infants learn to associate sensory inputs of warmth and satiation with suckling (breast or nipple), ingesting nutrients, visual cues, touch, and smells. While gazing into the eyes of their caregivers as they are held firmly and gently against a warm body and are fed, the infant begins to link these sensory experiences with satiation which sets the early feelings of pleasure. As the infant matures and experiences these basic senses (i.e., cognitive, visual, emotional, sensory, and kinesthetic), and gets his or her needs met in a timely fashion, that infant will learn how to get access to pleasurable events and avoid or minimize negative events. This infant learns to control his or her environment and develops a healthy sense of self and is one step closer to having the requisite components of healthy sexuality for a lifetime.

The same process continues through adolescence. The adolescent who learns to love himself, to be flexible in his view of others, to be patient with others, and to know how to be comforted and soothed by stable caregivers will be better able to adjust to the stresses of growing up as well as the rejection and conflict that may occur with peers.

Through this process youth also learn about the function, roles, sensations, and emotions connected to their body parts. Youth are naturally curious about sexuality and often experiment widely, especially during mid-adolescence. They become keenly aware of their bodies, the accompanying sensations to stimuli that occur in their bodies, and their associations to their sense of sexually. Adolescents may find some sensations they experience to be more pleasurable than others. They are attracted to some types of individuals and may fear or reject other types of people. These feelings of attraction are refined as youth grow and their exposure to pleasurable and aversive stimuli is broadened.

Female adolescents generally become more self conscious about their bodies as they make the critical journey through puberty. As their bodies develop breasts and their hips become full, female adolescents may become concerned about being fat and may fear being objects of sexual harassment [15]. Males who do not develop masculine characteristics are more likely to be more self conscious about their bodies [15]. Youth are often concerned about being too thin or too short. Female adolescents may be concerned about not developing large enough breasts or having breasts that are too small; male adolescents may be more concerned about musculature and penis size [16].

Other gender differences in sexuality development include developmental milestones. For example, females tend to develop most of their self esteem based on their physical attractiveness. This attitude corresponds roughly with Erikson's developmental task of "identity vs role confusion" in which she attempts to integrate her many roles, including that of being a sexual person, into a healthy self-image within the context of peer pressure and role models. Males base their sense of self-esteem on their ability to accomplish things. This corresponds with Erikson's developmental task of "industry vs inferiority" wherein he tries to develop a sense of self worth by refining skills [16]. Being different than one's peers is a major contributor to body dissatisfaction [15].

Expressions of sexual behaviors such as affection are initially learned in the adolescent's family. This family sets the rules, mores, and level of acceptance for what expressions of sexuality (sexual behavior [such as masturbation, kissing, hugging], emotions, and affection are acceptable or unacceptable. As the adolescent's environment broadens to include others (i.e., communities, schools, and peer groups) they learn more about sexuality and may have specific physiological responses to the emotion of affection and arousal. Adolescents may become concerned about whether their cognitions, emotions, and physiological reactions make them heterosexual or homosexual, especially if they are experiencing feelings of strong emotions towards a same sex person. Youth may also become confused by some of the thoughts they have about themselves and others. They are often hypersensitive to feedback from others about their physical characteristics, physical performance, and social skills (especially from peers). These experiences of hypersensitivity are normal and natural processes of normal maturation during adolescence, along with oral language and physical awkwardness.

Adolescents who develop low self-esteem, negative body image, doubts involving future self-sufficiency, and questions about their value may become easy prey for peers who criticize and bully others for their own advantage [17]. They may seek intimate relationships that are not mutually satisfying and healthy. Some of these youth may engage in high risk behaviors as a means of gaining peer approval, acceptance, and affection.2 As the individual moves into puberty, cognitive processes begin to focus on body image issues as growth patterns begin to accelerate rapidly and body contours change dramatically [2].

Female sexuality researchers and educators in sexuality often note considerable differences in how both sexes view sexuality [2]. Several studies on adolescent body and self esteem found that issues such as BMI, acne, and height each are related to an adolescent having lower self esteem and seeing themselves as being less sexually attractive. Although African Americans females in one study had more favorable body self esteem than Caucasians, they had higher BMIs. Additionally BMI was associated with overall body esteem and weight concerns but not with feelings of sexual attractiveness [15,17,18].

Males tend to learn their early concepts of sexuality in the context of social relationships. American males may learn early in their development to define masculinity as synonymous with such destructive concepts as dominance, competition, performance, and achievement. Males lacking extended contact with their fathers for appropriate role model patterns are especially vulnerable to such misogynic cues from the media. Males are taught from early life and throughout life to be more distrustful and insecure than females. Males are taught to control their sexual thoughts in regard to males and to use homophobia as a guiding principle. Males are more likely to carry negative attitudes about their bodies from their childhood throughout adolescence and adulthood. Though males tend to masturbate earlier than females, they are more likely to avoid group masturbation due to societal homophobic attitudes. The issue of whether or not females engage in group masturbation was not addressed in our review [2].

Self-esteem and Sexuality

Self esteem refers to how an individual feels about his or her physical attributes and instrumental effectiveness. Adolescents develop healthy self esteem that is positive and self-sustaining for a lifetime when they have been nurtured and reared in a cultural environment that has consistently taught them from infancy through adolescence that they are worthy, have intrinsic value, and are competent in all areas of life, including sexual realms. Females tend to develop most of their self esteem based on physical attractiveness or how pretty they are. Males tend to develop their self esteem based on their instrumental effectiveness or based on their ability to accomplish things.16

The female adolescent's self esteem is based on how happy they are with their bodies which translates into how attractive they may see themselves. During early adolescence, girls tend to base their body dissatisfaction on how well their physical attributes match or do not match those of their age appropriate peers. One researcher found that among their American subjects, Latinos and Asians, who were among the leanest 25 percent of girls, reported significantly more body dissatisfaction than did Caucasians [15]. Caucasian girls who were shorter in height and Asian girls who were taller in height than their peers were also more likely to be unhappy with their body type [15,19]. Adolescents who have learned to be satisfied with their bodies are less likely to experience body dissatisfaction even if their body mass index increases [20].

Impact of Obesity on Sexuality

Overweight adolescents may be viewed as unattractive and assumed to be sexually maladjusted. They may also develop poor self esteem, poor self image, unhealthy or unrealistically negative body images, and ineffective social skills. Overweight adolescents and those who view themselves as being overweight may experience social rejection, harassment, and mental health problems. There are no substantial clinical data at this point to support the psychological theory that obesity is a defense against sexuality [18,21].

Research supports the concept that overweight adolescents are more victimized, date less, and are less satisfied with their dating status, than are their non-overweight peers [17]. Because adolescents rely on their peers for the development and maintenance of their self-image, self-acceptance, and sense of belonging, the rejection that obese youth experience from their peers can have devastating effects on their overall social and psychological health [17]. Being overweight can result in an adolescent (except for African American females) experiencing negative social and psychological health through maladaptive peer experiences [17,22].

Studies of the impact of adolescent obesity and sexual activity were not found in our literature search. However, one study on the topic with adult males concluded that significantly obese adult males found that they had a) body image dissatisfaction, b) lacked desire for sexual activity, c) lacked erotic fantasies and d) lacked motivation in sexual advances.23 Extreme (morbid) obesity in an adolescent might present problems that interfere with the actual physical expression of sexuality. These youth may have difficulty consummating the act of sexual intercourse. They may feel inadequate compared with "normal" peers and therefore may feel a need to perform well sexually. This performance pressure may predispose to sexual dysfunction [25].

In order to gain peer acceptance and approval overweight or obese adolescents may become involved in high risk sexual activities to prove that they are normal and able to engage in the sexual activities they see modeled in the media by their thin peers. However, this same reaction can occur in adolescents who have physical disabilities, mental illness, chronic illness, or poor social relationships from various causes.

Conclusions

Primary care clinicians should understand and appreciate the importance of sexuality in the lives of their adolescent patients. All of the critical components to healthy child and adolescent development are equally important to the development of healthy sexuality. Sexuality is a critical part of normal growth and development. Adolescents need knowledgeable health care professionals who can a) help parents understand what healthy sexuality is about, and b) supplement parental teaching about human sexuality in a confidential and sensitive manner.

Obesity impacts healthy sexuality development if it impedes an adolescent's body image, self esteem, self confidence, self worth, and emotional health as well as peer relations. Not all overweight adolescents experience severe negative outcomes because of their obesity. But for those who do experience negative sexuality issues, the sensitive and caring clinician can help direct them to appropriate resources to address these issues. The clinician who is not biased against obesity and remains non judgmental while presenting helpful information on human sexuality is more likely to have an adolescent patient who is in compliance with recommended medical regimes.

References

[1] Lewis M. Overview of infant, child and adolescent development. In: Wiener JM, ed. Textbook of child and adolescent psychiatry, 2nd ed. Washington, DC: Am Psychiatr Press, 1997:39-66.

[2] Greydanus DE. National Institute of Health conference on disability through the lifespan. Peers and sexuality. Bethesda, MD, 21-22 Jul 2003.

[3] Pratt HD, Greydanus DE. Normal psychological development. In: Greydanus DE, Patel DR, Prat HD, eds. Behavioral pediatrics vol I. New York: Universe, 2006:5-36.

[4] Piaget J. Intellectual evaluation from adolescence to adulthood. Hum Dev 1972;15:1-12.

[5] Piaget J, Inhelder B. The psychology of the child. New York: Basic Books, 1969.

[6] Piaget J. The language and thought of the child. New York: Harcourt Brace, 1932.

[7] Flaherty T. Maria Montessori (1870-1952). Women's intellectual contributions to the study of mind and society. http://www.webster.edu/~woolflm/montessori.html

[8] Freud S. The origin and development of psychoanalysis. Am J Psychol 1910;21:181-218.

[9] Freud S. Collected works. Standard edition. London: Hogarth, 1954.

[10] Boeree CG. Personality theories. 1997. http://www.ship.edu/~cgboeree/perscontents.html

[11] Erikson EH. Childhood and society, 2nd ed. New York: WW Norton, 1963.

[12] Erickson E. Identity, youth and crisis. New York: WW Norton, 1968.

[13] Greydanus DE, Patel DR, Pratt HD,eds. Essential adolescent medicine. New York: McGraw-Hill Med, 2006.

[14] Center for Disease Control and Prevention. CDC growth charts: United States - Body mass index-for-age percentiles: Boys and girls ages 2 to 20 years.3rd, 5th, 10th, 25th, 50th, 75th, 85th, 90th, 95th, 97th percentiles. National Health and Nutrition Examination Survey. Hyattsville, MD: US Department of Health and Human Services, CDC, National Center for Health Statistics. 2000. Available at http://www. cdc.gov/nchs/data/nhanes/growthcharts/set1/chart03.pdf http://www.cdc.gov/nchs/data/nhanes/growthcharts/set1/chart04.pdf

[15] Kornblau IS, Pearson GC, Breitkopf CR. Demographic, behavioral, physical correlates of body esteem among low income female adolescents. J Adolesc Health 2007; 41(4):566-70.

[16] Dorian L, Garfinkel PE. Culture and body image in Western society. Eat Weight Disord 2002;7(1):1-19.

[17] Pearce MJ, Boergers J, Prinstein MJ. Adolescent obesity, overt and relational peer victimization, and romantic relationships. Obes Res 2002;10(5):386-93.

[18] Grabe S, Hyde JS, Lindberg SM. Body objectification and depression in adolescents: the role of gender shame, and rumination. Psychol Women Q 2007;31:164-75.

[19] Robinson TN, Killen JD, Litt IF, Hammer LD, Wilson DM, Haydel, et al. Ethnicity and body dissatisfaction: Are Hispanic and Asian girls at increased risk for eating disorders. J Adolesc Health 1996; 19:384-93.

[20] van den Berg P, Neumark-Sztainer D. Fat 'n happy 5 years later: Is it bad for overweight girls to like their bodies? J Adolesc Health 2007;41(4):415-7.

[21] 2Bess BE. Human sexuality and obesity. Int J Mental Health 1997; 26(1):61-7.

[22] Nichter M. "Fat talk": What girls and their parents say about dieting. Cambridge, MA: Harvard Univ Press, 2000.

[23] Jagstaidt V, Golay A, Pasini W. Relationships between sexuality and obesity in male patients. New Trends Exp Clin Psychiatry 1997;13(2):105-10.

[24] Pearce MJ, Boergers J, Prinstein MJ. Adolescent obesity, overt and relational peer victimization, and romantic relationships. Obes Res 2002;10:386-93.

[25] Greydanus DE, Pratt HD, Baxter T. Sexual dysfunction and the primary care physician. Adolesc Med State Art Rev 1996;7(1):9-26.

In: Obesity and Adolescence: A Public Health Concern ISBN: 978-1-60692-821-9
Editors: H.A. Omar, D.E. Greydanus et al.

Chapter VII

Obesity and Contraception

Donald E. Greydanus[1,*], Hatim A. Omar,[2] and Artemis K. Tsitsika[3]

[1]Pediatrics and Human Development, Michigan State University College of Human Medicine, Michigan State University/Kalamazoo Center for Medical Studies, Kalamazoo, Michigan, United States of America

[2]Adolescent Medicine and Young Parents Program, University of Kentucky, Kentucky Clinic, Lexington, Kentucky, United States of America

[3]Adolescent Health Unit, Second Department of Pediatrics, University of Athens-Greece, Children's Hospital, Athens, Greece

Abstract

All sexually active youth, whether obese or normal weight, should be offered counseling regarding contraception and appropriate contraceptive methods. However, obese youth who are sexually active may be less likely than their normal weight peers to use contraceptives correctly. Methods of contraception for obese adolescents are reviewed in this discussion. Combined oral contraceptives (COCs) and the contraceptive patch have higher failure rates in obese versus normal weight females, though failure rates are lower than noted with barrier contraceptives. The risk for venous thrombosis is higher in obese youth on COCs. Progestin-only pills and the levonorgestrel intrauterine system appear to be safe and effective methods in obese females. Depot-medroxyprogesterone acetate, intravaginal ring, and implants are also considered.

* Correspondence: Professor Donald E Greydanus, MD, Pediatrics and Human Development, Michigan State University College of Human Medicine, Pediatrics Program Director, Michigan State University/Kalamazoo Center for Medical Studies, Kalamazoo, MI 49008-1284 United States. Tel: 269-337-6450; Fax: 269-337-6474; E-mail: Greydanus@kcms.msu.edu

Introduction

Sexually active adolescents whether chronically ill or not, should be offered contraception if they are not willing to accept abstinence [1-7]. Adolescents who are obese are at risk for unwanted pregnancy with its well-known risks and thus, should also be offered safe and effective contraceptives. However, overweight or obese females are less likely to use contraception than their normal weight peers, despite their higher risk for pregnancy-related complications [8]. This chapter reviews contraception in obese youth. In general, contraception is much safer than risks posed because of obesity and pregnancy. Effective methods that the clinician should consider include combined oral contraceptives, mini-pills, depo-medroxyprogesterone aceate, intravaginal ring, implantable contraception, and levonorgestrel intrauterine device (see table 1). Barrier methods are not generally effective in youth.

Combined Oral Contraceptives (COCs)

Females with obesity have some decreased efficacy with COCs due to higher basal metabolic rates, higher hepatic metabolism of enzymes, and drug sequestration that is higher in adipose tissue; however, efficacy is higher than noted with barrier methods [9-13]. There are over 145 brands of combined oral contraceptives (COCs) used throughout the world, which generally contain both synthetic estrogen and synthetic progestin. In the United States, birth control pill brands are various combinations estrogen and progestin. The usual estrogen is ethinyl estradiol as the estrogen, though a few brands use mestranol. Various progestins are used including norgestrel, levonorgestrel, ethynodiol diacetate, norethindrone acetate, norethindrone, desogestrel, norgestimate, norethynodrel, drospirenone, and gestodene (not available in the US). The pill has been shown to be a safe and effective contraceptive for reproductive women – especially for those of the adolescent age group. Thus, motivate adolescent females who are obese can still be encouraged to use the COC despite the reported higher failure rates, mainly because of the overall efficacy of COCs and the known adverse pregnancy outcomes.

Current recommendations are to begin with a monophasic pill, which has 30-35 mcg of estrogen and 0.15 to 1.5 mg of progestin, or a triphasic pill. Triphasic pills are also recommended due to their low dose of estrogen and progestin. Careful monitoring and selection of patients for birth control pill use will reduce complications of the pill to a considerable extent. Contraindications to oral contraception are reviewed in table 2. Sexually active youth who are on combined oral contraceptives are advised to use condoms as well.

Table 1. Contraceptive methods

Abstinence
Combined Oral Contraceptives (COCs)
Contraceptive patch
Mini-pills (Progestin-only pills; POPs)
Emergency contraceptives
Injectable Contraceptives
Depo-Provera® (Depo-medroxy-progesterone acetate
Lunelle® (estradiol cypionate and medroxyprogesterone acetate)
Implants
Norplant I (withdrawn from the US market in 2000)
Implanon (one rod system with etonogestrel)
Jadelle (Norplant II: two silastic rods with levonorgestrel)
Intravaginal ring (NuvaRing)
Intrauterine Devices
Progestasert® IUD (with progesterone)
ParaGard® (Copper T380A IUD)
Mirena® (IUD with levonorgestrel)
Vaginal barrier contraceptives
Cervical cap (Prentif Cavity-rim®)
Condoms (male)
Contraceptive sponge (vaginal)
Diaphragm
Female condom (Reality®)
Spermicides (vaginal)

Ortho Evra Patch

The contraceptive patch provides contraceptive efficacy similar to COCs but may have an increased risk for cardiovascular complications due to delivery of increased hormonal levels in contrast to oral COCs [14]. As noted with the birth control pill, obesity (weight over 90 kg [198 pounds]) leads to reduced contraceptive efficacy, but still levels better than noted with barrier contraceptives [12,13,15,16]. Dermatitis can occur as well with patch technology. Females with a history of skin allergy or exfoliative dermatological disorders may not be good candidates for the patch. There is also an increased incidence in breast symptoms, though most are reported to be mild or moderate [14,17]. Causes of increased risk of contraceptive failure include having the patch on over seven days, patch detachment, and failure to start a new patch after seven days of being off the patch.

Contraindications to OCPs

The World Health Organization has published a list of medical eligibility guidelines to provide clinicians with guidelines for COC use in those with various chronic illnesses that place users at increased risk of complications (see table 2) [18,19]. Those in WHO Category 1 have no restrictions to OCP use, while those in Category 2 present with some increased risk, though the risks of pregnancy exceed them. Category 3 conditions have risks that are further increased, such that the pill is not used unless risks for pregnancy are even higher and no alternative contraceptive is available. Conditions found in Category 4 present risks that are so high that OCPs are not prescribed.

Cardiovascular Complications

Research has indicated an increased risk of cardiovascular complications in females on COCs [7,20,21]. Obese females on birth control pills have an increased risk for pulmonary emboli, thrombophlebitis, and vascular thromboses. Some studies note a greater incidence of myocardial infarction and subarachnoid hemorrhage as well [21]. An absolute OCP contraindication is a past history of venous thrombosis (VT) and the risk of VT is more significant for the adolescent or young adult than arterial thrombosis. Significant obesity is a VT risk factor and the risk is increased in obese COC users [12,13,22].

Cardiovascular deaths from venous and arterial complications in non-smoking females aged 20-24 years is 2-6 per million per year. There is a 3-6 fold increased risk factor for VT development in COC users and the risk for VT is higher with desogestrel versus levonorgestrel [7,20]. The VT risk in the general population is 0.8 per 10,000 women per year, 3-4 for those on COCs, and 6-12 for females who are pregnant or postpartum [20,23,24]. Most who develop venous thrombosis do not have identified VT risk factors. Table 3 lists screening questions to use when considering OCPs for contraception. In general, if there is no overt positive family history for VT, one does not need to screen for factor V Leiden or other prothrombotic mutations.

Table 2. WHO medical eligibility categories for OCPs. Used with permission [3]

Category one (no restrictions)	
	Antibiotics
	Benign breast disease
	Benign ovarian tumors
	Cervical ectropion
	Dysmenorrhea,
	Endometriosis
	Epilepsy
	Family history of breast cancer
	Gestational trophoblastic disease (benign or malignant)
	Headaches (mild)
	History of ectopic pregnancy or abortion (postabortion after first or second trimester),
	History of gestational diabetes
	Increased STD risk

Iron deficiency anemia
Irregular menstrual bleeding
Obesity
Ovarian or endometrial cancer
Past pelvic surgery
Pelvic inflammatory disease
Postpartum at or over 21 days
Thyroid disorders (as hypo/hyperthyroidism, simple goiter)
Varicose veins
Various infections :malaria, tuberculosis, others)
Sexually transmitted diseases
Viral hepatitis carrier

Category two (caution)

Cervical cancer
Diabetes mellitus (uncomplicated)
Headaches (severe and if they start after beginning OCPs)
Hypertension at 140-159/100-109 mm Hg
Major surgery without prolonged immobilization
Migraine headaches without focal neurologic involvement.
Patients who have a hard time taking the OCP correctly:
- drug or alchohol abuse
- mental retardation
- persistent history as poor OCP takers
- severe psychiatric disorders

Sickle cell disease or sickle C disease
Undiagnosed breast mass

Category three (Usually no OCP given)

Gallbladder disease
Lactating (6 weeks to 6 months),
Less than 21 days postpartum
Medications that interfere with OCP efficacy
Undiagnosed abnormal vaginal/uterine bleeding.

Category four (OCP contraindicated)

Breast cancer
Cerebrovascular accident (active or history)
Complicated structural heart disease (with pulmonary hypertension, atrial fibrillation or history of subacute bacterial endocarditis)
Coronary (or ischemic) heart disease (active or history)
Deep vein thrombosis or pulmonary embolism (active of history)
Diabetes mellitus (complicated with retinopathy, neuropathy, nephropathy)
Headaches (including migraine headaches) with focal neurologic symptoms
Hypertension (severe: (160+/110+ mm Hg or with vascular complications)
Lactation under 6 weeks postpartum
Liver disease (including liver cancer, benign hepatic adenoma, active viral hepatitis, severe cirrhosis)
Pregnancy, complicated
Surgery (involving the lower extremities and/or prolonged immobilization

Table 3. Screening questions about personal/family history of thromboembolism

1. Is there a history of blood clots in legs or lungs in close family members, including uncles and aunts?
2. Have any of your close family members been in the hospital for leg/lung blood clots?
3. Have you and/or close family members ever taking blood thinners?
4. What were the circumstances that led to blood clot (s), as for example while as a result of traveling by airplane?

The pill should be stopped before situations arise requiring prolonged bed rest as with some surgeries. Hypertension and hyperlipidemia may be complications of obesity. Blood pressure should be regularly checked since it may rise in some patients.25 If there is a family or personal history of hyperlidemia, OCPs may still be prescribed if low-density lipoprotein (LDL)levels remain < 160 mg/dl and triglycerides < 250. COCs are not recommended for adolescents (obese or not) if they have congestive heart failure, cardiac shunts, or low output heart disorders.5,26

Diabetes Mellitus

Diabetes mellitus may be a complication of or occur incidental of obesity. Current evidence suggests that combined oral contraceptives are safe for obese females with well-controlled diabetes mellitus types 1 and 2 [12]. COCs do not worsen the metabolic status in diabetic females [12,13,27]. Care is needed because of concern over worsening metabolic status due to progestins and increased risk for thromboembolic events due to estrogen [28]. COCs should not be offered if they are in poor metabolic control or have hypertension, nephropathy, or retinopathy. Other contraceptive methods that are safe and effective in females with diabetes include progestin-only pills and the intrauterine device (IUD) [13]. There may be an increase in recurrent, treatment-resistant vaginal yeast infections in diabetic youth with an IUD [28]. The use of depo-medroxyprogesterone acetate or levonorgestrel implant may worsen the metabolic status in diabetic females.

Migraine Headaches

Caution is advised when prescribing the birth control pill to an individual with a history of migraine headaches and the COC should be stopped if the migraine aura or headache pattern worsen on COCs [1-4]. If the individual has a history of severe migraines or migraines with prolonged auras (as with the hemiplegic or ophthalmoplegic types) the pill should not be given. If the migraine headache and/or the aura worsen while on the pill, it should be stopped immediately. Careful monitoring is advised when placing women with migraines on the pill. It is not known if obesity presents a greater risk for migraine-related cerebrovascular accidents that may be increased by the COCs or patch.

Other Conditions

Females with active liver disease should not be placed on OCPs. The effect of obesity-related NASH (nonalcoholic steatohepatitis) on COCs not clear at this time. Youth with obesity may be at risk for depression and no obesity-related complications with SSRIs are reported. Tricyclic antidepressants can reduce estrogen levels with increased BTB but not reduced contraceptive efficacy. St. John's wart is used to treat depression and can lead to increased break-through bleeding and anecdotal reports of reduced OC efficacy [1-4]. Some females with obesity are at increased risk for fungal infections and some anti-fungal agents are potent hepatic enzyme inducers with resultant decreased contraceptive efficacy; these agents include griseofulvin, ketoconazole and itraconazole. Other drugs can interfere with contraceptive efficacy, such as rifampin. Table 4 lists management principles for miscellaneous side effects of COCs.

Progestin-only Pills (POPs) (Mini-Pills)

POPs contain 0.35 mg of norethindrone (Micronor®; Nor-Q.D®) and 0.075 mg of norgestrel (Ovrette®). Obesity may be associated with reduced contraceptive efficacy [13]. POPs are typically used in those individuals having disorders where estrogen may be contraindicated – such as sickle cell anemia, cyanotic heart disease, severe hypertension, diabetes mellitus, and others (see table 2). Some clinicians have not recommended the mini-pill for teenagers because of its increased pregnancy rate as well as frequent breakthrough bleeding and amenorrhea noted in some females on the mini-pill [1-4]. POPs are avoided in those with a history of ectopic pregnancy and those taking certain medications (as anticonvulsants, griseofulvin and rifampin). There is no increase in VT in obese females on progestin-only pills [12,13].

Table 4. Management of some oral contraceptive related problems

Problem	Management
Acne	Anti-acne measures and medications
Acute/Chronic monilial vaginitis	Anti-fungal agents (as fluconazole); persistent infections: Look for underlying factors, as diabetes mellitus, other endocrinopathies, use of antibiotics, infected male genital tract, others. Oral nystatin may reduce gastrointestinal reservoir; use anti-fungal agents for a protracted period of treatment.
Breakthrough bleeding	Usually a transient condition; ensure patient is taking the pill each day; higher estrogen pill or supplemental estrogen may help; evaluate for underlying pathology
Suspected pregnancy	COCs are not teratogenic but should be stopped as soon as the pregnancy is identified.
Weight gain or edema	Use a lower estrogen pill

Depot-Medroxyprogesterone Acetate (DMPA)

The main injectable contraceptive available in the US is depomedroxy-progesterone acetate (Depo-Provera®). It is given in a dose of 150 mg intramuscularly every three months and DMPA has a better contraceptive efficacy than the COC with a failure rate of 0.3%. No decreased contraceptive efficacy is noted in obese females versus normal weight females [13]. Its mechanism of action includes an induction of a low FSH/LH level, low LH surge, production of an atrophic endometrium, and thickening of the cervical mucus. Side effects include irregular menses, amenorrhea, acne, breast tenderness, weight gain (with bloating), decrease in bone density, decrease in high-density lipoprotein levels, and some behavioral changes such as irritability and depression.

It is useful where a highly effective contraceptive is needed and where the side effects of an estrogen-type contraceptive must be avoided. Thus, it has been used for individuals with cyanotic heart disease, sickle-cell anemia, thrombophlebitis, and others. Internationally, psychotic and retarded individuals who are at risk for pregnancy have been prescribed this injectable contraceptive. It is considered to be a very effective hormonal contraceptive for obese females, despite the reported change in body composition towards fatness and central redistribution of fat following its use.

Another injectable contraceptive, Lunelle® (5 mg estradiol cypionate and 25 mg medroxyprogesterone acetate [MPA/E2C]), was approved by the FDA in 2000. Estrogen is added to allow a better menstrual period rhythm than seen with Depo-Provera. Less weight gain is noted and overall adverse effects are similar to COCs [29]. Lunelle® is given intramuscularly every 28-30 days and it has a high contraceptive efficacy rate [30]. One study noted that there was a weight gain of 0.9 kg to 1.8 kg if the female weighed under 68 kg versus a weight gain of 1.4 to 3.6 kg if over 68 kilograms [30]. There is no overt contraindication in females with obesity.

Emergency Contraceptives

Emergency contraceptives (EC) are among the most controversial and under prescribed contraceptive methods (seee table 5)[31]. Obesity is not a contraindication to use of ECs. Anti-emetics can be given to prevent the frequent occurrence of nausea and emesis that occurs with high dose estrogen; thus, an antiemetic should be taken an hour before taking these pills. In 1999, the US Food and Drug Administration (FDA) approved of Plan B®, a progestin-only method with two tables of 0.75 mg of levonorgestrel. The first tablet is taken immediately and the second tablet is taken two hours later. Because Plan B® contains no estrogen, nausea and vomiting is uncommon and there is no need to obtain a pregnancy test before administation. Thus, Plan B may be better tolerated than those with estrogen [32]. Though the official recommendation is that they must be used within three days of coitus, they may be effective in pregnancy prevention within five days.

Table 5. Emergency contraceptives

- Ovral® : 2 tablets followed by 2 tables in 12 hours
- Lo/Ovral®, Nordette® or Levlen® : 4 tabs and 4 more in 12 hours
- Plan B®: levonorgestrel, 0.75mg followed by 0.75 mg in 12 hours
- Preven® Emergency Contraceptive Kit
- Ovrette®: 20 tabs and 20 more in 12 hours
- TriPhasil® or Tri-Levlen® (yellow tabs only): 4 tabs, and 4 more in 12 hours

Nuvaring® (Vaginal Ring)

This is a soft, flexible, transparent vaginal ring made of a ethylene vinyl acetate copolymer; it has an outer diameter of 54 mm and a cross-section of 4 mm [2,4]. There are two steroid reservoir cores that provide a daily hormonal release of 15 mcg of ethinyl estradiol and 120 mcg of etonogestrel (an active metabolite of desogestrel) [30,33]. Side effects include extended withdrawal bleeding, vaginal discomfort, nausea, headache, nervousness, acne, breast tenderness, leukorrhea, reduced libido, and slight weight gain. There is an increased risk of thrombotic diseases [34]. There is usually less irregular bleeding than seen with COCs. Extremely overt weight females may have trouble inserting the ring. Obesity itself does not effect the contraceptive efficacy of the NuvaRing and it is considered as one of the most effective hormonal contraceptive methods for obese females.

Implanon®

Norplant® was the first implantable contraceptive developed and was very effective as a contraceptive. It contains six silastic levonorgestrel-containing rods; however, it was withdrawn from the United States market in 2000 [2,4]. The Jadelle® implant (Norplant II) contains two silastic rods with levonorgestrel and Implanon® contains one rod (vinyl ethylene acetate polymer) with etonogestrel [7,35]. Both Jadelle® and Implanon® are approved by the FDA for three years and are not contraindicated in obesity, though both may induce some weight gain. Though obese females have been found to have lower serum etonogestrel levels, there is no reduced efficacy noted with Implanon in obese female [13,36].

Intrauterine Device (IUD)

There are three IUDs which currently are used in the United States: Progestasert IUD®, the ParaGard® (Copper T380A) and the Mirena IUD [2,4,37-39]. Previous controversial IUD links with pelvic inflammatory disease (PID) have limited its application to adolescents. However, the IUD is an excellent contraceptive method with no contraindication in obese women. The Mirena® IUD (Levonorgestrel-containing IUD; LNG-IUD) was FDA-approved in 2001 for five years and contraindications are active PID, prosthetic heart valves, history of subacute bacterial endocarditis, and distorted uterine cavity. The most common side effect is menstrual bleeding; there is increased bleeding and spotting during the first 3-6 months after insertion that usually decreases after this time. Obese females have an increased incidence of dysfunctional uterine bleeding and endometrial hyperplasia, making the Mirena IUD a good contraceptive choice for obese females needing contraception [12]. No reduced contraceptive efficacy has been noted because of obesity [13,40]. In diabetic patients, an increase in vaginal yeast infections should be taken under consideration.

Conclusions

Contraceptive efficacy is reduced in obese females on the combined oral contraceptive and the contraceptive patch; however, the efficacy is still above that noted with barrier contraceptives. COCs are safe with obese females with diabetes mellitus if they are in good control and do not have nephropathy, retinopathy, neuropathy, or hypertension. Progestin-only pills are safe in obese females but decreased contraceptive efficacy is noted in all females on this contraceptive method. Obesity is not a contraindication to use of depo-medroxyprogesterone acetate, IUD, and intravaginal ring. The mini-pill and levonorgestrel IUD may be the safest for obese females needing contraception [12].

References

[1] Greydanus DE, Patel DR, Rimsza ME. Contraception in the adolescent: An update. Pediatrics 2001;107(3):562-73.

[2] Greydanus DE, Patel D. Contraception in the adolescent: Preparation for the 1990's. Med Clin North Am 1990;74(5):205-24.

[3] Greydanus DE. Contraception. In: Greydanus DE, Patel DR, Pratt H, Bhave S, eds. Course manual for adolescent health. Kalamazo, MI: Michigan State Univ Coll Hum Med, 2002:309-24.

[4] Greydanus DE, Rimsza ME, Matytsina L. Contraception for college students. Pediatr Clin North Am 2005;52:135-61.

[5] Gittes EB, Strickland JL. Contraceptive choices for chronically ill adolescents. Adolesc Med 2005;16(3):635-44.

[6] Rimsza ME. Contraception in adolescents. In: Greydanus DE, Patel DR, Pratt DH, eds. Essentials of adolescent medicine. New York: McGraw-Hill Med Publ, 2005:27.

[7] Klein JD, Barratt MS, Blythe MJ, et al. Contraception and adolescents. Pediatrics 2007;120:1135-48.

[8] Chuang CH, Chase GA, Bensyl DM, Weisman CS. Contraceptive use by diabetic and obese women. Women's Health Issues 2005; 15:167-73.

[9] Holt VL, Cushing-Haugen KL, Kaling JR. Body weight and risk of oral contraceptive failure. Obstet Gynecol 2002; 99(5 Pt 1): 820-7.

[10] Holt VL, Scholes D, Wicklund KG, et al. Body mass index, weight, and oral contraceptive failure risk. Obstet Gynecol 2005;105(1):46-52.

[11] Brunner Huber LR, Hogue CJ, Stein AD, et al. Body mass index and risk for oral contraceptive failure: a case-cohort study in South Carolina Ann Epidemiol 2006;16(8):637-43.

[12] ACOG Practice Bulletin. Use of hormonal contraception in women with coexisting medical conditions. Clinical Management Guidelines for Obstetrician-Gynecologists. Obstet Gynecol 2006;107:1453-72.

[13] Teal SB, Ginosar DM. Contraception for women with chronic medical conditions. Obstet Gynecol Clin North Am 2007;34:113-26.

[14] Sicat BL. Ortho Evra, a new contraceptive patch. Pharmacotherapy 2003; 23:472-80.

[15] Ortho Evra. A contraceptive patch. Med Lett 2002; 44:8.

[16] Zieman M, Guillebaud J, Weisberg E, et al. Contraceptive efficacy and cycle control with the Ortho Evra/Evra transdermal system: the analysis of pooled data. Fertil Steril 2002;77(2 Suppl):S13-8.

[17] Sibai BM, Odlind C, Meador ML, et al. A comparative and pooled analysis of the safety and tolerability of the contraceptive patch (Ortho Evra/Evra). Fertil Steril 2002;77(Suppl 2):S19-26.

[18] World Health Organization. Medical eligibility criteria for contraceptive use, 2ed. Geneva: WHO, Reprod Health Res, 2000.

[19] World Health Organization. Medical eligibility criteria for contraceptive use, 2ed. Geneva: WHO, Reprod Health Res, 2002.

[20] Vandenbrouke JP, Rosing J, Bloemenkamp KWM, et al.: Oral contraceptives and the risk of venous thrombosis. N Engl J Med 2001;344:1527-35.

[21] Sheldon T. Venous thromboembolism and oral contraceptives. BMJ 2002;324:869.

[22] Sidney S, Petitti DB, Soff GA, et al. Venous thromboembolic disease in users of low-estrogen combined estrogen-progestin oral contraceptives. Contraception 2004;70(1):3-10.

[23] Greer IA. Thrombosis in pregnancy: maternal and fetal issues. Lancet 1999;353:1258-65.

[24] Kujovich JL. Hormones and pregnancy: thromboembolic risks for women. Br J Haematol 2004;126:443-54.

[25] Mottram Hall Guidelines. Evidence-guided prescribing of the pill. Carnforth: Parthenon Publ, 1996.

[26] Heroux K. Contraceptive choices in medically ill adolescents. Semin Reprod Med 2003;21(4):389-98.

[27] Garg SK, Chase HP, Marshall G, et al. Oral contraceptives and renal and retinal complications in young women with insulin-dependent diabetes mellitus. JAMA 1994;271:1099-1102.

[28] Owens K, Honebrink A. Gynecologic care of medically complicated adolescents. Pediatr Clin North Am 1999;46:631-42.

[29] Freeman S. Contraceptive efficacy and patient acceptance of Lunelle. J Am Acad Nurs Pract 2002;14:241-346.

[30] Keder LM. Tips for clinicians: New developments in contraception. J Pediatr Adolesc Gynecol 2002;15:179-81.

[31] Trussell J, Ellertson C, Steward F, et al. The role of emergency contraception. Am J Obstet Gynecol 2004;190(Suppl 4):S30-8.

[32] Emergency contraception OTC. Med Lett 2004;46:10-11.

[33] Mulders TM, Dieben TO, Bennick HJ. Ovarian function with a novel combined contraceptive vaginal ring. Hum Reprod 2002; 17:2594-9.

[34] Murphy NA, Elias ER. Council on children with disabilities. Sexuality of children and adolescents with developmental disabilities. Pediatrics 2006;118:398-403.

[35] Glasier A. Implantable contraceptives for women: effectiveness, discontinuation rates, return of fertility, and outcome of pregnancies. Contraception 2002;65:29-37.

[36] Huber J, Wenzl R. Pharmacokinetics of Implanon: an integrated analysis. Contraception 1998;58(6 Suppl):85S-90.

[37] Arias RD. Compelling reasons for recommending IUDs to any woman of reproductivde age. Int J Fertil 2002;47:87-95.

[38] A progestin-releasing intrauterine device for long-term contraception. Med Lett 2001;43:7-8.

[39] Baldaszti E, Wimmer-Puchinger B, Loschke K. Acceptability of the long-term contraceptive levonorgestrel-releasing intrauterine system (Mirena): a 3-year follow-up study. Contraception 2003;67:87-91.

[40] Mansour D. Implications of the growing obesity epidemic on contraception and reproductive health. J Fam Plann Reprod Health Care 2004;30(4):209-11.

IV. Physical Activities

In: Obesity and Adolescence: A Public Health Concern
Editors: H.A. Omar, D.E. Greydanus et al.
ISBN: 978-1-60692-821-9

Chapter VIII

Obesity and Sport

Dilip R. Patel*[*], and Donald E. Greydanus
Department of Pediatrics and Human Development, Michigan State University College of Human Medicine, Kalamazoo Center for Medical Studies, Kalamazoo, Michigan, United States of America

Abstract

Obesity is increasingly prevalent in adolescents with significant lifelong medical complications. The exact prevalence of obesity among adolescent athletes is not known; however, there is research that suggests obesity prevalence varies by the type of sports. A few studies suggest that youth sport participation can be an effective tool in the management of obesity in children and youth. Regular physical activity and sport participation that is fun is strongly recommended. This discussion considers the role of sports in helping obese adolescents and also what physical activity is recommended. It is concluded that sports participation can be an important part of effective management of obese youth and setting the stage for a lifelong pursuit of physical activity to control and/or reduce obesity in the adolescent and adult population.

Introduction

The prevalence of obesity is estimated to be 20% in the United States and other developed countries [1-8]. Over the past 25 years there has been a 75% relative increase in obesity in American adolescents. The number of adolescents who are overweight or obese has doubled during the same period in children between 6 and 11 years of age and tripled in adolescents between 12 and 17 years of age.

* Correspondence: Professor Dilip R Patel, MD, Department of Pediatrics and Human Development, Michigan State University College of Human Medicine, Kalamazoo Center for Medical Studies, 1000, Oakland Drive, Kalamazoo, MI 49008 United States. E-mail: patel@kcms.msu.edu

The exact prevalence of overweight and obesity in adolescents regularly participating in various sports is not known. In a recent study, Malina et al looked at the prevalence of overweight and obesity among participants between ages 9 and 14 years in American football. The cross-sectional study of 653 participants found that overall 45% of participants were overweight and 42.6% were obese [9]. The prevalence of overweight and obesity was highest among early maturing boys, and relatively higher in offensive and defensive linemen. The authors concluded that the prevalence of overweight and obesity was relatively higher among young football players compared to national samples of American boys [9]. These adolescents are at a higher risk for becoming obese adults. The very nature of American football in which a high value is place on large body mass of players is a risk factor for overweight and obesity among these adolescents.

The long term adverse effects of obesity on health have been well documented in published literature. The causes of increased prevalence of obesity in children and adolescents are multi-factorial that includes a complex interplay of genetic and environmental factors [10-12]. A sedentary lifestyle and lack of regular physical activity are major factors contributing to the increasing prevalence of obesity. The role of sports participation in the management of obesity in adolescents is now considered.

Role of Sport Participation in Prevention and Treatment of Obesity

Lifestyle modification is an essential component of management of obesity. In order to effectively loose weight the adolescent needs to expend more calories than what he or she consumes. Appropriate dietary modification combined with regular physical activity has been shown to be effective in achieving steady weight loss over a long period of time; however, the role of behavior modification therapy, pharmacotherapy, and bariatric surgery in the treatment of adolescent obesity is not clear at this time [13-23].

Role of regular physical activity in weight management and other benefits of exercise have been well known (see table 1) (24]. Structured exercise programs have been shown to have a favorable impact on body composition of adolescents, especially when combined with reduced total caloric intake. One study has shown than obese children improve their lipid profiles if placed on a low fat diet and exercise program of moderate intensity (i.e., heart rate at 60-80% of maximum) for eight weeks with progressively increased duration of activities such as aerobic dancing, swimming, walking, or jogging [25]. Programs that include regular exercise tend to have lasting effects on weight reduction and may prevent later development of obesity. Reasons for adolescents not engaging in regular physical activities are many and include lack of opportunity at school, exercise related injuries, inappropriate exercises, and psychosocial environment that is conducive to sedentary as well as isolated lifestyle [26].

Obesity itself may play a role in discouraging exercise because of some inherent biomechanical and physiological factors that impede exercise performance [27]. Obese adolescents often have increased friction between their thighs, arms, and torso. They also may have suboptimal level of pulmonary function because of the need to move a heavier body mass and increased need for oxygen relative to more thin adolescents. These factors may affect effective participation in certain activities such as running and jumping. Excessive weight may also impose demands on weigh bearing exercises.

Korsten-Reck et al looked at motor abilities and aerobic fitness of obese children [28]. Data were collected on 49 obese children ages 8-12 years and compared with age-matched control group before and after an intervention program that consisted of a combination of organized sports, behavior therapy, and nutritional counseling. Before the intervention program, aerobic capacity of obese subjects was found to be significantly below the control group. Similarly the obese subject performed relatively poorly on motor abilities measured by medicine-ball toss. The investigators noted that following intervention, performance in motor abilities improved and the difference in strength between obese and control group decreased [28].

Weintraub et al have evaluated the feasibility, acceptability, and efficacy of an after-school team sports program for reducing weight gain in low-income overweight children in a trial called the Stanford Sports to Prevent Obesity Randomized Trial (SPORT) [29]. The subjects were children in 4th and 5th grade with BMI at or above the 85th percentile. The intervention consisted of participation in after-school soccer play and the reference group intervention consisted of health education program. The study found that all 21 participants in soccer group had decreased BMI at 3 and 6 months and increased levels of physical activity at three months [29].

Recommendations for Sports

Fun activities whether they are part of organized sports or not should be recommended to all adolescents [16,30-32]. Children and adolescents generally do better with exercise if the fun aspect is emphasized in contrast to the health benefits. Such activities may include walking, dancing, cycling, swimming, and other aerobic activities (see table 2). A variety of different activities should be encouraged and tried while activities should be periodically changed. Children and adolescents should be actively and regularly encouraged to engage in regular physical activities. School-based programs should be strongly encouraged. Sport participation and physical activity should be viewed as a lifelong recommendation while such activities as golf, tennis, swimming, and running should be encouraged. Parents should consistently encourage their children and adolescents to engage in various physical activities on a regular basis. Appropriately supervised weight training is safe and children as well as adolescents should be allowed to participate in such programs.

A summary of recommended activities is provided in table 3. Adolescents should generally participate in physical activities of moderate intensity for 30 minutes daily. Sport participation should be tailored to the abilities of the child or adolescents. For examples, obese adolescents may be taller and stronger than some of their peers and may do better at sports requiring strength and or height such as throwing events, football or basketball. A number of obese adolescents may prefer water sports because adipose tissue provides more buoyancy in water and tends to hide their increased size.

Table 1. Positive effects of exercise

Decrease	
	Body mass
	Percentage body fat
	Visceral fat
	Blood pressure (arterial)
	Triglycerides
	LDL cholesterol
Increase	
	Insulin sensitivity
	HDL cholesterol
	Physical fitness
	Self esteem

Table 2. Aerobic activities for obese youth [31]. Used with permission

Indoor activities tailored for aerobic exercise	
	Dance
	Treadmill
	Rowing machine
	Stationary bike
	Others
Outdoor activities for aerobic exercise	
	Jogging
	Bicycling
	Long distance running
	Roller blading
	Power walking
	Others

Conclusions

Obesity is increasingly prevalent in children and adolescents with significant lifelong medical complications. The exact prevalence of obesity among athletes is not known, though some studies suggest that it varies by the type of sports. American football players have been shown to have higher prevalence of overweight and obesity. The role of exercise and increased physical activity in general as an essential component of management of obese youth is well accepted; however, the role of sport participation in the management of obesity is not so clear. A few studies suggest that youth sport participation can be an effective tool in the management of obesity. Regular physical activity and sport participation is that is fun is strongly recommended.

Table 3. Recommendations for physical activity for obese children/youth [27,31]. Used with permission

Overweight Children: <150% IBW; >85-95 percentile BMI

Aerobic Activities: Weight bearing:

- Brisk walking
- Treadmill or stair climber
- Field sports, roller blading, hiking
- Racquetball or tennis
- Martial arts
- Skiing, jump rope
- Indoor sports: swim, dance, play tag, aerobic dance

Obese Children: 150-200% IBW; >95-97 percentile BMI

Aerobic activities: Non-weight bearing

- Swimming
- Cycling
- Strength or aerobic circuit training
- Arm-specific aerobic dancing
- Arm ergometer (crank)
- Interval walking with rest as necessary; gradually work up to longer walks with fewer rest stops

Severely Obese Children: >200% IBW; >97 percentile BMI

Weekly supervision by trained exercise professional

Only non-weight-bearing aerobic physical activity:

- Swimming
- Recline biking
- Arm ergometer
- Seated (chair) aerobics
- Seated or lying circuit training

References

[1] Rowlett JD Obesity in the adolescent. In: Greydanus DE, Patel DR, Pratt HD, eds. Essential adolescent medicine. New York: McGraw-Hill Med Publ, 2006:651-65.

[2] Dietz WH. Overweight in childhood and adolescence. N Engl J Med 2004;350:855-7.

[3] Eneli I, Davies HD. Epidemiology of childhood obesity. In: Davies HD, ed. Obesity in childhood and adolescence. Westport, CT: Praeger, 2008:3-23.

[4] Kohn M, Booth M. The worldwide epidemic of obesity in adolescents. Adolesc Med 2003;14:1-9.

[5] World Health Organization. Obesity: Preventing and managing the global epidemic. Geneva: WHO, 1997.

[6] Kiess W, Boettner A. Obesity in the adolescent. Adolesc Med 2002;13:181-90.

[7] Livingstone MB. Epidemiology of childhood obesity in Europe. Eur J Pediatr 2000;159(Suppl): S14-S34.

[8] Seidell JC. Obesity: A growing problem. Acta Paediatr 1999;88 (Suppl) 46-50.
[9] Malina RM, Morano PJ, Barron M, et al. Overweight and obestiy among youth participants in American football. J Pediatr 2007;151:378-82.
[10] Strauss RS, Knight J. Influence of the home environment on the development of obesity in children. Pediatrics 1999;103:127.
[11] Hill J, Peters J. Environmental contributions to the obesity epidemic. Science 1998;280:1371-4.
[12] Hofmann AD. Obesity. In: Hofman AD, Greydanus DE, eds. Adolescents medicine, 3rd ed. Stamford, CT: Appleton Lange, 1997:663-82.
[13] Guide to clinical preventative services, 3rd ed. Report of the US Preventative Services Task Force. Philadelphia, PA: Lippincott Williams Wilkins, 2002:219-29.
[14] Lowry R, Galuska DA, Fulton JE, et al. Physical activity, food choice and weight management goals and practices among US. college students. Am J Prev Med 2000;18:18-27.
[15] Hill JO, Trowbridge FL, eds. Symposium on the causes and health consequences of obesity in children and adolescents. Pediatrics 1998;101(3:Suppl):497-574.
[16] Greydanus DE, Bhave S. Editorial. Obesity in adolescence. Indian Pediatrics 2004;41:545-50.
[17] Berkowitz RI, Wadden TA, Tershakovec AM, Cronquist JL. Behavioral therapy and sibutramine for the treatment of adolescent obesity. A randomized controlled trial. JAMA 2003;289:1805-12.
[18] Yanovski SZ. Pharmacotherapy for obesity. Promise and uncertainty. N Engl J Med 2005;353:2187-9.
[19] Yanovski SZ, Yanovski JA. Obesity. N Engl J Med 2002;346:591-602.
[20] Sugerman HJ, Sugarman EL, DeMaria EJ, et al. Bariatric surgery for severely obese adolescents. J Gastrointest Surg 2003;7:102-8.
[21] Barlow SE: Bariatric surgery in adolescents: for treatment failures or health care system failures? Pediatrics 2004;114:252-3.
[22] Steinbrook R. Surgery for severe obesity. N Engl J Med 2004;350:1075-9.
[23] Himes JH, Dietz WH. Guidelines for overweight in adolescent preventive services: Recommendations from an expert committee. The Expert Committee on Clinical Guidelines for Overweight in Adolescent Preventive Services. Am J Clin Nutr 1994;59(2):307.
[24] Berkey CS, Rockett HRH, Gillman MW, et al. One-year changes in activity and inactivity among 10- and 15-year old boys and girls: Relationship to change in body mass index. Pediatrics 2003; 111:836-43.
[25] Becque M, Katch V, Rocchini A, et al. Coronary risk incidence of obese adolescents: Reduction by exercise plus diet intervention. Pediatrics 1988;81:605-12.
[26] Amisola RB, Jacobson MS. Physical activity, exercise, and sedentary activity: relationship to the causes and treatment of obesity. Adolesc Med 2003;14:23-35.
[27] Sothern MS. Childhood and adolescent obesity: Exercise as a modality in the treatment of childhood obesity. Pediatric Clin North Am 2001;48:1-17.
[28] Korsten-Reck U, Kaspar T, Korsten K, et al. Motor abilities and aerobic fitness of obese children. Int J Sports Med 2007;28(9):762-7.

[29] Weintraub DL, Tirumaldi EC, Haydel F, et al. Team sports for overweight children: The Standford Sports to Prevent Obesity Randomized Trial (SPORT). Arch Pediatr Adolesc Med 2008; 162(3):232-7.

[30] Watts K, Jones TW, Davis EA, Green D. Exercise training in obese children and adolescents. Sports Med 2005;35(5):375-92.

[31] Greydanus DE, Bricker LA, Patel DR. The benefits of sports participation in childhood and adolescents to prevent obesity in adolescents and adults. Asian J Ped Pract 2006;9(4):1-7.

[32] Eneli I, Mantinan KD. Managing the overweight child In: Fitzgerald HE, Mousouli V, eds. Obesity in childhood and adolescence. Westport, CT: Praeger, 2008:191-225.

In: Obesity and Adolescence: A Public Health Concern
Editors: H.A. Omar, D.E. Greydanus et al.
ISBN: 978-1-60692-821-9

Chapter IX

Health, Sleeping Habits and Physical Activity

Marie Alricsson[1,2,*], Debra Domalewski[2], Ulla Romild[3] and Ragnar Asplund[4,5]

[1]Department of Health Sciences, Mid Sweden University, Östersund, Sweden
[2]Griffith Abilities Research Program, Research Centre for Clinical and Community Practice Innovation, Griffith University, Logan Campus, Australia
[3]Department of Information Technology and Media, Mid Sweden University, Östersund, Sweden
[4]The Centre of Family Medicine, Karolinska Institute, Huddinge, Sweden
[5]The Research and Development Unit, Jämtland County Council, Östersund, Sweden

Abstract

Adolescents are becoming less physically active and are increasingly adopting a sedentary life-style in front of computers and television screens. In this chapter we look at self-related health, physical activity, sleeping habits, the prevalence of overweight and body complaints in two senior high schools with questions about weight and height, health, physical activity, type of physical activity/sport, intensity, sleeping habits and possible injuries or complaints during the last three months. Seventy seven percent % of the high school students participated in sports on a regular basis. In academic programs compared to vocational programs, more males and females in academic programs participated in sports (71% and 80% respectively). Males reported significantly better health than females, but 65% reported body complaints during the last three months. A higher number of females than males reported back and hip complaints. Good sleep was reported in 82.1% of the males (76.6% of the females). In males 44.3% were often sleepy in the daytime (females 56.6%). Underweight, physical activity and good sleep were

* Correspondence: Associate Professor, Marie Alricsson, Department of Health Sciences, Mid Sweden University, SE-831 25 Östersund, Sweden. Tel: +46 63 165603; Fax: +46 63 165626; E-mail: marie.alricsson@miun.se

found to be factors with significant positive effect on good health, whereas overweight was a negative factor. Proper sleep habits and higher physical activity levels should be promoted among high school students and TV viewing time and video game use restricted. Additionally, schools should provide opportunities for young people to participate in a wider range of physical activities that address their individual needs, while promoting the health benefits of engaging in regular exercise.

Introduction

Physical activity in adolescence is becoming less attractive and a sedentary life-style in front of computers and television screens is adopted [1]. Recent reports have shown a strong correlation between the amount of physical activity and health in grown-up individuals. Physical inactivity and obesity have emerged as an important risk factor for many chronic diseases [2-3]. Furthermore, it is reported that physical inactivity during growth might lead to impaired health later on in life [4]. An alarming trend is the increase in childhood and adolescent obesity and this global trend shows no signs of abating in the near future. In Australia, obesity and overweight levels are reported to be between 19 % and 23 % among children and adolescents [5]. Overweight children are more likely to become overweight in adulthood than are underweight/normal children. Furthermore, children who are overweight or obese are more prone to impaired health and well-being problems, in both the short and long terms [6]. Since physical activity is an important factor related to weight control there is renewed interest in the relationship between physical activity and body composition of children and adolescents, as well as in the importance of physical activity in maintaining good health and well-being [6].

Attitudes to sport and the socio-demographic factors that impact on physical activity habits and fitness in adults are complex [4]. Wendell et al [7] found that experiences that relate to participation in physical activity during childhood and adolescence may positively influence physical activity during adulthood. Similarly, Telama et al [8] reported that persistent and especially when regular participation in sport at the ages between 9 to 18 years, significantly predicted a higher level of physical activity later in life. Therefore understanding how activity levels and body composition of children and adolescents relate to a healthy lifestyle is a growing area of research.

The aim of the present investigation was to study self-related health, physical activity, sleeping habits, the prevalence of overweight as well as body complaints in Australian senior high school students. More specifically, the data also aimed to compare female and male students, students in academic programs with those in vocational programs.

Our Experience from an Australian Study

High Schools were identified using the internet school directory, and then permission was sought from Education Queensland to approach the principals of the selected schools and invite them to participate in the research. Information letters and consent forms explaining the project were distributed directly by the school to students or distributed by the researchers to the students during project information seminars requested by the school. Questionnaires were completed at school during school hours. Willing students present at this particular time that had obtained written legal consent from their guardians where invited to answer the questionnaire. The research team distributed and then collected the questionnaires which were used. Students filling out the questionnaires were supervised by the researchers and class teachers. Four hundred and sixty-six out of 799 (60 %) Australian state high school students, 185 males and 281 females, from two Queensland high school communities, voluntarily participated in the study. Mean age of the students was 16.2 (± 0.8) years. In Queensland, Australia, high school students in the targeted age group of 15-17 years are in Grades 10, 11 and 12.

The survey was based on a Swedish questionnaire [9] and translated from the Swedish to the English language according to the 'Guidelines for the Process of Cross-Cultural Adaptation of Self-Reported Measures' [10]. The questionnaire included questions about weight and height, self-related health, physical activity behavior, type of physical activity/sport, intensity, duration, sleeping habits, and possible injuries or complaints during the last three months.

Self-related health was determined based on the following questions: 1) 'How do you judge your general health?', and 2) 'How do you rate your health?' To investigate the sleeping habits the students reported: 1) if they sleep well at night, 2) if they often wake up at night, 3) if it is difficult to fall back to sleep once they have woken up during the night, 4) if they are tired when they wake up in the morning, 5) if they are often sleepy in the daytime, 6) what time they generally fall in asleep at night, 7) what time they generally wake up in the morning, 8) how many times they go to the toilet at night.

To investigate physical activity the students reported how often they performed physical activity at a high, medium or low level of effort. A high level was defined as increased pulse rate, breathlessness and sweating. A medium level was defined as being able to talk with somebody during the physical performance and a low level was defined as walking and/or cycling at a slow pace. The students were asked to report the types of sport/physical activities they performed and the frequency of these activities during the last six months.

Possible symptoms or complaints during the last three months were determined based on the following questions: 'Have you during the last three months had any symptoms from any part of the body?' If answered 'yes', the students were further asked to specify which body part was symptomatic. Body Mass Index (BMI) was used for prevalence of overweight in the adolescents. The same cut off points were used as in Cole et al's standard definition for child overweight and obesity worldwide [11]. Three categories were used in the study: I. Underweight /normal weight (BMI > 23.5), II. Risk for overweight (BMI 23.5-24.19), III. Overweight/obesities (BMI 24.2>).

Table 1. Main characteristics of the subjects n=466, (10 missing in schooling)

	Subjects		
Characteristics	Male (%)	Female (%)	Total (%)
Academic program	121 (37)	207 (63)	328
Vocational program	57 (45)	71 (55)	128
Body pain last 3 months	115 (62)	187 (66.5)	302 (65)
Active in sports	138 (77.5)	216 (77.7)	354 (77)

What did we Find?

The questionnaire was completed initially by 185 males (39.8%) and by 281 females (60.2%). Thus there were 466 valuable questionnaires. The mean ages; (SD) of the male and female participants were 16.3; (0.8) and 16.2; (0.8) years, respectively.

Main characteristics of the participants are shown in table 1, which shows that 77 % of the high school students participated in sports on regular basis. There was a significant difference between students in academic programs compared to vocational programs, more students in academic programs participated in sports (71% and 80% respectively) (p=0.036). There was also significant difference between females in academic and vocational programs, females in academic programs were more active in sports than females in vocational programs, 81.6% and 66.2 % respectively (p=0.007). The most popular sports among males were (in order of popularity): walking, gym/fitness, soccer, rugby, swimming, tennis, cricket, volleyball. Among females the most popular sports were: walking, swimming, gym/fitness, volleyball, netball, athletics, cycling, horseback riding. A great deal of those who did not perform any sport spent time with friends, used the computer, played video games, listened to music or read books or magazines.

A significantly higher number of females than males (25% and 17% respectively) participated in physical activities at a low level of effort one to three times/week or more and also a higher number of females than males did not perform any physical activity at all (12 % and 5 % respectively) (p=0.001). On the other hand, a significantly higher number of males than females trained at a medium and high level of effort one to three times per week or more (p=0.001). There were significant differences between vocational and academic programs, 16% of the students in vocational and 7 % in academic programs did not participate in any physical activity at all (p=0.001). The opposite was reported in the high level of physical activity, where students in vocational programs compared to students in academic programs, participated in physical activity at a high level were 8 % and 18 % respectively (p=0.001). Among females in academic and vocational programs who reported no level of physical effort were 8 % in academic and 25 % in vocational programs (p=0.0001). We found that 17.4 % of the students suffer from overweight or obesity and that almost 45 % are in risk (BMI=23.5-24.19) for overweight (see table 2).

Table 2. Prevalence of overweight in adolescents (15 – 17 years old) (n=403, 63 people missing)

	Subjects		
BMI	Male (%)	Female (%)	Total (%)
>23.5	130 (74.3)	185 (81.1)	315 (78.2)
23.5-24.19	10 (5.7)	8 (3.5)	18 (4.5)
24.2 >	35 (20)	35 (15.4)	70 (17.4)
TOTAL	175 (100)	228 (100)	403 (100)

Males reported significantly better health than females ($p<0.0001$). Thirty-six percent of males and 18 % of females reported their health to be very good. There were no differences between students in academic programs compared to those in vocational programs.

As shown in table 1, 65 % of the study group reported body complaints during the last three months. There were no differences between students in academic programs compared to those in vocational programs. The most common body parts for complaints were the back, knees, neck, ankle and shoulders (see table 3). A higher number of females than males reported complaints from the back ($p=0.007$) and the hip ($p=0.05$) and a higher number of males than females reported complaints from the hand ($p=0.0001$) and the elbow ($p=0.0001$) (see table 3).

The mean sleep time was 8.4 (sd = 1.1) hours in both males and females. Good sleep was reported in 82.1% of the males and in 76.6% of the females (NS). There was no sex difference in the occurrence of frequent awakenings (30.6% vs. 37.8%; NS), but males reported more seldom than females (23.5% vs. 33.5%; $p < 0.05$) that they had difficulty in falling asleep after nocturnal night-time awakenings. The occurrence of tiredness in the morning showed no sex difference. In males 44.3% were often sleepy in the daytime and the corresponding percentage number in females was 56.6% ($p < 0.01$).

Table 3. Students who reported body pain during the last three months (n=302)

Location	**Male** n (%)	**Female** n (%)	**P-value** p
Back	64 (34.6)	133 (47.3)	0.007
Knee	56 (30.3)	82 (29.2)	n.s
Neck	45 (24.3)	85 (30.2)	n.s
Ankle	45 (24.3)	78 (27.8)	n.s
Shoulder	39 (21.1)	81 (28.8)	n.s
Hand	36 (19.5)	22 (7.8)	0.0001
Hip	11 (5.9)	32 (11.4)	0.05
Elbow	21 (11.4)	8 (2.8)	0.0001

Table 4. Logistic regression analysis of general health

variables	B	p-value	Odds Ratio	95% Confidence interval *Lower*	*Upper*
BMI		0.000			
BMI<20	1.042	0.018	2.834	1.196	6.715
BMI >24	-.963	0.008	0.382	0.187	0.781
Activity		0.003			
Activity low	1.137	0.03	3.118	1.118	8.699
Activity medium	1.374	0.002	3.950	1.630	9.574
Activity high	2.483	0.001	11.983	2.871	50.018
Good sleep	1.407	0.001	4.083	1.803	9.245
Constant	0.207	0.622	1.230		

Health perception was more favorable in males than in females. Thirty-six percent of the males who reported poor health had poor sleep, and the corresponding amount in males reported relatively good or very good health were 17.7% and 10.8%, respectively ($p < 0.05$). The corresponding percentages in females were 30.8%, and reported relatively good or very good health 22.2% and 22.0% respectively (NS).

Medium or high physical activity (vs. none or low) was reported by 22.3% of the males and 13.1% of the females ($p < 0.05$). In the whole group of males and females no difference in sleep variables was observed in groups with different degrees of physical activity but the statement "I am often sleepy in the daytime" was answered affirmatively more often (53.3% vs. 32.4%; $p < 0.01$) in those who reported low or no physical activity than in those with medium or high physical activity.

Bodily complaints, most prevalent in the locomotor system, were present in 58.3% of the males and in 60.6% of the females. Poor sleep occurred in 10.0% and 22.8% of males without and with bodily complaints, respectively ($p < 0.05$) and, correspondingly, in 10.6% and 29.9% of the females ($p < 0.0001$). BMI was 21.8 (sd = 3.7) in males and 21.1 (sd = 3.2) in females (p =0.04). Reports on poor sleep in males with BMI < 20; 20.0-23.9 and = 24.0 occurred in 5.4%, 21.1% and 26.2%, respectively ($p < 0.01$). The corresponding percentages in females were 20.7%, 26.5% and 21.1%, respectively (NS). In males, BMI = 24.0 were present in 15.2% of those without daytime sleepiness and in 27.0% of those who were troubled by sleepiness in the daytime ($p < 0.05$). The corresponding percentages in females were 13.4% and 16.3%, respectively (NS).

Logistic regression analysis was used to estimate a model for good health (see table 4). Underweight, physical activity and good sleep was concluded to be factors with significant positive effect on good health, whereas overweight was a negative factor. Gender, type of program, sleep hours per night and complaints were non significant and therefore excluded from the model.

Our Findings in Context

In the present study, 77 % of the high school students participated in sports on a regular basis comprising no gender differences. There was a significant difference between males and females in vocational and academic programs, more males and females in academic programs participated in sports. These findings are similar to Westerståhl et al [12] study, which found that the difference between the educational programs (vocational and academic) correlated with physical activity levels and that vocational programs were associated to lower socio-economic status, and lower perceived positive influence from parents to be physically active among the students in vocational programs.

The American College of Sports Medicine (ACSM) and the American Heart Association (AHA) physical activity guidelines have updated, stating to promote and maintain health, all healthy people need moderate-intensity aerobic (endurance) physical activity for a minimum of 30 minutes on five days each week or vigorous-intensity aerobic physical activity for a minimum of 20 minutes on three days each week. Combinations of moderate and vigorous intensity activity can be performed to meet this recommendation [13]. In a study of 16 to 18 year old Finnish youths, Aarnio et al [14] found that those who participated in organised sports were more likely to be fit than those who did not. The Finnish study also reported that 24 to 28 % of the girls and 32 to 36 % of the boys to be extremely physical active, 4-5 times a week [14]. This is somewhat more than in the present study and a Norwegian study by Alricsson et al [15], but similar to a Swedish study [9]. This could indicate that some students have reported physical activity when they have performed non organised activities such as when they had probably walked or went by bike to school for instance. Furthermore, the present Australian study supported findings that identified [15] that a higher number of females participated in physical activities at a low level of effort (one to three times per week or more) than males.

Males were not fitter than females, but males participated in activities at a higher level of effort (one to three times or more weekly) than females. This may suggest that males were more likely to take part in competitive sports whereas females were more likely to be involved in recreation sports [9,15]. This finding is similar to Sirard et al [16], who found that gender-specific motivational factors exist for middle school youth. Boys are more attracted to the competitive aspects of sports whereas girls are motivated by the social opportunities that sports provide. Allender et al [17] found that fun, enjoyment and social support for aspects of identity were reported more often as predictors of participation and non-participation in sports than perceived health benefits for teenage girls. Furthermore, a dialectic approach can be seen between girls wanting to be physically active and at the same time feminine [17]. Pfeiffer et al [18] found that girls who played sports for a longer number of years were more active than nonparticipants, suggesting that adolescent girls who participated in sports in eighth, ninth, and 12th grades have higher odds probability of being vigorously active in their 12th grade. Additionally, three-year sport participants maintain consistent activity patterns over time [18]. One of the most important barriers to increased physical activity of youth is the recent reduction in physical education programs in schools. This global trend might well be reversed if studies demonstrate that physical activity contributes to improving classroom behaviour and performance [19].

The present study showed that males reported significantly better health than females. Recent studies have indicated that gender is a powerful predictor of self-related health as often males rate their health higher than females [9,15,20]. Congruent with other research findings, females consistently rated their health lower than males. Furthermore, physical activity and body mass weight also influence adolescent self-related health [20]. The consistency of results across different studies is impressive, even though the studies differ with regard to their design, population and the way in which self-related health is assessed.

The most common argument is that young people's lack of participation in sport and physical activity is directly equated with a dramatic rise in childhood obesity. In the present study 22 % of the students suffer from overweight/obesity or are at risk of being overweight. Janssen et al [21] showed in a review article that overweight and obesity prevalence was particularly high in countries located in North America, Great Britain and South-Western Europe. Within most countries physical activity levels were lower and television viewing times were higher in overweight youths compared to normal weight youths. Increasing physical activity participation and decreasing television viewing should be the focus of strategies aimed at preventing and treating overweight and obesity in youth [21]. A significant share of the study group (63 of 466) did not answer the question about their own weight. The researchers were unable to find any literature to support the finding that overweight students prefer not to give information about their own weight. On the contrary, underestimation of self-reported weight was usual. Tsigilis [22] showed that students in secondary schools significantly underestimated their weight. Those at risk of being overweight/obese underestimated their weight to a greater extend than their 'normal weight' counterparts [22]. Elgar et al [23] showed that a sample of 418 high school students in year 11 underreported their body weight by an average of .52 kg. This fact influenced our decision to analyze the material in three different groups (underweight/normal weight, risk for overweight, overweight/obesities) was based on this knowledge. No significant differences were noted in the present study regarding prevalence of overweight in relation to self-related health or body complaints. On the contrary, Vinglis et al. showed that physical activity and BMI influenced self-related health [20]. Several other studies show that there is no strong relation between BMI and low back pain [15,24].

In the present study, 65 % of the students reported body complaints during the last three months. Most common body parts for complaints were the back, knees, neck, ankle and shoulder. Smedbråten et al [25] showed that about 50 % of the 15 year old adolescents reported body complaints and that knee and back pain were most frequently reported. These findings are in line with previous studies of Alricsson et al [9,15]. Back problems have been reported to occur as early as 16 years of age for both males and females. Symptoms in childhood, particularly if they are frequent, may have important consequences for chronic pain in adulthood [26].

Evidence is growing that sleep problems in adolescents are significant impediments to learning and negatively affect behaviour, attainment of social competence and quality of life [27]. A growing body of epidemiological evidence suggests an association between short sleep duration and obesity [28] In the present study the mean sleep time was 8.4 hours in both males and females. Gaina et al [29] found that prevalence of sleepiness did not significantly differ among groups who had 7.5 hours sleep or more. Good sleep was reported in 82.1% of the males and in 76.6% of the females. The occurrence of tiredness in the morning showed no sex difference. In males 44.3% were often sleepy in the daytime and the corresponding percentage number in females was 56.6% and significant. This is somewhat less than Gibson et al [27] whose study identified that 58-68 % of Canadian high school students reported that they were "really sleepy" between 8 and 10 A:M. Furthermore, Gaina et al [29] showed regarding sex difference, a higher proportion of girls reported sleepiness in comparison to boys (79 % vs 66 %). In our study we couldn't find any gender differences, but the statement "I am often sleepy in the daytime" was answered affirmatively more often (53.3% vs. 32.4%) in those who reported low or no physical activity than in those with medium or high physical activity. Proper sleep habits, high physical activity level, and limited TV viewing time and limited video game use should be promoted among school children and high school students [1,29].

The most common argument is that young people's lack of participation in sport and physical activity is directly equated with a dramatic rise in childhood obesity. Accumulated evidence suggests that overweight youths become overweight adults, and inactive youths also become inactive adults.

Underweight, physical activity and good sleep were concluded to be factors with significant positive effect on good health, whereas overweight was a negative factor. Proper sleep habits and higher physical activity levels should be promoted among high school students and TV viewing time and video game use restricted. Additionally, schools should provide opportunities for young people to participate in a wider range of physical activities that address their individual needs while promoting the health benefits of engaging in regular exercise.

Acknowledgments

This research was supported by the Swedish National Center for Research in Sport (CIF), Stockholm, Sweden and by Professor Elizabeth Kendall, Griffith Abilities Research Program, Research Centre for Clinical and Community Practice Innovation, Griffith University, Logan Campus, Australia. This chapter is a adapted version of our paper Alricsson M, Domalewski D, Romild U, Asplund R. Physical activity, health, body mass index, sleeping habits and body complaints in Australian senior high school students. Int J Adolesc Med Health 2008;20[4].

References

[1] Olds T, Ridley K, Dollman J. Screenieboppers and extreme screenies: the place of screen time in the time budgets of 10-13 year-old Australian children. Aust NZ J Public Health 2006;30:137-42.

[2] Paffenbarger RS, Blair SN, Lee IM. A history of physical activity, cardiovascular health and longevity: the scientific contributions of Jeremy N Morris. Int J Epidemiol 2001;30:1184 -92.

[3] Hardman AE. Physical activity and health: current issues and research needs. Int J Epidemiol 2001;30:1193-7.

[4] Barnekow-Bergkvist M, Hedberg G, Janlert U, Jansson E. Prediction of physical fitness and physical activity level in adulthood by physical performance and physical activity in adolescence – An 18-year follow–up study. Scand J Med Sci Sports 1998;8:299-308.

[5] Booth ML, Wake M, Armstrong T, Chey T, Hesketh K, Mathur S. The epidemiology of overweight and obesity among Australian children and adolescents, 1995-97. Aust NZ J Public Health 2001;25:162-9.

[6] Wang Y, Lobstein T. Worldwide trends in childhood overweight and obesity. Int J Pediatr Obes 2006;1:11-25.

[7] Wendell CT, Blair SN, Cummings SS, Wun CC, Malina RM. Childhood and adolescent physical activity patterns and adult physical activity. Med Sci Sports Exerc 1999;31:118-23.

[8] Telama R, Yang X, Viikari J, Valimäki I, Wanne O, Raitakari O. Physical activity from childhood to adulthood. A 21-Year tracking study. Am J Prev Med 2005;28(3):267-73.

[9] Alricsson M, Landstad BJ, Romild U, Werner S. Self-related health, physical activity and complaints in Swedish high school students. ScientificWorldJournal 2006;6:816-26.

[10] Beaton DE, Bombardier C, Guillemin F, Ferraz MB. Guidelines for the process of cross-cultural adaptation of self-reported measures. Spine 2000;25(24):3186-91.

[11] Cole TJ, Bellizzi MC, Flegal KM, Dietz W. Establishing a standard definition for child overweight and obesity worldwide: international survey. BMJ 2000;320:1240-3.

[12] Westerståhl M, Barnekow-Bergkvist M, Jansson E. Low physical activity among adolescents in practical education. Scand J Med Sci Sports 2005;15:287-97.

[13] Haskell WL, Lee I-M, Pate RR, Powell KE, Blair SN, Franklin BA, Macera CA, Heath GW, Thompson PD, Bauman A. Physical activity and public health: Updated recommendation for adults from the American College of Sports Medicine and the American Heart Association. Med Sci Sports Exerc 2007;39(8):1423-34.

[14] Aarnio M, Winter T, Peltonen J, Kujala UM, Kaprio J. Stability of leisure-time physical activity during adolescence – a longitudinal study among 16-, 17- and 18-years-old Finnish youth. Scand J Med Sci Sports 2002;12:179-85.

[15] Alricsson M, Landstad B, Romild R, Gundersen KT. Physical activity, health, BMI and body complaints in high school students. Minerva Pediatr 2008;60(1):19-25.

[16] Sirard JR, Pfeiffer KA, Pate RR. Motivational factors associated with sports program participation in middle school students. J Adolesc Health 2006;38:696-703.

[17] Allender S, Cowburn G, Foster C. Understanding participation in sport and physical activity among children and adults: a review of qualitative studies. Health Educ Res 2006;21:826-35.

[18] Pfeiffer KA, Dowda M, Dishman RK, McIver KL, Sirard JR, Ward DS, Pate RR. Sport participation and physical activity in adolescent females across a four-year period. J Adolesc Health 2006;39(4):523-29.

[19] Dietz WH. Physical activity recommendations: where do we go from here? J Pediatr 2005;146:719-20.
[20] Vingilis ER, Wade TJ, Seeley JS. Predictors of adolescent self-rated health. Can J Public Health 2002;93(3):193-7.
[21] Janssen I, Katzmarzyk PT, Boyce WF, Vereecken C, Mulvihill C, Roberts C, Currie C, Pickett W. Comparison of overweight and obesity prevalence in school-aged youth from 34 countries and their relationships with physical activity and dietary patterns. Obes Rev 2005;6:123-32.
[22] Tsigilis N. Can secondary school students' self-reported measures of height and weight be trusted? An effect size approach. Eur J Public Health 2006;16(5):532-35.
[23] Elgar FJ, Roberts C, Tudor-Smith C, Moore L. Validity of self-reported height and weight and predictors of bias in adolescents. J Adolesc Health 2005;37(5):371-5.
[24] Deyo RA, Bass JE. Lifestyle and low back pain: the influence of smoking and obesity. Spine 1989;14:501-506.
[25] Smedbråten BK, Natvig B, Rutle O. Self-reported bodily pain in schoolchildren. Scand J Rheumatol 1998;27:273-76.
[26] Brattberg G. Do pain problems in young school children persist into early adulthood? A 13-year follow-up. Eur J Pain 2004;8:187-99.
[27] Gibson Es, Powles AC, Thabane L, O´Brien S, Molnar DS, Trajanovic N, Ogilvie R, Shapiro C, Yan M, Chilcott-Tanser L. "Sleepiness" is serious in adolescence: two surveys of 3,235 Canadian students. BMC Public Health 2006;(2)6:116.
[28] Kohatsu ND, Tsai R, Young T, VanGilder R, Burmeister LF, Stromqvist AM, Merchant JA. Sleep duration and body mass index in a rural population. Arch Intern Med 2006;166:1701-5.
[29] Gaina A, Sekine M, Hamanishi S, Chen X, Wang H, Yamagami T, Kagamimori S. Daytime sleepiness and associated factors in Japanese school children. J Pediatr 2007;151(5):518-22.

In: Obesity and Adolescence: A Public Health Concern
Editors: H.A. Omar, D.E. Greydanus et al.
ISBN: 978-1-60692-821-9

Chapter X

Obesity and Lack of Physical Activity

Hatim A. Omar**, Efrat Merrick-Kenig, and Joav Merrick
Section of Adolescent Medicine, Department of Pediatrics, University of Kentucky, Lexington, Kentucky, United States of America, National Institute of Child Health and Human Development, Office of the Medical Director, Division for Mental Retardation, Ministry of Social Affairs, Jerusalem, Israel

Abstract

Lack of physical activity and overweight status continues to be a significant health problem in the United States. To assess the actual prevalence of these problems, we reviewed data from the School-based Health Promotion Centers in one middle school, and one high school in central Kentucky. A total of 232 6th graders and 607 9th graders were included. A total of 92% of 6th graders and 45% of 9th graders reported complete lack of regular exercise. 37% of 9th graders and 59% of 6th graders had inappropriate nutrition, 47% of 9th graders and 33% of 6th graders had Body Mass Index over the 85th percentile for age. Among overweight adolescents, only 16% of 9th graders and 1% of 6th graders thought they were overweight. Since the body mass index data is derived from actual objective measurement, we conclude that overweight status is a significant problem in Kentucky and that the actual numbers may be higher than those reported for the State based on surveys and estimates. Furthermore, many adolescents are not aware of their weight problem and most of them do not participate in regular exercise.

Introduction

* Correspondence: Hatim Omar, MD, Professor of Pediatrics and Obstetrics/Gynecology, Department of Pediatrics, Kentucky Clinic, Rm. J422, Lexington, KY 40536-0284, USA. Tel. 859-323-5643; FAX. 859-257-7706; Email: haomar2@uky.edu

Overweight and obesity among adolescents have been referred to as a worldwide epidemic [1]. The World Health Organization (WHO) defines overweight as a body mass index (BMI) of over 25 kg/m2 and obesity as a BMI of over 30 kg/m2 [2]. The 2003 Youth Risk Behavior Survey (YRBS) found that 13.5% of American students were overweight. Overall, the prevalence of being overweight was higher among male (17.4%) than female (9.4%) students, and higher among black (17.6%) than white (12.2%) students. 29.6% of students described themselves as slightly or very overweight and 43.8% reported they were trying to lose weight. Overall, the prevalence of trying to lose weight was higher among female (59.3%) than male (29.1%) students and highest among white females (62.6%) [3].

The United States Department of Agriculture (USDA) and the United States Department of Health and Human Services (HHS) recommend that children and adolescents engage in at least 60 minutes of physical activity per day [4]. However, according to the 2003 YRBS, 33.4% of students nationwide participated in insufficient physical activity in the previous week and 11.5% had not participated in either vigorous physical activity or moderate physical activity at all [5].

57.1% of students nationwide had exercised to lose weight or to keep from gaining weight during the 30 days preceding the survey. 42.2% of students had eaten less food, fewer calories, or foods low in fat to lose weight or to keep from gaining weight and 13.3% had gone without eating for over 24 hours to lose weight or to keep from gaining weight. During the 30 days preceding the survey, 9.2 % of students had taken diet pills, powders, or liquids without advice from a physician and 6% had vomited or taken laxatives to lose weight or to keep from gaining weight [3].

Only 22.0% of American students reported eating fruits and vegetables over five times/day during the seven days preceding the survey [5], as recommended by the USDA and HHS [6]. The health risks of overweight and obesity are significant, including cardiovascular disease [7], type II Diabetes [8], orthopedic issues such as slipped capital femoral epiphysis, pulmonary issues such as obstructive sleep apnea, and psychosocial pathology such as depression and poor self-esteem [9].

Poor nutrition and decreased levels of activity are widely touted as the causes of the epidemic of overweight and obesity in the United States. In this study, we evaluated weight, nutrition, weight perception and exercise status in middle and high school students in Central Kentucky.

What Is the Situation in Kentucky?

School-Based Health Promotion Centers (SBHC) in one middle school and one high school in Central Kentucky were utilized for this study. SBHC screen all students entering middle (6th grade) and high (9th grade) school for all risk taking behaviors. Students are excluded if their parents do not give consent for confidential screening. Data from these screenings were collected from the years 2002 and 2003. Body Mass Index (BMI) was calculated by dividing the actual weight in kilograms by the height in square meters. The rest of the information was obtained by interviewing the students using the Perkins Adolescent Risk Screen (PARS) [10,11].

During the years 2002 and 2003, a total of 232 6th graders (105 females and 127 males) and 607 9th (306 females and 301 males) graders were screened. Only 23% of females and 9% of males among 9th graders and 1% of females and 1.5% of males of 6th graders perceived themselves as overweight. 51% of 9th graders and 53% of 6th graders reported spending more than four hours on non-school days and more than two hours on school days on sedentary activities (watching television or using computers or video games). Poor nutrition was defined as eating mostly fast food, not eating fruit and vegetables and/or consuming too many unhealthy snacks and carbonated beverages. Exercise was defined as a minimum 20 minutes of vigorous physical activity at least five days every week. The prevalence of abnormal BMI, poor nutrition and lack of exercise is shown in table 1.

This study was a simple descriptive one that did not address causes or management of obesity. It did not look at ethnic or socioeconomic differences. The goal was to assess the extent of obesity and lack of physical activity among middle and high school students in the area. Most available data is usually derived from subjective surveys, which may overstate or understate facts. Adolescents responding to written surveys may sometimes fail to understand the questions. In our SBHC, adolescents were interviewed one on one by the same trained professional, allowing for more consistency. Objective measurement of weight and height were also obtained. Our results showed a similar percentage of obese adolescents (16.5%) to that reported by CDC (14.6%) for Kentucky [12] in high school students. In this study, an additional 31% were at risk for obesity with BMI>85%. Among middle school students these numbers were slightly better (see table 1). One disturbing result in the study was the low percentage of students in both groups who correctly perceived their weight as inappropriate. When exact parameters for exercise were explained to students, the majority in both groups showed lack of regular exercise (see table 1). A similar percentage of students had poor nutrition habits.

Based on these results we conclude that sedentary life-style, lack of regular exercise and poor nutrition are very prevalent in Kentucky adolescents. Furthermore, many adolescents do not recognize their weight problem as such. Education of adolescents, their parents, teachers, and the community is needed to help prevent further increases of these problems.

Table 1. BMI, nutrition and exercise among Kentucky adolescents

	9th Graders		6th Graders	
	Males	Females	Males	Females
BMI 85%-95%	32%	30%	21%	22%
BMI >95%	13%	20%	13%	9%
Poor nutrition	24%	50%	61%	57%
No exercise	37%	54%	92%	92%

References

[1] Kohn M. The worldwide epidemic of obesity in adolescents. Adolesc Med 2003;14(1):1-9.

[2] Website: http://www.who.int/dietphysicalactivity/media/en/gsfs_obesity.pdf

[3] Centers for Disease Control and Prevention. Surveillance Summaries, May 21, 2004. MMWR 2004;53:25-7.

[4] United States Departments of Agriculture and Health and Human Services. Nutrition and Your Health: Dietary Guidelines for Americans, Fifth Edition. Washington, DC: Authors, 2000:13-4.

[5] Centers for Disease Control and Prevention. Surveillance Summaries, May 21, 2004. MMWR 2004;53:21-4.

[6] United States Departments of Agriculture and Health and Human Services. Nutrition and Your Health: Dietary Guidelines for Americans, Fifth Edition. Washington, DC: Authors, 2000:16-7.

[7] Smith JC. The current epidemic of childhood obesity and its implications for future coronary heart disease. Pediatr Clin North Am 2004;(51) 6:1679-95.

[8] Goran MI. Obesity and risk of Type 2 diabetes and cardiovascular disease in children and adolescents. J Clin Endocrin Metabol 2003;88(4):1417-27.

[9] Brown WM. Obesity in children and adolescents. Clin Fam Pract 2002; 4(3):603-13.

[10] Perkins K, Ferrari N, Rosas A, Bessette R, Williams A, Omar H. You won't know unless you ask: the biopsychosocial interview for adoles¬cents. Clin Ped 1997;36:79-86.

[11] Adams C, Perkins K, Lumley V, Hughes C, Burns J, Omar H. Vali¬dation of the Perkins Adolescent Risk Screen (PARS). J Adolesc Health 2003;33:462-70.

[12] Centers for Disease Control and Prevention. Surveillance Summaries, May 21, 2004. MMWR 2004;53: Figure 8.

V. Psychological Aspects

In: Obesity and Adolescence: A Public Health Concern
Editors: H.A. Omar, D.E. Greydanus et al.
ISBN: 978-1-60692-821-9

Chapter XI

The Psychology of Obesity

Helen D. Pratt*
Division of Behavioral and Developmental Pediatrics, Pediatrics Program, Michigan State University/Kalamazoo Center for Medical Studies, Kalamazoo, Michigan, United States of America

Abstsract

Obesity has been deemed a public health epidemic, which carries with it high financial and psychological stakes, social consequences, and ethics of public, mental, and medical health care research pushing for all adolescents, who are "obese" to lose weight. This article reviews the psychological aspects of overweight in adolescents. No single factor has been shown to cause obesity; most researchers agree that the causes of obesity are multifaceted and complicated. Adolescents who are overweight may experience the deleterious effects of obesity on psychological functioning. Concepts of beauty, perceptions of body image and satisfaction all contribute to the psychological attitudes and beliefs about personal value, worthiness, self image, body satisfaction, and dieting. Not all adolescents who are at-risk-for-overweight or are overweight are unhealthy. Clinicians should consider that just as they warn the obese about the risks of obesity, they must expend as much energy evaluating the risks of successful weight loss. They must also remember that there are other standards of beauty and body size among ethnic groups and other cultures. The weight for height by body type tables that are used to calculate BMI should be changed to reflect the body types and fat distributions of Latino- and African-Americans.

---

* Correspondence: Helen D Pratt, PhD, Pediatrics Program, MSU/KCMS, 1000 Oakland Dr, Kalamazoo, MI 49008 United States. Tel: 269 337-6450; Fax 269-337-6474; E-mail: pratt@kcms.msu.edu

Introduction

Obesity has been deemed a public health epidemic which carries with it high stakes financial, psychological, and social consequences [1,2]. Approximately 14% of adolescents (ages 12 to 19 years) are overweight [3,4]. The CDC reported the cost of care for overweight adolescents has not been calculated [3] however, costs for adult obesity were estimated to be approximately 100 billion dollars for which sixty percent of those costs are for inpatient, outpatient, and laboratory services [2,4,5]. Although the literature supports that the costs for obesity add a burden to the costs of health care, the profits from the obesity industry are rarely discussed. Treatment of obesity in the United States has produced a 46 billion dollar weight loss industry; promoters of weight loss products and bariatric surgery focus on the negative emotions of being "fat" and concentrate on poor physical health, social isolation and rejection, and feelings of sadness and depression [4].

Table 1. Factors that influence risk and prevalence of obesity

• Age • Certain medical conditions • Sedentary life styles • Physical inactivity • Diet high in calories • Diet low in nutrient dense foods • Smoking cessation • Food is seen as entertainment versus sustenance • Increase use of TV, video games, computers	• Genetic susceptibility • Social Economic Status (SES) (higher SES for non Hispanic Caucasians, lower SES for African-Americans and youth of Hispanic-ancestry • Race/ethnicity • Family history – Eating patters – Food choices – Attitudes about obesity or "fat" – Eat out more often – Have fewer family meals	**Schools:** • Physical education no longer mandatory in schools • Vending machines high calorie dense food choices are money makers for schools and do not support goals of providing healthy nutrition in meals and snacks • Cafeteria foods often high calorie foods that offer little choice to select balanced foods **Communities** • Limited access to safe places to engage in physical activity • Access to fresh fruit and vegetables limited • Cost higher for healthier foods in urban areas

Table 2. Changes in behavior that influence risk and prevalence of obesity

- Exercise is no longer a part of one's daily functioning and must be artificially introduced.
- Youth have difficulty incorporating physical exercise into normal, everyday mandatory activity (walking to school; playing in safe areas in their communities in the out of doors)
- Youth have little control over what they have access to eat at home and school
- Youth, especially minority youth are subjected to targeted marking of high fat low nutrition low fiber foods
- Most fast food and restaurant have changed to larger portion sizes
- Food is viewed as and used for entertainment or as therapy
- View that one can eat drink as much as one wishes to have a good time and have fun.

Ethiology

No single factor has been shown to cause obesity (see table 1)[2,4,5]. Several controversial views have been put forth to account for increases in weight in children or adolescents.5, 6 Current views hold that when children and adolescents gain weight, many complementary changes have simultaneously increased the individual's energy intake and decreased his/her energy expenditure (see table 2) [5,7].

Obesity in the Adolescent Population

The term "obese" is no longer applied to children or adolescents; instead, the terms "at risk of overweight" and "overweight" are designated by the Centers for Disease Control and Prevention (CDC) in Atlanta, Georgia, as appropriate descriptions that are not based on health outcomes or risk but take into account the age and gender of an individual [7]. These terms are defined in other articles of this issue on obesity.

Social Consequences of Obesity

Obesity puts adolescents at risk for physical health problems and negatively impacts their social and psychological health. Adolescents also have an increased likelihood they will experiencing feelings of cultural isolation as a result maladaptive family, peer, and healthcare provider experiences (see table 3)[2,4,8-13]. Adolescent females who see themselves as overweight are prone to dieting, exercising to lose weight, using pills, and vomiting to lose weight. Caucasian female adolescents are almost two times more likely than African-American females to a) perceive themselves as overweight and b) engage in unhealthy weight management practices [14]. The stigma of obesity is so strong that adolescents may face biases in all aspects of their lives [11,14,15].

Psychological Aspects of Obesity

Adolescents who are overweight may experience the deleterious effects of obesity on psychological functioning (see table 3)[12,13]. Psychological aspects of overweight during adolescence include how an adolescent a) thinks about him or herself, b) views the feedback about him or her, and c) how that feedback is interpreted; these issues all combine with the adolescents' temperament and cultural environment. An adolescent's views of self-image, values about body-shape, body-mass, beauty, and weight begin to develop during childhood and are shaped within the context of his or her cultural environment [10,11,14].

Prior to age 11 years, children are primarily influenced by their families and intimate environment. As their world expands, adolescents' perceptions of how others view them become increasingly more important. These factors (family and cultural environments) have great influence over how a person develops his or her views of self perception and attitudes about body size, weight, body fat, and beauty; however, peers, teachers, physicians, and the media can exert significant influence such that they can provide negative factors that can often exacerbate an adolescent's psychological (i.e., cognitive, affective, and social) distress.16 Peers, teachers, and the media can also provide protective factors to promote or sustain an adolescent's psychological well being [10,14,16].

Adolescents are usually resilient and can overcome harsh environmental events with family and community support. Despite this resilience, adolescents are still vulnerable from a developmental point of view; they lack a history of interpersonal relationship successes to offset negative views about obesity expressed by family members and peers. Based on feedback from their cultural environment, adolescents develop their views of who they are, discover why they are unique, and determine their strengths and weaknesses.

Table 3. Associated psychological outcomes for overweight and obesity in adolescents

- perpetrating or being a victim of bullying behavior
    - boys reported more overt victimization
    - girls
        - reported more problems with
            - intimate peer relations with other girls
                - refusal to spend time with subject
                - silent treatment
                - refusal to sit near subject at lunch or in class
                - verbal teasing
        - have less supportive and more antagonistic friendships
        - are less likely to date than their peers
        - have fewer opportunities to develop intimate romantic relationships
        - may experience more self-consciousness and anxiety depression and low self-esteem.
- Obese boys and girls reported being more dissatisfied with their dating status compared with average-weight peers.

Based on these discoveries they develop healthy or unhealthy self-esteem and negative or positive perceptions of their value and self-worth. If that environment provides negative feedback, the adolescent may develop poor self esteem, unhealthy self image, and develop body dissatisfaction. The combination of these negative cognitive emotions and multiple sources of insults (i.e., family, peers, health care providers, and the media) regarding obesity result in negative affective states that can erode the adolescent's ability to be resilient. Adolescents need protection and nurturance from parents, other family members, and peers to withstand these negative situations. Without this support they can develop profound sadness, distress, or even depression as a result of harassment, bullying, and peer rejection [10,11,15].

Perceptions of Beauty

Standards of beauty in Western cultures and in the United States in particular, exclude many adolescents who do not exemplify the "thin ideal." Thinness is associated with attractiveness, fitness, worthiness, access (i.e., friendship, dating, and special favors) and health; in contrast, obesity/overweight is associated with unattractiveness, poor health, being food-obsessed, being physically unfit, being lazy, not having will power or self-control, and potentially costing society an unfair share amount of money for health care [2,10,12,13,17].

These negative views of overweight may result in social biases which may expose the adolescent to stigmatizing experiences and promote unhealthy weight loss practices [7]. Such biases can help overweight youth become victims of peer rejection, harassment or bullying. Although not the common outcome of obesity bias, some overweight youth become perpetrators of harassment or bullying [11]. Yet, in some cultures where the "Western Ideal" has not been adopted, there is greater acceptance of higher body weights. Fatness or plumpness may be considered a sign of beauty or is accepted without bias [17].

Adolescents, especially ethnic girls (African-, Asian, Hispanic-, Native-Americans, and Alaskan/Pacific Island Native-Americans) are keenly aware of differences between Western standards of beauty and their own physical characteristics; perhaps this is why they tend to describe beauty in terms of personality traits instead of physical attributes (i.e., intelligence, social skills, altruism, grooming, and having a good sense of humor) [18]. Caucasian adolescents are more likely to attempt to diet to lose weight, engage in compensatory behaviors (i.e., purging, excessive exercise, calorie restriction). African American girls perceive beauty as flexible, fluid, and as exceeding physical characteristics. They judged beauty on the basis of how one moved rather than how much one weighed -- even in light of society's beliefs and media portrayals of the "western ideal as the standard of beauty [18].

Youth who express biases and prejudices about overweight adolescents can learn to have more positive views of their overweight peers if they receive education directed at the causes of obesity [15]. Based on exposure to peer views of overweight as positive and not a moral defect, others can view youth who have larger body types, as healthy and not representing examples of medical or psychological pathology.

Body Dissatisfaction

Individuals who do not like the physical characteristics of their bodies can be said to experience some aspect of body dissatisfaction (i.e., height, weight, size, and shape of face, nose, or mouth, eye shape or color, type of hair, others). Body dissatisfaction as used when talking about the issue of obesity is generally focused on a more narrow aspect of body mass, and how fat is deposited over the body. Body dissatisfaction may be pervasive among adolescents and not just a problem of obesity. Robinson, et al [19] compared body dissatisfaction between 6th and 7th grade American females (African-, Asian- and Caucasian-American) and found that even adolescents who are very lean/short/tall, will report body dissatisfaction. They further found that BMI was the strongest independent predictor of increased body dissatisfaction for all subjects [19]. The researcher concluded that African-

American girls had the highest body satisfaction. Girls with high body satisfaction were more likely to report parental and peer attitudes that encouraged healthy eating and exercising to be fit versus dieting [19].

Baskin, Aluwalia and Resnicow [18] offered that the positive body images of African American girls need not be viewed as problematic or abnormal. In fact, it could be argued that majority culture has a dysfunctional view of body image and obesity. Body dissatisfaction may result in an adolescent developing a low self-esteem, feeling bad about his or herself, questioning his or her personal value and uniqueness, and feeling bad about his or her physical characteristics. Such negative cognitions can lead to adolescents developing a poor self image.

Self Image

In a recent survey approximately 35% described themselves as being overweight (Males-25% and females-38%)[6]. Research on body image with African- and Caucasian-American concluded that media influences on self-perceptions of body images are different for each group. When exposed to mainstream media, Caucasian subjects reported poorer body image, while African American subjects did not. When exposed to African American media Caucasian subjects reported no impact. African American subjects who were also exposed to African American oriented television had healthier body image while viewing mainstream television. Ethnic identity also predicted healthier body image among black women [20].

Relationship between Overweight and Depression

The psychological correlates between overweight and depression with the resulting consequences are not well understood [21-23]. An adolescent's relative weight is associated with depressive symptoms for girls (but not boys) and was stronger among adolescents in lower grades [23]. A recent study concluded that the behavioral, cognitive, physiological, and social mechanisms that form the pathway between obesity and depression is bidirectional [23,24].

Depression and obesity in teens have been linked to family income, educational level, and socioeconomic status. Researchers found about a third of the cases of depression and obesity among those teens could be attributed to being from families with low incomes or having parents with low levels of education. Lower parental education was associated with 40 percent of depression and 39 percent of obesity among these teens.21-23 Obesity rates are about 50% higher in families below the poverty line when compared to youth whose family income is at or above it. These rates are higher for ethnic females (i.e., African Americans, Hispanics and Native Americans) than among Caucasian-Americans [21-23].

Impact of Weight Re-gain after Treatment

Although adolescents may successfully lose weight, they may suffer other negative side effects post intervention or post surgery which includes unhealthy eating and physical activity obsessions [24]. A search of web based publications shows that questions regarding the development of addictive behaviors (i.e., gambling, sex addition, and other impulse control disorders) resulting from bariatric surgery. A review of the literature using First Search, Medline, and Psych Info did not yield any empirical studies linking bariatric surgery, weight loss, and the development of impulse control disorder symptoms.

A meta-analytic review of 64 obesity prevention programs yields that 21% produced significant prevention effects that were typically pre- to post treatment intervention effects [25]. Larger effects emerged for programs that targeted children and adolescents (vs. preadolescents) and females. The researchers concluded that effective prevention had the following components: a) the programs were relatively brief; b) they solely targeted weight control versus other health behaviors (e.g., smoking); c) they had been evaluated during pilot trials; and d) the participants self-selected into the intervention. Other factors, including mandated improvements in diet and exercise, sedentary behavior reduction, delivery by trained interventionists, and parental involvement, were not associated with significantly larger effects [25].

Controversies that Impact the Psychology of Obesity

Fleck and Petersmarch [4] questioned the right of public health and medical organizations, physicians, and other health care clinicians to push or encourage adolescents to "lose weight." The authors contended that dieting and weight loss carry with them their own health risks. They also reminded clinicians that patients should set their own goals, even if that means they chose not to lose weight. Many health care professionals inform their patients about the risks of being overweight, but do not discuss the risks of their recommended interventions. For example, clinicians do not discuss complications that often result from weight loss (i.e., gall stones), nor do they present the risks of extreme weight loss interventions (i.e., starvation, severe food restriction, and bariatric surgery). Some health and psychological risks may exceed the risks of being overweight for some patients. Therefore, they ask physicians to adhere to their ethical duty to "do no harm" [4].

Other researchers [23,25] also support Flech Petersmarch's findings [4] that most patients do not maintain their weight loss post intervention, and may regain the lost weight; the increase in weight gain can result in the adolescent experiencing increased negative physical and psychological outcomes. Weight regain can result in the adolescent feeling like he or she is a failure, especially after accepting the negative aspects about their obesity from the agency, health care professional or surgeons who have helped them to be successful in weight loss. The adolescent who loses weight works hard not to be a representative of the negative stereotypes and works hard to please the clinical and weight loss professionals who help them with their efforts. Not only may the adolescent experience feelings of personal failure because of the weight re-gain, but now they have the added burden of no longer meeting the expectations of those professionals.

Another issue concerning the ethics of interventions to address overweight involves issues with minority populations. Fat distribution for African- and Latino-Americans is different than for their non-Hispanic Caucasian. The tables of ideal weights derived from non-Hispanic populations are not applicable to African- and Latino Americans.14 Research suggests that Latino American appeared to tolerate higher body weights without an adverse impact on their mortality experience and therefore, support the notion that new tables should be derived from prospective data specific to African- and Latino-American populations [18]. Assessment and treatment interventions should also take into account the cultural and ethnic issues related to providing health care that meets the general and specific needs of these populations [4].

Conclusions

Adolescent overweight has significantly increased over the past 20 years while most researchers agree that the causes of obesity are multifaceted and complicated; however the exact causes of the significant increases in the prevalence of overweight have not been clearly identified. Some researcher offers that many changes in the adolescent's physical activity, types and quality of foods they ingest, and use of food as entertainment contribute to the overall problem of overweight and obesity. In a society where thinness is one of the signs of beauty and health, being overweight can contribute to psychological distress in adolescents who are not thin. It is important that clinicians remember that there are other standards of beauty and body size among ethnic groups and other cultures.

Psychopathology (i.e., depression, sadness, feelings of isolation, and sense of rejection) that has been associated with overweight has not been shown to result from just being overweight. Researchers have found that these affective states can also be present in adolescents without the presence of overweight or obesity. Problems with self-image, body satisfaction, self-esteem also occur during adolescence with those who are both too thin (males), too short, or who do not look like the "thin ideal" of the perfect body. The relationship between depression and overweight has been show to be bidirectional. Clinicians must consider that even though overweight is associated with a number of adverse consequences, treatment to lose weight and actual weight loss also have adverse consequences. Further, not all overweight individuals are unhealthy or exhibiting medical or mental pathology. The acceptance of Western ideals of thinness as the only form of beauty can create conflicting cultural demands for people who do not fit this body type.

References

[1] Dietz WH, Robinson TN. Overweight children and adolescents. N Engl J Med 2005;352:2100-9.

[2] Gortmaker SL, Must A, Perrin JM, Sobol AM, Dietz WH. Social and economic consequences of overweight in adolescence and young adulthood. N Engl J Med 1993;329(14):1008-12.
[3] CDC. Prevalence of overweight among children and adolescents: United States, 1999--2002. National Health and Nutrition Examination Survey. Hyattsville, MD: US Department of Health and Human Services, CDC, National Center for Health Statistics, 2007. Available http://www.cdc.gov/nchs/products/pubs/pubd/hestats/overwght99.htm
[4] Fleck LM, Petersmarch KA. Ethical Considerations related to obesity intervention. In: Davies HD, Fitzgerld HE, ed. Obesity in childhood and adolescence: Understanding development and prevention, vol 2. Westport, CT: Praeger, 2008:271-303.
[5] Center for Disease Control and Prevention, University of North Carolina at Chapel Hill School of Public Health. North Carolina Institute for Public Health. Public Health Grand Rounds: The epidemic of obesity: Personal choice or environmental consequence? Available: http://www.publichealthgrandrounds.unc.edu/obesity/webcast.htm.
[6] Fitzgibbon ML, Stolley MR. Environmental changes: May be needed for prevention of overweight in minority children. Pediatric Ann 2004;33(1):45-9.
[7] Center for Disease Control and Prevention. CDC Growth Charts: United States - Body mass index-for-age percentiles: Boys and girls ages 2 to 20 years.3rd, 5th, 10th, 25th, 50th, 75th, 85th, 90th, 95th, 97th percentiles. National Health and Nutrition Examination Survey. Hyattsville, MD: US Department of Health and Human Services, CDC, National Center for Health Statistics, 2000. Available at http://www.cdc.gov/nchs/data/nhanes/growthcharts/set1/chart03.pdf http://www.cdc.gov/nchs/data/nhanes/growthcharts/set1/chart04.pdf
[8] Gordon-Larsen P, Adair LS, Popkin BM. The relationship of ethnicity, socioeconomic factors, and overweight in US adolescents. Obes Res 2003;11(1):121-9.
[9] Pearce MJ, Boergers J, Prinstein MJ. Adolescent obesity, overt and relational peer victimization, and romantic relationships. Obes Res 2002;10(5):386-93.
[10] Erermis S, Cetin N, Tamar M, Bukusoglu N, Akdeniz F, Goksen D. Is obesity a risk factor for psychopathology among adolescents? Pediatr Int 2004;46(3):296-301.
[11] Puhl RM, Latner JD. Stigma, obesity, and the health of the nation's children. Psychol Bull 2007;133(4):557-80.
[12] Griffiths LJ, Wolke D, Page AS, Horwood JP the ALSPAC Study Team. Obesity and bullying: different effects for boys and girls. Arch Dis Child 2006;91:121-5.
[13] Eisenberg ME, Neumark -Sztainer D, Story M. Associations of weight-based teasing and emotional well-being among adolescents. Arch Pediatr Adolesc Med 2003;157(8):733–8.
[14] Neumark-Sztainer D, Story M, Faibisch L. Perceived stigmatization among overweight African-American and Caucasian adolescent girls. J Adolesc Health 1998;23(5):264-70.
[15] Puhl RM, Schwartz MB. Brownell KD. Impact of perceived consensus on stereotypes about obese people: A new approach for reducing bias. Health Psychol 2005;24(5):517-25.

[16] Fulkerson JA, Strauss J, Neumark-Sztainer D, Story M, Boutelle K. Correlates of psychological well-being among overweight adolescents: The role of family. J Consul Clin Psychol 2007;75(1):181-6

[17] Kelly AM, Wall M, Eisenberg ME, Story M, Neumark-Sztainer D. Adolescent girls with high body satisfaction: who are they and what can they teach us? J Adolesc Health 2005;37(5):391-6.

[18] Baskin ML, Ahluwalia HK, Resnicow K. Obesity intervention among African-American children and adolescents. Pediatr Clin North Am 2001;48(4):1027-39.

[19] Robinson TN, Killen D, Litt IF, Hammer LD, Wilson DM, Haydel F, Hayward D, Taylor CB. Ethnicity and body dissatisfaction: Are Hispanic and Asian girls at increased risk for eating disorders. J Adolesc Health 1996;19(16):384-93.

[20] Schooler D,Ward ML, Merriwether A, Caruthers A. Who's that girl: Television's role in the body image development of young white and black women. Psychol Women Q 2004;28(1):38-47.

[21] Kostanski M, Fisher A, Gullone E. Current conceptualization of body image dissatisfaction: have we got it wrong? J Child Psychol Psychiatry 2004; 45(7):1317-25.

[22] Cunningham MR, Roberts AR, Barbee AP, Druen PB, Wu CH. Their ideas of beauty are, on the whole, the same as ours: Consistency and variability in the cross-cultural perception of female physical attractiveness. J Personality Soc Psychol 1995;68:261-79.

[23] Needham BL, Crosnoe R. Overweight status and depressive symptoms during adolescence. J Adolesc Health 2005;36(1):48–55.

[24] Markowitz S, Friedman M A, Arent SM. Understanding the relation between obesity and depression: causal mechanisms and implications for treatment. Clin Psychol Sci Pract 2003;15(1):1-20.

[25] Stice E, Shaw H, Marti CN. A meta-analytic review of obesity prevention programs for children and adolescents: The skinny on interventions that work. Psychol Bull 2006;132(5):667-91.

In: Obesity and Adolescence: A Public Health Concern ISBN: 978-1-60692-821-9
Editors: H.A. Omar, D.E. Greydanus et al.

Chapter XII

Psychological and Social Development

Kimberly K. McClanahan, Marlene B. Huff, and Hatim A. Omar*

Division of Adolescent Medicine, Department of Pediatrics, Kentucky Children's Hospital, University of Kentucky, Lexington, United States of America

Abstract

The global epidemic of childhood and adolescent overweight has become a major public health concern. Not only are these youth more likely to become obese as adults, and thus more prone to obesity-related diseases than their non overweight peers, they are also likely to suffer emotional and social effects associated with overweight. Overweight in youth has been linked to depression, low self-esteem, eating disorders, negative body image, and stigma. It appears to be bi-directional in nature, with overweight sometimes predicting certain psychological effects and psychosocial issues sometimes predicting overweight. Effective assessment and treatment of psychological and mental health issues in overweight youth will help overweight youth deal more effectively with their social and psychological milieus. Additionally, interventions for mental health concerns may have the added health benefit of increasing weight loss, thus decreasing obesity-related disease for which the overweight adolescent is prone.

Introduction

Adolescence is defined most simply by the word 'change'--physical, cognitive, emotional, and social. As physical and cognitive changes occur, so do changes in the domains of emotional/psychological development and social interaction/relationships. Psychological health and social adequacy are important components of mental health, but adolescence

* Correspondence: Hatim Omar, MD, FAAP, Professor of Pediatrics and Obstetrics/Gynecology, Chief, Adolescent Medicine and Young Parent programs, J422, Kentucky Clinic, University of Kentucky, Lexington, KY 40536 United States. Tel: 859-323-6426 ext. 311; Fax: 859-257-7706; E-mail: haomar2@uky.edu

brings with it unique challenges, and interruption of development within any domain may occur. Disruptions in emotional and social development can be influenced by many things, including physical and/or medical problems [1].

Obesity has become one of the most common diseases and disease-associated conditions in the United States (US) and other countries. In the year 2000, it was estimated that obesity would soon surpass tobacco smoking as the leading cause of preventable death in the United States [2] and it has also been suggested that today's young people may, on average, live less healthy and ultimately shorter lives than their parents due to overweight and obesity; in fact, this epidemic may reverse the modern era's steady increase in life expectancy [3,4]. Further, it has been estimated that as this century progresses, more people will die from the complications of overnutrition than of starvation [5]. Pinhas-Hamiel [6] noted that "life-style-related diseases are no longer the exclusive domain of adult medicine." Furthermore, overweight has a bi-directional relationship with mental and psychological health in that psychosocial factors have been shown to predict overweight, but overweight also impacts psychosocial factors such as psychological development and social functioning [7,8].

Overweight in children and adolescents is usually defined as a body mass index (BMI) equal to or greater than the 95th percentile, compared to pediatric population reference data when plotted on the appropriate age and gender chart; children and adolescents with a BMI between the 85th and 95th percentile are considered to be at risk for overweight, according to the Centers for Disease Control and Prevention (CDC); the CDC does not use the term obesity for children and adolescents. Most overweight preadolescent children and at least 70% of overweight adolescents will remain obese into adulthood [9], significantly increasing the chances of obesity-related disease as well as psychological complications associated with overweight [7,8].

Between 1980 and 2002, overweight prevalence tripled in children and adolescents ages 6 to 19 years [10-12]. Comparing results obtained from the 1999-2000 National Health and Nutrition Examination Survey (NHANES) to results from the NHANES survey in 2003-2004, 13.9% vs. 17.1%, respectively, of US children and adolescents were overweight. For female children and adolescents, the percentage overweight increased from 13.8% in 1999-2000 to 16.0% in 2003-2004; for male children and adolescents, the increase went from 14.0% to 18.2% during the same time period [11]. More than 10% of school age children are overweight worldwide with the Americas reporting rates as high as 32% [9]. According to the 2005 Youth Risk Behavior Survey, a national probability sample of 9th – 12th graders which assesses risk behaviors and risk factors [13], approximately 16% of students in the US were at risk for overweight, and 13% were already overweight.

Childhood and adolescent overweight has some endogenous causes, but when those causes are ruled out, then behavioral and psychological factors, rather than biological ones, are primarily responsible for the upward trend in adolescent overweight.14 Behavioral factors such as lack of physical exercise, sedentary behavior, and poor dietary choices have been cited as common risk factors for weight gain, although psychological and mental health factors also factor into the equation [14,15].

Psychosocial Risks for Adolescents

In the realm of psychological and social development, today's youth often face challenges in mental health and wellness as they progress from childhood to adolescence to adulthood. Over the past 20 years, the proportion of pediatric patient visits in general pediatric practices with psychosocial problems has increased from 7% to 19% [16]. According to the 1999 US Surgeon General's report on children's mental health, 13% of children and adolescents have anxiety disorders, 6.2% have mood disorders, 10.3% have disruptive disorders, and 2% have substance use disorders, for a total of 20.9% having one or more mental health or substance abuse disorders [1]. Of those needing active mental health interventions, 11% were found to have significant functional impairment and 5% were found to have extreme functional impairment [1]. Other research has found that 27% of children ages 9, 11, and 13 years of age have mental impairment, and 20% have a diagnosable mental health condition [17]. Further, suicide is the third leading cause of death in the US for children ages 15-24 years and suicide attempts reach a peak during the midadolescent years [1,18,19] highlighting the psychological vulnerability adolescents experience.

Many children and adolescents have both physical and mental disorders, and it has been found that the majority of children and adolescents with medical problems have higher levels of mental disorders [20], suggesting that having a chronic health condition, such as overweight, may increase the likelihood of mental health issues and concerns. In fact, one recent study found serious adverse consequences of overweight on health-related quality of life (HRQOL) in a clinical sample of severely overweight (BMI: 34.7) children and adolescents 5 to 15 years of age [21].

Psycho-Social Risks for Overweight Adolescents

Depression

Several studies have documented a clear correlation between depression and overweight in adolescents [22-24]. Goodman et al [25] have shown in a nationally representative, longitudinal study of over 9,000 adolescents that depressed mood in non overweight individuals is associated with the development of overweight at one year and worsening overweight in baseline overweight participants, suggesting that depression may precede overweight. Other studies using community samples of overweight versus non overweight adolescents have found no differences in depressive symptoms between the two groups [26]. Swallen et al [27] found a statistically significant relationship between BMI and general physical health in adolescents from age 12 to 20 years, but only young adolescents [12-14 years) evidenced a deleterious impact on emotional health as reported by depression and/or low self esteem. Several studies, including a recent one by Daniels [22], failed to confirm a relationship between overweight and symptoms of depression in adolescents. Thus, the relationship between depressive symptoms and overweight in children and adolescents is not completely clear, although depression appears to play a role in the mental health of a certain subpopulation of overweight adolescents.

Self-Esteem

Studies on self-esteem in overweight children and adolescents also report inconsistent results. Some studies have shown moderately lower self-esteem in overweight children and adolescents than their non overweight peers [28, 29], while others have shown no difference between population-based groups of overweight children and their non overweight peers [30,31]. Studies also show that overweight females are at greater risk for self-esteem problems because body image is so important to self-image [28], perhaps because girls are expected to be thin, beautiful, flawless, sexy, cookie-cutter images of the super models and actresses they attempt to emulate. In clinical populations, there is a clear relationship between overweight and self-esteem in children and adolescents, with more heavily overweight children having lower self-esteem [31]. One hypothesis is that clinically referred children represent a subgroup of overweight children associated with especially low self-esteem [15].

Eating Disorders

The age of onset for 85% of all eating disorders is between 11 and 20 years [32] and eating disorders have been found to be associated with overweight in adolescents [33]. Overweight youth are stigmatized [34], predisposing them to unhealthy dieting practices and attempts to lose weight. Britz et al [35] reported that the rate of eating disorders was six times higher in an overweight patient group than a population-based control group. The disorders included bulimia nervosa, eating disorders not otherwise specified, and anorexia nervosa. Sixty percent of females and 35.5% of males reported binge eating episodes.

Body Image

Overweight in adolescents has been associated with negative body image [7]. Overweight children as young as age five can develop a negative body image [36]. A consistently replicated finding is that overweight children and adolescents have a more negative body image than their peers [37]. A 1994 study by Grilo et al [38] demonstrated that "the greater the frequency of being teased about weight and shape while growing up, the more negative one's appearance is regarded, and the greater the degree of body dissatisfaction in adulthood" (p. 448]. Studies have shown that overweight girls appear to have a more negative body image than overweight boys [29].

Stigmatization

Stigmatization of overweight children and adolescents is significant and has long been a part of western culture [39]. Studies have shown that children as young as three years of age begin to have negative attitudes toward overweight and obesity. When given different methods for assessing stigmatizing attitudes, these children ascribe negative characteristics to overweight targets, including mean, ugly, stupid, and sloppy, compared to non overweight targets [40]. These trends tend to worsen as children get older [41]. Such stereotypes are born out in real-life when studies show that US women who were overweight adolescents become adults with lower educational attainment, lower paying jobs, higher rates of poverty, and less likelihood of marriage in comparison to thinner women [42,43]. Stigma associated with overweight thought to be greater for girls than for boys [27].

Overweight impacts adolescents' relationships due to increased vulnerability to weight-related teasing and social isolation. Overweight adolescents may be socially marginalized among their peers and experience more weight-related stigmatization by peers and family members [7,44]. Overweight youth have greater difficulty in gaining admission to college, although there is no indication that they are less apt to be able to complete the course work [39].

Evaluation of Mental Health

Overweight adolescents should be thoroughly evaluated to identify any psychological conditions that may affect the course of medical treatment for weight loss or other medical co-morbidities [15]. However, most pediatric health care providers are not trained to assess mental health issues and may have limited experience in daily practice in addressing mental health related problems. Other factors, including limited visit time and lack of established office strategies [24], may also contribute to the lack of detection of the psychological and psychosocial factors leading to overweight or originating from it. Additionally, pediatricians may directly or indirectly express "fatism," which may contaminate the relationship with their young patients, and is particularly true with younger, overweight patients where parent-bashing or blaming is common [15].

Jonides et al [45] reporting results of a questionnaire to pediatricians asking about the routine evaluation of various psychological and emotional factors including self-esteem, eating disorders, concern about weight, family dynamics and history of abuse, showed that by far not every provider asks and elaborates on all of those important factors. Friedman [46] suggested that pediatricians are in an ideal position to detect psychological issues in young people, and they should be better trained to probe for and recognize signs of major mental illnesses. Weitzman and Leventhal [47] concluded that the pediatric practice setting is an optimal environment for behavioral health screening if the currently available tools are used effectively. However, training is lacking in these areas.

Given that most providers specializing in adolescent overweight are not trained in mental and behavioral health evaluations, having a team of providers, including mental health providers familiar with evaluation of and treatment options for various mental and behavioral health conditions in adolescents, would add significant value to the team caring for this particular patient subset. Evaluation and treatment of underlying psychological and behavioral problems by a health care provider trained in adolescent mental health will aid in the reduction of obesity-related psychological co-morbidity in adolescents.

Suggestions for Mental Health Evaluation

There is no consensus recommendation for the evaluation of mental health in overweight adolescents, and there are no studies comparing different methods for psychiatric assessment of affected children [15]. An expert committee recommendation on overweight evaluation and treatment by Barlow and Dietz [48] suggested that asking the right questions in "objective, non accusatory language" would help establish a basis of trust between family and provider, which is key to long-term, successful management. Additionally, the use of well-validated instruments for evaluation is important.

A thorough psychiatric, psychological and family history regarding the patient needs to be taken. As rapport is established, questions regarding the patient's weight, concerns about weight, weight gain or loss, eating issues, and psychosocial issues associated with being overweight (e.g., friendships, teasing, depression, low self-esteem) need to be broached. It is also important to assess readiness for change. When dealing with an adolescent, the family context is important, and the entire family must have some readiness for change for any to occur.

Paper and pencil assessment instruments can be useful in the initial assessment of psychological variables associated with overweight. As noted earlier, no specific guidelines have been established, but the following instruments are suggested as a potential assessment packet which assesses depressive symptoms, behaviors across a variety of domains, eating issues, and acute and characterological psychological concerns. A summary of the suggested instruments may be seen in table 1.

In order to assess level of depression, the Children's Depression Inventory (CDI), a 27-item, symptom-oriented scale for children ages 6 -17 years [49] may be utilized. The CDI is a highly reliable and valid measure [50] and has been used effectively in several studies with overweight children [51,52]. Since the CDI is a self-report measure, it can be supplemented by a parent-completed Child Behavior Checklist [53] in order to obtain corroborating or conflicting data from parents. Issues regarding eating can be measured through completion of a version of the Eating Attitude Test [54,55]. This is a 6-point, forced choice, self-report inventory that measures dieting behaviors, food preoccupation, anorexia, bulimia, and concerns about being overweight. Versions for teenagers and younger children (chEAT), have demonstrated concurrent and predictive validity as well as reliability [55]. Finally, for overall symptom assessment, younger children [9-12 years) can complete the Millon Pre-adolescent Clinical Inventory (M-PACI), and adolescents [13-19 years) can complete the Millon Adolescent Clinical Inventory (MACI). Both instruments are designed to quickly and accurately identify psychological problems and determine both emerging personality patterns and acute psychological symptoms.

Addressing mental health by correct and timely assessment and intervention can be of significant importance in improving the outcome of obesity-related problems in adolescents. Also, the correct diagnosis and therapy of mental health problems, if associated with overweight, can improve weight management and decrease medical complications.

Table 1. Psychological assessment instruments for overweight adolescents

Instrument	Age Group (yrs)	Measures	Method of report
Children's Depression Inventory (CDI)	6-17	Symptoms of depression	Self-report
Child Behavior Checklist (CBCL)	6-18	Child's activities, social relations, and school performance	Parent report
Children's Eating Attitude Test (chEAT)	7-14	Diet behaviors, food preoccupation, anorexia, bulimia, concerns about overweight	Self-report
Millon Pre-adolescent Clinical Inventory (M-PACI)	9-12	Emerging personality patterns and acute psychological symptoms	Self-report
Millon Adolescent Clinical Inventory (MACI)	13-19	Emerging personality patterns and acute psychological symptoms	Self-report

Conclusions

Overweight, obesity, and obesity-related diseases have become major problems in the developed and developing world in recent years. Adolescents are a high risk group for developing overweight, and most overweight teenagers will be unsuccessful in their attempts, should they make any, to lose weight; they move on to become an overweight or obese adult with the concomitant risk for medical disease. Along with obesity-related disease states, overweight adolescents are also likely to suffer from some psychosocial effects of overweight, such as depression, low self-esteem, eating disorders, negative body image, and stigmatization from peers, thus increasing the probability of obesity-related mental health co-morbidities.

The public health agenda with regard to overweight and obesity has shifted the focus toward primary prevention of overweight. Primary prevention is certainly the strategy for which to strive, but secondary and tertiary prevention are more reasonable strategies at this time since overweight and its potential complications are more prevalent than ever and need to be addressed aggressively and comprehensively.

To improve obesity-related morbidity and mortality in this age group, providers involved in their care need to develop a better understanding and increased focus on mental health in addition to physical health. One strategy is a comprehensive team approach, including a mental health specialist who not only addresses those issues in the patient and family but also teaches the pediatric provider better strategies for initial screening.

References

[1] Surgeon general. Mental health: A report of the surgeon general. Washington, DC: US Dept Health Hum Serv, 1999.

[2] Mokdad AH, Marks JS, Stroup DF, Gerberding JL. Actual causes of death in the United States, 2000. JAMA 2004;291(10):1238-45.

[3] Daniels SR. The consequences of childhood overweight and obesity. Future Child 2006;16(1):47-67.

[4] Olshansky SJ, Passaro DJ, Hershow RC, et al. A potential decline in life expectancy in the United States in the 21st century. New Engl J Med 2005;352:1135-7.

[5] Rossner S. Obesity: The disease of the twenty-first century. Int J Obes 2002;26(Suppl 4):S2-S4.

[6] Pinhas-Hamiel O, Zeitler P. "Who is the wise man?--The one who foresees consequences:". Childhood obesity, new associated comorbidity and prevention. Prev Med 2000;31(6):702-5.

[7] Jelalian E, Wember YM, Bungeroth H, Birmaher V. Practitioner review: Bridging the gap between research and clinical practic inpediatric obesity. J Child Psychol Psychiatry 2007;48(2):115-27.

[8] Hassink S. A clinical guide to pediatric weight management and obesity. Philadelphia, PA: Lippincott Williams Wilkins, 2007.

[9] Reilly JJ. Obesity in childhood and adolescence: evidence based clinical and public health perspectives. Postgrad Med J 2006;82(969):429-37.

[10] Hedley AA, Ogden CL, Johnson CL, Carroll MD, Curtin LR, Flegal KM. Prevalence of overweight and obesity among US children, adolescents, and adults, 1999-2002. JAMA 2004;291(23):2847-50.

[11] Ogden CL, Carroll MD, Curtin LR, McDowell MA, Tabak CJ, Flegal KM. Prevalence of overweight and obesity in the U.S., 1999-2004. JAMA 2006;295(13):1549-55.

[12] Ogden CL, Flegal KM, Carroll MD, Johnson CL. Prevalence and trends in overweight among US children and adolescents, 1999-2000. JAMA 2002;288(14):1728-32.

[13] Danice Eaton DK, Kann L, Kinchen S,Ross J, Hawkins J, et al. Youth risk behavior surveillance--United States, 2005. MMWR 2006;55(SS05):1-108.

[14] Stice E, Presnell K, Shaw H. Psychological and behavioral risk factors for obesity onset in adolescent girls: A prospective study. J Consult Clin Psychol 2005;73(2):195-202.

[15] Zametkin AJ, Zoon CK, Klein HW, Munson S. Psychiatric aspects of child and adolescent obesity: a review of the past 10 years. J Am Acad Child Adolesc Psychiatry 2004;43(2):134-50.

[16] Kelleher KJ, McIrney TK, Gardner WP, Childs GE, Wasserman RC. Increasing identification of psychosocial problems: 1979-1996. Pediatrics 2000;105:1313-21.

[17] Burns BJ, Costello EJ, Angold A, et al. Children's mental health services use across service sectors. Health Affairs 1995;14(3):147-59.

[18] Lubell KM, Kegler SR, Crosby AE, Karch D. Suicide tends among youths and young adults aged 10-24 years, United States, 1990-2004. MMWR 2007;56(35):905-8.

[19] Hoyert DL, kochanek KD, Murphy SL. Deaths: Final data for 1997. Nat Vital Stat Report 1999;47(9).
[20] Spady DW, Schopflocher DP, Svenson Lw, Thompson AH. Medical and psychiatric comorbidity and health care use among children 6 to 17 years old. Arch Pediatr Adolesc Med 2005;159:231-7.
[21] Schwimmer JB, Burwinkle TM, Varni Jw. Health-related quality of life of severely obese children and adolescents. JAMA 2003;289:1813-9.
[22] Daniels J. Weight and weight concerns: are they associated with reported depressive symptoms in adolescents? J Pediatr Health Care 2005;19(1):33-41.
[23] Heo M, Pietrobelli A, Fontaine KR, Sirey JA, Faith MS. Depressive mood and obesity in US adults: comparison and moderation by sex, age, and race. Int J Obes (Lond) 2006;30(3):513-9.
[24] Kabir AA, Whelton PK, Khan MM, Gustat J, Chen W. Association of symptoms of depression and obesity with hypertension: the Bogalusa Heart Study. Am J Hypertens 2006;19(6):639-45.
[25] Goodman E, Whitaker RC. A prospective study of the role of depression in the development and persistence of adolescent obesity. Pediatrics 2002;110(3):497-504.
[26] Wardle J, Williamson S, Johnson F, Edwards C. Depression in adolescent obesity: Cultural moderators of the association between obesity and depressive symptoms. Int J Obes 2006;30:634-43.
[27] Swallen KC, Reither EN, Haas SA, Meier AM. Overweight, obesity, and health-related quality of life among adolescents: the National Longitudinal Study of Adolescent Health. Pediatrics 2005;115(2):340-7.
[28] Pesa JA, Syre TS, Jones E. Psychosocial differences associated with body weight among female adolescents: The importance of body image. J Adolesc Health 2000;26:330-7.
[29] Strauss RS. Childhood obesity and self-esteem. Pediatrics 2000;105:1-5.
[30] Renman C, Engstrom I, Silfverdal SA, Aman J. Mental health and psychosocial characteristics in adolescent obesity: A poulation-based case-control study. Acta Paediatr 1999;88:998-1003.
[31] Rumpel C, Harris TB. The influence of weight on adolescent self-esteem. J Psychosomat Res 1994;38:547-56.
[32] Yager J, Andersen A, Devin M, Mitchell J, Powers P, Yates A. American Psychiatric Association proactice guidelines for eating disorders. Am J Psychiatry 1993;150:207-28.
[33] Neumark-Sztainer D, Story M, French SA, Falkner NH, Beuhring T, Resnick MD. Sociodemographic and personal characteristics of adolescents engaged in weight loss and weight/muscle gain behaviors: Who is doing what? Prev Med 1999;28:40-50.
[34] Pipher M. Reviving Ophelia. New York: Ballantine, 1994.
[35] Britz B, Siegfried W, Ziegler A, et al. Rates of psychiatric disorders in a clinical study group of adolescents with extreme obesity and in obese adolescents ascertained via a population based study. Int J Obes 2000;24:1707-14.
[36] Ebbeling CB, Pawlak DB, Ludwig DS. Childhood obesity: public health crisis, common sense cure. Lancet 2002;360:473-82.

[37] Buddeburg-Fisher b, Klaghofer R, Reed V. Associations between body weight, psychiatric disorders and body image in female adolescents. Psychother Psychosomat Med 1999;68:325-32.
[38] Grilo CM, Wilfley DE, Brownell KD, Rodin J. Teasing, body image, and self-esteem in a clinical sample of obese women. Addict Behav 1994;19:443-50.
[39] Puhl RM, Latner JD. Stigma, obesity, and the health of the nation's children. Psychol Bull 2007;133(4):557-80.
[40] Cramer P, Steinwert T. Thin is good, fat is bad: how early does it begin? J Appl Dev Psychol 1998;19:429-51.
[41] Wardle J, Volz C, Golding C. Social variation in attitudes to obesity in children. Int J Obes 1995;19:562-9.
[42] Dietz WH. Periods of risk in childhood for the development of adult obesity--what do we need to learn? J Nutr 1997;127(Suppl):1884S-6.
[43] Maffies C, Tato L. Long-term effects of childhood obesity on morbidity and mortality. Horm Res 2001;55SS(suppl 1):42-5.
[44] Neumark-Sztainer D, Falkner NH, Story M, Perry C, Hannan PJ, Mulert S. Weight-teasing among adolescents: correlations with weight status and disordered eating behaviors. Int J Obes 2002;26:123-31.
[45] Jonides L, Buschbacher V, Barlow SE. Management of child and adolescent obesity: psychological, emotional, and behavioral assessment. Pediatrics 2002;110(1 Pt 2):215-21.
[46] Friedman RA. Uncovering an epidemic - screening for mental illness in teens. N Engl J Med 2006;355(26):2717-9.
[47] Weitzman CC, Leventhal JM. Screening for behavioral health problems in primary care. Curr Opin Pediatr 2006;18(6):641-8.
[48] Barlow SE, Dietz WH. Obesity evaluation and treatment: Expert committee recommendations. The Maternal and Child Health Bureau, Health Resources and Services Administration and the Department of Health and Human Services. Pediatrics 1998;102(3):E29.
[49] Kovacs M. The Children's Depression Inventory (CDI). Psychopharmacol Bull 1985;21:995-8.
[50] Knight D, Hensley VR, Waters B. Validation of the Children's Depression Scale and the Children's Depression Inventory in a prepubertal sample. J Child Psychol Psychiatry 1988;29:853-63.
[51] Sheslow D, Hassink S, et al. The relationship between self-esteem and depression in obese children. Ann NY Acad Sci 1993;699:289-91.
[52] Wallace WJ, Sheslow D, Hassink S. Obesity in children: A risk for depression. Ann NY Acad Sci 1993;699:301-3.
[53] Achenbach TM, Ruffle TM. Child Behavior Checklist and related forms for assessing behavioral/emotional problems and competencies. Pediatr Rev 2000;21:265-71.
[54] Garner DM, Garfinkle PE. The eating attitudes test: An index of the symptoms of anorexia nervosa. Psychol Med 1979;9:273-9.
[55] Maloney MJ, McGuire JB, Daniels SR. Reliability testing of a children's version of the Eating Attitude Test. J Am Acad Child Adolesc Psychiatry 1988;27:541-3.

In: Obesity and Adolescence: A Public Health Concern
Editors: H.A. Omar, D.E. Greydanus et al.
ISBN: 978-1-60692-821-9

Chapter XIII

Cultural Aspects of Body Satisfaction

Chulanee Thianthai*

Department of Sociology and Anthropology, Faculty of Political Science, Chulalongkorn University, Bangkok, Thailand

This chapter in order to learn how female and male adolescents view their dissatisfaction body parts and to learn how gender-related body dissatisfaction parts of Thai adolescents differ from those studied in Western countries. We studies 400 Thai male and female adolescents in Bangkok, attending high school to freshmen level, and ranging from 16-19 years. Survey questionnaires containing questions related to the research objectives were distributed to every student. We also conducted in-depth follow-up interviews with 40 students to gain insightful data. We found that Thai female and male adolescents viewed their dissatisfaction body parts differently. While Thai female adolescents viewed their dissatisfied body parts individually and looked at their bodies in detail, Thai male adolescents tended to view their bodies as a whole and describe their dissatisfied body parts as problematic area(s). Moreover, some of the results in this study showed similarity with research conducted in the West. However, there were also differences that can be seen in detail that showed a variation on the gender-related dissatisfied body parts names, percentage to each body part/areas, and its beautified meanings. Like studies conducted in the West, female adolescents showed greater dissatisfaction with their bodies and felt more pressure to fix problematic parts than men.

* Correspondence: Assistant professor Chulanee Thianthai, Department of Sociology and Anthropology, Faculty of Political Science, Chulalongkorn University, Patumwan, Bangkok 10330, Thailand. Tel: (662) 218-7292; Fax: (662) 218-7300; E-mail: chulanee00@hotmail.com or chulane.t@chula.ac.th

Introduction

The term body dissatisfaction simply means the unpleasant feelings, attitudes, or actions resulting from negative evaluation of one's own figure or body parts. Currently, body dissatisfaction has received a lot of attention from health scientists. It is related to preoccupation with appearance, emotional distress, and unhealthy risk-taking measures as individuals attempt to alter the shape of unsatisfactory body parts, and undergo unnecessary cosmetic surgery [1,2]. Body dissatisfaction usually is caused by a complex combination of sociocultural, biological, and psychological factors, all of which will affect women and men differently [3-5].

Until recently, most of the studies concerning gender-related body dissatisfaction were conducted in Western societies. Many of these studies revealed that females, more than males, are likely to be dissatisfied with their bodies since females tend to experience more pressure from the sociological factors [6,7]. Generally, women tend to describe themselves as fat, weigh themselves often, diet more frequently than men, and perceive their bodies to be heavier than their actual weight [8]. Studies showed that men, on the other hand, tended to view their bodies positively regardless of their weight and were less obsessive about and dissatisfied with their body [9]. However, a closer review of these studies also showed, men and women have different body structure and patterns of fat distribution [10,11], therefore, they tend to focus on different problematic body parts. Studies in the West reported that women are often dissatisfied with body hair, chin, stomach, hips, thighs, legs, buttocks, and weight [12,13], while men are dissatisfied with their biceps, shoulders, and chest [5,13]. Over all, most Western women usually want to decrease their body size in order to be thin and slim, whereas Western men want to increase their body size to achieve a muscular V-shaped figure [14]. To date, however, few researchers have focused on non-Western populations and how they compare to the studies done in the West [15]. In this chapter information from a population of Thai adolescents will be provided, which can add to our knowledge of body image issues in non-western populations.

A Study from Thailand

Bangkok known as Krung Thep, the city of angles, the capital of Thailand, was selected to be the setting of this study. Since Bangkok is known for having the best educational institutions, which attract students from different regions in Thailand, it enabled the researcher to include students from various socio-economic backgrounds. Through permission from six public high schools and four universities located in central Bangkok, the researcher was able to recruit 500 Thai male and female high school and university freshmen students to voluntarily participate in this study. The researcher was particularly interested in choosing adolescents between 16-19 years of age. This group is defined by the World Health Organization as being in their later years of adolescence. This age group also coincides with Thai cultural definition of adolescence.

First, the researcher visited six public high schools and four universities located in central Bangkok and used convenience and snowball sampling techniques to recruit students.

A number of students were recommended by the teachers to meet with the researcher during break times or after school hours. This group of students then introduced the researcher to their network of friends, which helped the researcher establish a larger number of participants. In total, 500 survey questionnaires were equally distributed among students of each gender in each institution. However, only 400 questionnaires were considered complete.

Each questionnaire contained demographic questions (i.e. sex, age, level of education, etc.) and open-ended questions relating to satisfaction and dissatisfaction toward their body parts, including how they foresee taking measures to fix their problematic body parts. The students usually took from half an hour to an hour filling the questionnaires. One out of 10 students who returned the questionnaire was randomly selected for a follow up in-depth interview. 30 to 40 minutes of in-depth interview focused on talking to students about how they pictured their ideal body parts, the unsatisfying feelings they have towards their body parts, and plans, if any, to achieve their ideal body shape. Each interview was taped and later transcribed. A quantitative analysis was used to determine the percent of the population identifying specific body parts as problematic. The qualitative data based on the in-depth interview helped the researcher gain insights into gender differences in how adolescents viewed and felt toward their problematic body parts. The in-depth interview transcriptions were analyzed based on the content analysis technique—that is to analyze how words and sentences that each gender used in the conversations to describe their problematic body parts were similar or different from each other [18]. Additionally, in the in-depth interview transcripts were also used to reveal adolescents' desired body shape and the pressures to take measures in fixing their problematic body parts.

What did we learn from our study?

This study showed there were clear gender differences in how the Thai adolescents viewed their dissatisfaction with body parts. Like much of the research conducted in Western countries, Thai female adolescents in this study showed greater dissatisfaction with their bodies than males. Only 19 out of 200 female adolescents (~ 20%) said they were happy with the way that they looked or were satisfied with their bodies. The responses among those female who stated that they were dissatisfied with their body parts varied from having dissatisfying feeling toward one or more body parts to feeling pressured into taking measure(s) that would help them achieve their desired body shapes, such as going on a diet, using body slimming cream or body wrap procedures, taking laxatives, to the extreme of saving up money to have surgery when they get older. During the in-depth interviews, female adolescents usually described their dissatisfied body parts by listing each body part and its unwanted characteristics in detail.

Most Thai female adolescents reported that they were dissatisfied with their body parts, namely their noses, face structure, arms, shoulders, stomach, buttocks, waist, hips, legs, thighs, and calves because they were too large in size. In contrast, they wanted to enlarge their eyes and breasts. Moreover, the body parts female adolescents indicated would be more attractive if they were longer were the neck, fingers, and legs. Those female adolescents who reported that they were dissatisfied with their skin complexion often complained that they felt that their skin complexion was too dark and thus unattractive. They desired to have a lighter skin complexion, especially a white and glowing healthy skin color. Those body parts that were mentioned to be disliked because of their unattractive shapes were teeth, nails, belly buttons and noses. A few female adolescents showed interest in pursuing surgeries; particularly to widen their eyes and eye lid shape and to get a nose job when they get older. Overall, Thai female adolescents also felt that if they were able to gain height and lose more weight it would reduce a lot of their dissatisfaction with their body parts.

In contrast, the majority of male adolescents in this study were satisfied with their bodies, while only one in ten felt unsatisfied with their body part(s). These male adolescents did not feel pressure to fix their body dissatisfaction and thus, many choose to do nothing about it. Only three male adolescents in this study reported that they took the initiative in finding measures to achieve their desired body shapes by planning weekly sport activities or an intensive workout schedule. Moreover, the male adolescents often referred to the particular body part that they felt unsatisfied with by identifying them as problematic area(s), such as the upper body and the middle part of the body.

Thai male adolescents reports were more varied than the reports given by the females. The males were either dissatisfied with their body parts because they were too small in size or too large in size. Most male adolescents felt that they were too thin and wanted to increase the size of their upper body by broadening their chest and shoulders or by gaining weight. A few also mentioned that they have an unbalanced and disproportionate body—that is a tall body with small upper body parts. Some reported that they were dissatisfied with their lower body parts because they have non-muscular thighs and skinny chicken legs. They also indicated that they were dissatisfied with the middle part of their, particularly their abdominal area, because it was too large and out of shape. The trend of male in favoring the V-shaped figure, emphasizing large biceps, chest, and shoulders of gaining additional muscular look, is becoming more and more popular among young Thai male adolescents. However, no matter how dissatisfying their feelings were towards their bodies, this group of Thai male adolescents did not show that body-related concerns were serious. This is because they indicated the parts of their body that was problematic could be improved over time, and therefore, they did not feel the need to take drastic measures to reduce their body image-related problems.

Based on the analysis of the survey questions and the content analysis of the in depth interviews the findings from this study indicated Thai female and male adolescents viewed their dissatisfaction with body parts differently. Thai female adolescents viewed their dissatisfied body parts individually and looked at their bodies in detail, while Thai male adolescents tended to view their bodies as a whole and described their dissatisfied body parts in terms of problematic area(s). The data in this study showed how women displayed greater dissatisfaction toward their bodies and in response felt more pressure to take the initiative in fixing their dissatisfying body parts than men did. These findings are similar to those results in previous studies conducted among Western women and men. Furthermore, Thai adolescents of both gender showed a similar trend as in Western studies where the ideal body image favored a thin feminine ideal body and a robust masculine male body image.

After comparing this study with previous studies conducted in Western countries, the researcher found three areas of difference. First, the gender-related dissatisfying body parts

Thai adolescents described varied from those of Western adolescents. For example, Thai adolescents mentioned eye shape, fingers, and neck, whereas Western adolescents were not concerned with these body parts. Second, it is possible to assume that the percentage distribution of different dissatisfied body part would vary from culture to culture. For instance, Thai female adolescents were less concerned with breast size than female adolescents in Western countries and Thai male adolescents are more likely to be more concerned with height than Westerners. Lastly, the Thai definition of ideal beauty appears to be different from the Western definition. For example, an ideal skin complexion in the eyes of Thai female adolescents is fair, whereas, Westerners prefer a darker complexion.

The findings of this study can better explain why the dieting habits of females and males are different and why females have a greater risk of developing eating disorders. Due to the gender differences in body they take different paths to achieve their ideal body shapes. Thus, the understanding of gender-related body dissatisfaction differences is crucial to establishing preventive health interventions.

Since this study was not conducted over the participants' lifetime, as was done in some longitudinal studies, it is hard to detect changes occurred during those periods. The researcher strongly encourages future studies to replicate these findings with a larger representative sample, including a broader population of different age groups and various ethnic backgrounds. Such findings would provide a greater contribution to the study of body image, gender differences, cultural studies, adolescents' health, as well as to the health sciences as a whole.

Acknowledgments

The author wishes to thank the students, teachers, and participating schools, the Thailand Research Fund (TRF) and Commission on Higher Education Grant for making this study possible and for Dr. Geraldine Moreno-Black and Raksaya Aunsnunta for contributing valuable comments. This chapter is based on an earlier published paper Thianthai C. Do male and female adolescents view their dissatisfaction body parts in the same way? Int J Adolesc Med health 2008;20(1):33-9.

References

[1] Hoffman JM, Brownell KD. Sex differences in the relationship of body fat distribution with psychosocial variables. Int J Eating Disord 1997;22:139-45.

[2] Thompson JK, Heinberg LJ, Altabe M et al. Exacting beauty: Theory, assessment, and treatment of body image disturbance. Washington DC: Am Psychol Assoc, 1999.

[3] Mickalide AD. Sociocultural factors influencing weight among males. In: Andersen AE, ed. Males with eating disorders. New York: Brunner/Mazel, 1990:30-40.

[4] Monteath SA, McCabe MP. The influence of societal factors on female body image. J Soc Psychol 1997;137:708-27.

[5] Grogan S. Body image: Understanding body dissatisfaction in men, women and children. New York: Routledge, 1999.

[6] Presnell K, Bearman SK, Stice E. Risk factors for body dissatisfaction in adolescent boys and girls: A prospective study. Int J Eating Disord 2004;36:389-401.

[7] Lokken K, Ferraro FR, Kirchner T et al. Gender differences in body size dissatisfaction among individuals with low, medium, or high levels of body focus. J Gen Psychol 2003;130:305-10.

[8] Furnham A, Badmin N, Sneade I. Body image dissatisfaction: Gender differences in eating attitudes, self-esteem, and reasons for exercise. J Psychol 2000;136:581-96.

[9] Demarest J, Allen R. Body image: Gender, ethnic, and age differences. J Soc Psychol 2000;140:465-72.

[10] Fallon A, Rozin P. Sex differences in perceptions of desirable body shape. J Abn Psychol 1985;94:102-5.

[11] Bjorntorp P. The importance of body fat distribution. In: Brownell, KD, Fairburn CG, eds. Eating disorders and obesity: A comprehensive handbook. New York: Guilford Press, 1995:445-9.

[12] McCabe MP, Ricciardelli LA. Parents, peer, and media influences on body image and strategies to both increase and decrease body size among adolescent boys and girls. Adolescence 2001;36:225-40.

[13] Furnham A, Greaves N. Gender and locus of control correlates of body image dissatisfaction. Eur J Pers 1994;8:183-200.

[14] Furnham A, Badmin N, Sneane I. Body image dissatisfaction: Gender differences in eating attitudes, self-esteem, and reasons for exercise. J Psychol 2002;136:581-96.

[15] Bunnell DW, Cooper PJ, Hertz S et al. Body shape concerns among adolescents. Int J Eating Disord 1992;11:79-83.

In: Obesity and Adolescence: A Public Health Concern
Editors: H.A. Omar, D.E. Greydanus et al.
ISBN: 978-1-60692-821-9

Chapter XIV

Self-Perception of Body Weight

Randy M. Page**, *Ching-Mei Lee and Nae-Fang Miao
Department of Health Science, Brigham Young University, Provo, United States of America, Department of Health Education, National Taiwan Normal University, Taipei, Taiwan and College of Nursing, Taipei Medical University, Taipei, Taiwan

Abstract

This chapter will describe the self-perception of body weight and other weight-related factors among 2,665 Taipei high school students. A high percent of the girls (70.7%) and boys (42.2%) reported that they were too fat and these percentages were much higher than those reported by US students in a recent Youth Risk Behavior Survey. In addition, only 13.2% of girls and 22.0% of boys reported being completely satisfied with their weight and the level of dissatisfaction with weight appeared to be greater than among US students. Yet, in comparison to US students, the Taiwanese students were considerably less likely than their US counterparts to engage in weight management practices (e.g., dieting, eating less food, using diet pills). Taiwanese students with a self-perception of being too fat were more likely than those with perceptions of being just right or too thin to engage in weight management practices, to be dissatisfied with their weight, feel that they were unattractive, estimate that their same-sex peers were trying to loose weight, and have a higher body mass index. The findings from this study showed a relationship between self-perception of body size and engaging in weight control behaviors was consistent with other research. It suggested that self-perception of body weight, more so than objective weight status, was predictive of weight loss behavior and also negative psychological outcomes associated with poor body weight image. As a result, self-perception of weight may be an important point of focus for the design and implementation of clinical and public health initiatives targeted at this adolescent population as well as others.

* Correspondence: Professor Randy M. Page, PhD, Department of Health Science, Brigham Young University, 221 Richards Building, Provo, UT 84602 United States. Tel: 801-422-1131; Fax: 801-422-0273; E-mail: randy_page@byu.edu

Introduction

Overweight and obesity has increased in many areas of the world and is often referred to as a "global epidemic" [1,2]. Taiwan appears to be no exception with studies that indicate a rising prevalence of overweight and obesity among both children and adults [3,4]. Public health reports in Taiwan indicated that for the general population, the availability of a high-fat and high-energy diet has steadily increased over the past few decades [5,6]. This is compounded by the fact that the lifestyle has also become more sedentary and physically inactive [7]. In addition to an increase in overweight/obesity, the occurrence of eating disorders in Asian countries is becoming more common [8,9]. Research in Western nations indicates that eating disorders are especially prevalent during adolescence and early adulthood, yet children as young as nine years are concerned about and dissatisfied with their weight [10]. A study of 10-14 year old Taiwanese girls found that one-third of those classified in the acceptable weight category perceived themselves as overweight and 11% perceived themselves as obese [11]. This study also found that 71% of girls of "acceptable" weight desired to be thinner as well as one-fourth of girls classified as underweight. Overestimations of body weight were also found in studies of female [12] and male [13] Taiwanese college students.

Studies in other Chinese contexts reveal that concern about weight and getting fat is a salient issue for Chinese adolescents and young adults. Results from a study of female junior and senior high school students across mainland China showed a high level of weight-related concern [14]. Wang et al [15] also reported that a considerable proportion of Chinese Singaporean youth are dissatisfied with their body size/shape and have a preference for thinness even among those considered underweight. Only 36% of females and 40% of males were satisfied with their current weight and high proportions also reported that they think they are too heavy, dislike their body shape, worry about their weight, think their stomach is too big, and think about dieting. A study of high school students in Hong Kong, Shenzen, and Hunan showed that female students were very aware of matters pertaining to fat concern and dieting, despite the fact that in general they were far from being overweight [16]. A substantial proportion of female students in Hong Kong (74%), Shenzen (61%), and Hunan (44.3%) desired lower body weight. The gradient of fat concern across these three sites suggests that fat concern and possibly disordered eating may be linked to modernity, westernization, or socioeconomic factors. It is interesting that in one study, an even higher percentage of Hong Kong students than female college students in the United States desired to lose weight [17]. Lee and Lee [16] comment that greeting young women with "you have put on weight" (*fafu*), which used to be regarded as a compliment, may now be considered as an offensive remark in Hong Kong.

The effect of Chinese and East Asian culture on body weight issues is an important concern. Traditionally in Chinese culture, thinness was believed to be not highly prized because of the inherent biological tendency of Chinese people toward leanness. However today, problematic eating attitudes and behaviors pertaining to concern about becoming fat are now commonly found among young females in high-income East Asian societies such as Japan, Singapore, Hong Kong, the Republic of Korea, and Taiwan [18,19]. The increase of eating disorders in non-Western societies after the introduction of Western ideas, fashion and media, supports the belief that culture plays an important role in the development of eating disorders, since their prevalence in Western societies is high. Based on a study of Chinese-born undergraduates in Hong Kong, Lee [20] argued that Chinese females share a similar ideal of slimness as Western females, but dieting and eating disorders remained rare in comparison. However, research by Lake et al. [21] suggests that Western criteria for eating disorders may not take into account cultural differences to help with diagnosis and the low number of reported cases of eating disorders is probably related to inadequate diagnosing tools in Chinese cultural contexts.

The purpose of this chapter is to assess self-perception of body weight among a selected sample of Taipei, Taiwan high school students and other weight-related factors such as weight management practices, weight management goal, weight satisfaction, perception of physical attractiveness, and normative perceptions of schoolmates regarding weight loss. The association between self-perception of body weight and body mass index was examined as was the relationship between self-perception of body weight and the other weight-related factors. Data about self-perception of body weight, weight management goals and practices, and the other variables investigated in this study are important because they give guidance to health professionals designing interventions which focus on helping young people develop/maintain healthy body weight and body weight image. This is particularly true in countries, such as Taiwan, where overweight/obesity is rising rapidly and there appears to also be an increase in eating disorders and concern about weight gain.

How Is Adolescent Self-perception in Taiwan?

We looked at tenth-to-twelfth grade students enrolled in senior high schools and vocational high schools in the Taipei, Taiwan areas (Taipei City and Taipei County) with a population of students in Taipei City at 134,164 students, while the population in Taipei County was 69,204 students. Twenty-one schools were randomly selected as sampling schools (14 schools in Taipei City and seven schools in Taipei County) out of a total of 114 senior and vocational schools in the Taipei area. Within each selected school, one class in each grade (tenth, eleventh, and twelfth grade) was randomly selected to be included in the sample. This yielded a total of 63 classes consisting of 2,820 students. From this number, survey instruments were collected from 2,665 students. Surveys from 155 students were either not obtained due to absence or from failure to participate. The mean age for students participating in the study was 16.72 (SD = 1.06). The range of reported ages ranged from 15 to 21, however 98% were between the ages of 15 and 18. The sample was fairly evenly distributed in tenth (34.9%, n = 912), eleventh (33.0%, n = 864), and twelfth (32.1%, n = 839) grades. The sample included 1564 males and 1026 females. The number of subjects not reporting their gender was 25. These subjects were excluded from the analysis.

The survey instrument for this study included items assessing self-perception of body weight, current height, current weight, weight satisfaction, perceived attractiveness, weight management practices, weight management goal, perceived peer weight management goal norm, normative peer estimation of schoolmates trying to loose weight, and going on a diet. Self-perception of body weight was assessed by asking respondents "How do you rate your body?" Response options included much too thin, a little too thin, just right, a little too fat, or much too fat. Subjects were asked to self-report their present weight and height. Weight satisfaction was assessed by having subjects indicate how they feel about their current weight on a 5-point scale ranging from completely dissatisfied [1] to completely satisfied [5]. Perceived physical attractiveness was assessed in a manner consistent with other research using this construct [14] by using a 9-point rating scale ranging from extremely unattractive [1] to extremely attractive [9]. Weight management goal was assessed by asking "Which of the following statements best describes your feelings about your weight?" and providing the following response options: I am completely satisfied with my weight; I would like to loose between 1 and 5 pounds; I would like to loose between 6 and 10 pounds; I would like to loose more than 10 pounds; and I would like to gain some weight. Perceived peer weight management goal norm was ascertained in a similar fashion by asking "Which one following statements best describes the feelings of most *boys* at your high school?" and "Which one of the following statements best describes the feelings of most *girls* at your high school?" Response options were: most are completely satisfied with their weight; most would like to loose between 1 and 5 pounds; most would like to loose between 6 and 10 pounds; most would like to loose more than 10 pounds; and most would like to gain some weight. Normative peer estimation of trying to lose weight was measured by asking respondents to indicate the percent of male and female students in their high school they say are trying to loose weight. The items to assess weight management practices were identical to the items used in the US Centers for Disease Control and Prevention's Youth Risk Behavior Survey and have widely been used in youth risk behavior surveillance studies [23]. Respondents were asked to identify weight management practices that they engaged in to lose weight or keep from gaining weight in the past 30 days. Weight management practices included: going without eating for 24 hours of more (fasting); eating less food, fewer calories, or foods low in fat; taking any diet pills, powders, or liquids without a doctor's advice; vomiting; taking laxatives; exercise; and going on a diet.

The psychometric properties of the items used in this study were not evaluated in the present study. However, studies confirm that the concept of measuring aspects of adolescent health using self-report is well-established. The Youth Risk Behavior Survey, which provides some of the items in the present study, has a kappa statistic reliability of 61-80% or higher and an alpha reliability of 0.79 [24,25]. Further, the items in this study to measure weight perception, weight satisfaction, and perceived physical attractiveness are similar to those items in other studies investigating these issues in adolescent populations in other Chinese contexts.

Table 1. Self-perception of body weight, weight management practices, weight management goal and perceived weight management goal norms of schoolmates

	Boys % (f) N=1564&	Girls % (f) N=1026&	Chi-Square χ2
Self-perception of body weight			226.38***
Much too thin	8.1% (127)	2.4% (25)	
A little too thin	22.5% (351)	7.9% (81)	
Just right	27.2% (426)	19.0% (195)	
A little too fat	31.5% (492)	55.1% (565)	
Much too fat	10.7% (168)	15.6% (160)	
Weight management practices past 30 days			
Fasting	3.4% (53)	6.3% (64)	11.75**
Eat less	39.2% (612)	63.9% (654)	150.84***
Diet pills	1.1% (17)	5.3% (54)	40.49***
Vomit	1.3% (21)	3.8% (39)	16.60***
Laxatives	0.3% (5)	2.1% (21)	18.63***
Exercise	68.0% (1064)	71.9% (737)	4.38*
Went on a Diet	9.6% (150)	23.0% (236)	87.81***
Weight management goal			294.99***
Completely satisfied	22.0% (344)	13.2% (135)	
Want to loose 1-5	14.2% (222)	19.7% (202)	
Want to loose 6-10	11.5% (179)	23.8% (244)	
Want to loose > 10	23.8% (372)	37.4% (383)	
Want to gain weight	28.5% (445)	5.9% (61)	
Perceived weight management goal norm for boys at your school			16.39**
Completely satisfied	36.7% (573)	44.3% (391)	
Want to loose 1-5	29.2 % (455)	26.9% (238)	
Want to loose 6-10	20.8% (324)	17.6% (156)	
Want to loose > 10	7.3% (113)	5.0% (44)	
Want to gain weight	6.0% (94)	6.2% (55)	
Perceived weight management goal norm for girls at your school			64.22***
Completely satisfied	9.6% (137)	2.7% (28)	
Want to loose 1-5	18.7% (266)	17.2% (176)	
Want to loose 6-10	35.8% (510)	46.3% (474)	
Want to loose > 10	34.6% (493)	33.4% (342)	
Want to gain weight	1.3% (18)	0.4% (4)	

* Boys and girls differed significantly on Chi-square test of difference, *p* < .05*, *p* < . 01**, *p* < .001***.

& Sample sizes vary from item to item because of missing data.

The survey instrument used in this study was translated from English to Chinese by two faculty members representing the Department of Health Education, National Taiwan Normal University. These two faculty members also traveled to schools and administered the surveys in the selected classes. Surveys were passed out to students in class by these faculty members and they instructed students not to place their names on the survey forms, that their participation was voluntary, and to answer the questions honestly and accurately. Students were also informed that if they had any questions or difficulty understanding questions to raise their hands for assistance. This allowed for the faculty members to assist students when questions or difficulties arose. The survey took 10-15 minutes for most students to complete and took about 20 minutes of class time for the administration of the survey. Coding and entry of the data was performed in Taiwan and managed by these faculty members.

Descriptive statistics were used to describe self-perception of body weight and other survey responses. Body mass index (kg/m^2) was calculated from self-reported height and weight [26]. Chi-square and *t*-tests were used to test for differences between boys and girls on each survey response. Self-perception of body weight was the independent variable of primary concern in this study. Analysis of covariance (ANCOVA) was used to test whether self-perception of body weight groups (much too fat, a little too fat, just right, a little too thin, or much too thin) differed in terms of body mass index, weight satisfaction, perceived attractiveness, and normative peer estimation of trying to loose weight. Age was statistically controlled for and least squares means were calculated to determine how groups differed from each other. Chi-square testing was used to test whether self-perception of weight appropriateness groups differed with respect to weight management practices (e.g., fasting, using diet pills, going on a diet, etc.). These ANCOVA and chi-square tests were run separately for boys and girls. Least squares means and percentages were also calculated separately for boys and girls. All analyses were performed using SAS Version 8.02.

Table 1 displays the percentages and frequencies of boys and girls for all of the categorically-scaled variables used in this study. Also included in the table are chi-square results showing that boys and girls differed significantly on the following variables of interest: self-perceptions of body weight; each of the weight management practices (fasting, eating less, using diet pills, vomiting, using laxatives, exercise, and going on a diet); weight management goal; and perception of weight management goal norm for schoolmates (both boys and for girls). Table 2 shows means for the continuously-scaled variables. ANCOVA results showed that boys and girls differed significantly on body mass index, weight satisfaction, perceived attractiveness, and estimation of the percent of female students tying to loose weight. There was no gender difference in the estimation of the percent of male students trying to loose weight.

Table 3 displays the percentages and frequencies of boys and girls in each self-perception of body weight group reporting specific weight management practices. Chi-square results reported in the table show that self-perception of body weight groups for both boys and girls differ significantly in terms of each of the weight management practices (fasting, using diet pills, vomiting, using laxatives, exercising, eating less, and going on a diet) except for vomiting and using laxatives.

Table 2. Means for body mass index (BMI), weight satisfaction, perceived attractiveness and estimation of the percent of same-sex schoolmates trying to loose

	Boys *M* (*SD*) N=1564[&]	**Girls *M (SD)* N=1026**[&]	***t* value**	**Effect Size Cohen's d**
Body mass index (BMI)	21.7 (5.0)	20.4 (3.5)	7.10***	.30
Weight satisfaction	2.8 (1.08)	2.4 (1.0)	8.37***	.38
Perceived attractiveness	5.3 (1.7)	5.1 (1.5)	3.09**	.12
Estimation of the percent of male students in your school trying to loose weight	25.4 (21.82)	25.0 (22.2)	0.45	.01
Estimation of the percent of female students in your school trying to loose weight	45.2 (30.1)	57.5 (26.6)	10.67***	.43

[&] Sample sizes vary from item to item because of missing data.
* Boys and girls differed significantly on *t* test, $p < .05$*, $p < .01$**, $p < .001$***.

Table 3. Weight management practices by self-perception of body weight

	Boys % (*f*) N=1564[&]	**Girls % (*f*) N=1026**[&]	**Chi-Square χ^2** [±]Boys [I]Girls
Fasted to lose weight			[H]41.92*** [I]19.39**
Much too thin	0.8 %(1)	0.0% (0)	
A little too thin	0.6% (2)	1.2% (1)	
Just right	1.9% (8)	3.1% (6)	
A little too fat	5.1% (25)	6.6% (37)	
Much too fat	10.2% (17)	12.6% (20)	
Used diet pills, powders, or liquids to lose weight			[H]12.61* [I]30.04***
Much too thin	0.0% (0)	0.0% (0)	
A little too thin	0.0% (0)	0.0% (0)	
Just right	0.7% (3)	1.0% (2)	
A little too fat	2.0% (10)	5.7% (32)	
Much too fat	2.4% (4)	12.6% (20)	

Table 3. Continued

	Boys % (f) N=1564&	Girls % (f) N=1026&	Chi-Square χ^2 $^{\pm}$Boys ^{I}Girls
Vomited to lose weight			^{H}0.05 ^{I}7.20*
Much too thin	1.6% (2)	0.0% (0)	
A little too thin	1.1% (4)	2.5% (2)	
Just right	1.2% (5)	2.1% (4)	
A little too fat	1.4% (7)	3.9% (22)	
Much too fat	1.8% (3)	6.9% (11)	
Use laxatives to lose weight			^{H}4.75 ^{I}13.35**
Much too thin	0.0% (0)	0.0% (0)	
A little too thin	0.3% (1)	0.0% (0)	
Just right	0.2% (1)	1.6% (3)	
A little too fat	0.2% (1)	1.6% (9)	
Much too fat	1.2% (2)	5.7% (9)	
Exercised to lose weight			^{H}206.18*** ^{I}59.41***
Much too thin	37.0% (47)	32.0% (8)	
A little too thin	52.1% (183)	55.6% (45)	
Just right	62.0% (264)	61.0% (119)	
A little too fat	86.2% (424)	76.2% (430)	
Much too fat	86.9% (146)	84.4% (135)	
Ate less food, fewer calories, or foods low in fat to lose weight			^{H}422.68*** ^{I}182.22***
Much too thin	7.1% (9)	12.0% (3)	
A little too thin	12.5% (44)	22/2% (18)	
Just right	25.9% (110)	41.2% (80)	
A little too fat	66.7% (328)	76.2% (430)	
Much too fat	72.0% (121)	76.9% (123)	
Went on a diet to lose weight			^{H}172.92*** ^{I}66.80***
Much too thin	0.0% (0)	0.0% (0)	
A little too thin	1.1% (4)	4.9% (4)	
Just right	3.1% (13)	8.8% (17)	
A little too fat	16.9% (83)	30.0% (158)	
Much too fat	29.9% (50)	35.6% (57)	

* Self-perception of body weight groups differed significantly on Chi-square test of difference, $p < .05$*, $p < .01$**, $p < .001$***. [&]Sample sizes vary from item to item because of missing data.

Table 4 presents the means and ANCOVA results for body mass index, weight satisfaction, perception of attractiveness, and percent of same-sex peers estimated as trying to loose weight according to self-perception of body weight categories. For both boys and girls, self-perception of body weight groups differed significantly on each of these variables.

Discussion

Body Weight Perceptions and Feelings

More than two-thirds of girls (70.7%) in this sample reported that they were too fat and less than one-fifth (19.0%) rated themselves as just right. Boys were more likely to rate their weight as just right (27.2%) and less likely to report being too fat (42.2%). The perception of being too thin was more common in boys (30.6%) than girls (10.3%). These perceptions differ substantially from those reported by U.S. high school students on 1999 national Youth Risk Behavior Survey (YRBS) which showed a much higher percent of girls (50.5%) and boys (56.5%) reporting that their weight was about right and lower percent reporting their weight as overweight (36.3% of US girls, 23.7% of U.S. boys) [27]. Taiwanese students were also more likely than U.S. students to rate themselves as too thin.

High proportions of Taipei girls expressed desire to loose weight and feeling unsatisfied with their weight. The tendency for a high proportion of girls, including those of normal weight, to perceive themselves to be too fat, to feel dissatisfied with their weight, and desire to lose weight is consistent with other studies of adolescents [11,28]. In fact, most research shows self-perception of weight correlates poorly with actual weight status and that adolescent girls often misperceive themselves as overweight [29]. A study of 10- to 14-year-old girls attending elementary schools in Taichung City, Taiwan found that 65.5% of these young girls desired to be thinner including 8.8% of girls objectively measured as "severely underweight," 25.0% of those measured as "underweight", and 71.0% of those measured as "acceptable weight."

This underscores the potential influences of social norms that equate thinness with attractiveness and social approvals in Taiwan. The fact that a higher proportion of the Taiwanese students than US high school students held the perception that they were too fat was puzzling, given the fact that the Taiwanese boys in our sample have similar BMIs to U.S. boys and that Taiwanse girls have BMIs lower than US girls. The mean BMI among our sample of Taiwanese students was 21.7 for boys and 20.4 for girls. By comparison, the median BMI for US adolescents range from 20.9 to 21.8 for boys and 21.1 to 22.2 for girls aged 15 to 17 [30]. The pursuit of a slim physique appears to have become an important ideal among Taipei high school students and further research is needed to elucidate what might account for the inclination of adolescents of viewing themselves as too fat. Socio-cultural factors including pressures from peers, relatives, media, and other elements of the social environment may affect these adolescents' weight norms. Taiwan, and particularly Taipei, is one of the most economically developed and most modernized areas in Asia. Along with experiencing economic development and modernization, adolescents in Taipei are exposed to pervasive imported Western media, advertising, fashion, and lifestyle. These may account for the sense of body dissatisfaction found among boys and girls in Taipei.

Table 4. Body mass index (BMI), weight satisfaction, perception of attractiveness and estimation of percent of same-sex peers trying to loose weight by self-perception of body weight

	Boys *M (SD)* N=1564	Girls *M (SD)* N=1026	*F* value ^{H}Boys ^{I}Girls	Effect Size ω^2
Body mass index			^{H}153.35*** ^{I}125.91***	^{H}.33 ^{I}.37
Much too thin	18.1^{a}	16.6^{a}		
A little too thin	19.2^{b}	17.5^{a}		
Just right	20.6^{c}	18.6^{b}		
A little too fat	23.0^{d}	20.4^{c}		
Much too fat	28.5^{e}	24.7^{d}		
Weight satisfaction			^{H}221.53*** ^{I}205.27***	^{H}.41 ^{I}.49
Much too thin	1.9^{a}	2.7^{a}		
A little too thin	2.9^{b}	3.3^{b}		
Just right	3.7^{c}	3.5^{c}		
A little too fat	2.4^{d}	2.2^{d}		
Much too fat	1.6^{e}	1.3^{e}		
Perception of attractiveness			^{H}24.21*** ^{I}21.87***	^{H}.07 ^{I}.09
Much too thin	5.1^{a}	5.3^{a}		
A little too thin	5.6^{b}	5.5^{a}		
Just right	5.7^{b}	5.5^{a}		
A little too fat	5.2^{a}	5.2^{a}		
Much too fat	4.1^{c}	4.1^{b}		
Percent of same-sex peers estimated as trying to loose weight			^{H}11.76*** ^{I}9.36***	^{H}.02 ^{I}.09
Much too thin	21.1^{a}	56.7^{a,b,c}		
A little too thin	21.7^{a}	49.0^{a}		
Just right	22.3^{a}	48.7^{a}		
A little too fat	29.1^{b}	59.6^{b}		
Much too fat	32.4^{b}	65.0^{c}		

Note. Means in the same column for each variable with the same superscript letter are not significantly different.

* Self-perception of body weight groups differed significantly on ANCOVA test controlling for age, $p < .05$*, $p < .01$**, $p < .001$***.

Xie et al [28], point out that having a filled-out physique has traditionally been an important symbol of family wealth and fertility in Chinese culture and this belief may still predominate in rural and less economically developed areas. However, this belief is being replaced by a preference for a slim body physique in urban areas and among adolescents and youth, in particular girls.

Weight-Management Practices

Consistent with feeling dissatisfied with weight and the perception of being too fat, Taipei girls were more likely than boys to engage in most of the weight management practices investigated in this study. Girls were much more likely than boys to fast, eat less, use diet pills, vomit, use laxatives, and go on a diet to lose weight. Compared to US high school students taking the 1999 YRBS survey, lower percentages of Taipei boys and girls reported fasting, eating less, using diet pills, vomiting or using laxatives, and going on a diet to lose weight. It is interesting that while this study found that students in Taipei were more dissatisfied with their weight and more likely to perceive themselves as fat than U.S. students, they were, at the same time, much less likely to engage in the weight management practices assessed in this study. Because behaviors such as dieting, fasting, using diet pills, vomiting, and using laxatives to lose or maintain weight are lower, it appears that the level of eating disorders seen in the US has not yet emerged into this population of adolescents. However, the high level of body weight dissatisfaction, desire for thinness, and distorted sense of body weight among Taipei students may be a warning sign that disordered eating may be on the rise

Relationship between Self-Perception of Body Weight and Weight-Related Variables

It is not surprising that students with a self-perception of being too fat were more likely than those with perceptions of being just right or too thin to engage in the following weight management practices to lose weight: fasting; using diet pills, powders, or liquids; vomiting; using laxatives; exercising; eating less food, fewer calories, or foods low in fat; and going on a diet. Serious long-term adverse health consequences may result from unhealthy weight loss behaviors among youth (e.g., dieting, using diet pills, vomiting or using laxatives). Nutritional self-deprivation by recurrent weight fluctuations in children and adolescents may increase the likelihood of weight gain and obesity in adulthood. In addition, unhealthy weight loss behaviors may be associated with nutritional deficiencies, decreases in growth, and delays of pubertal and psychosocial development [31].

Self-perception of body weight was also related to body mass index, weight satisfaction, perception of attractiveness, and estimation of the percent of same-sex peers trying to loose weight. In general, as students with a perception of being too fat had higher BMI, lowered weight satisfaction and perception of physical attractiveness, and lower estimations of the percent of same-sex peers trying to loose weight.

Perception of Body Weight as a Point of Focus

Previous research has identified that self-perception of body weight often differs from both public health and normative cultural standards of weight appropriateness [32]. Furthermore, self-perception of body weight, also termed as self-perceived weight status, is often not predictive of actual body size. Our findings showing a relationship between self-perception of body size and engaging in weight control behaviors is consistent with other studies finding this same relationship, often independently of objective weight status [29,33]. In other words, it is the perception of being too fat that appears to drive attempts at weight loss, more so than one's objective weight status. Furthermore, research among Chinese [28] and US [34,35] adolescents make it clear that it is weight-related body image concern and perception of body weight, not objective BMI or actual weight categories that significantly predicts such adverse effects as anxiety symptoms, depressive symptoms, and perceived peer isolation. These results suggest that body image or weight perception may have a mediating effect on the relationship between actual body weight and depressive psychological symptoms. Therefore, Xie et al [28] suggest that because weight-related body image transcends actual body weight as a predictor of detrimental psychological effects, that body image or weight perception plays a more important role than body fat itself in predicting negative psychological outcomes associated with weight. Given the important role of perception of body weight as a predictor of weight loss behavior and adverse psychological effects, Chang and Christakis [32] point out that self-perception of weight may an important point of focus for the design and implementation of clinical and public health initiatives.

Further research is needed to determine why such a high percent of the students in Taipei had the perception that their weight was too fat and there was so much dissatisfaction with weight, particularly in light of the fact that they do not appear to be heavier than other adolescent populations (e.g., US high school students). There is concern that distorted weight perception, may potentially influence adolescents to adopt unhealthy weight control strategies such as unhealthy eating habits and cigarette smoking to regulate their weight [28]. There is also concern that distorted weight perception can lead to negative psychological outcomes. Health professionals in Taiwan and elsewhere need to help adolescents establish health-based standards for normative weight perceptions. However, to be able to effectively do this, more research is needed to understand how to target the socio-cultural factors that may positively influence weight perceptions norms [28].

There are several important issues and limitations of this study that need mentioning. It is highly likely that the constructs investigated in this study such as self-perception of weight, weight satisfaction, and weight management practices manifest very different meanings across Chinese culture and Western culture. For example, the perception of being too fat may represent very different cultural meanings for an adolescent in Taiwan than for an adolescent in the U.S. or another Western nation. Qualitative research methods might be applied to better understand the cultural contexts of these constructs among Taiwanese and other Chinese adolescent populations.

This study is limited by the fact that the psychometric properties of survey items were not evaluated. It is recommended that future research involve assessing the stability of these items (e.g., test-retest reliability) over a two or three week time period.

Another limitation is the lack of ability to test how well the sample reflects the population. The fact that schools were randomly selected and classes selected for inclusion were stratified by grade level increases the likelihood of similarity. The addition of additional demographic variables to the survey instrument (e.g., indicators of socioeconomic status) would increase the ability to match sample characteristics with population characteristics. This would increase the generalizability of this study's findings and also would have allowed us to determine the relationship between weight-related variables and socioeconomic status.

Given the cross-sectional nature of this study and the challenge of gaining insight into such complex human behaviors related weight-related concerns and behavior, readers need to exercise caution in interpreting the results. In looking at the relationships between self-perception of body weight, body mass index, and other weight-related factors, it is important not to assign directionality or casuality to these relationships.

Acknowledgments

This chapter is based on an earlier published paper: Page RM, Lee C, Miao N. Self-perception of body weight among high school students in Taipei, Taiwan, Int J Adolesc Med Health 2005;17(2):123-36.

References

[1] Caballero B, Popkin BM. The Nutrition Transition: Diet and Disease in the Developing World. London: Academic Press, 2002.

[2] Ebbeling CB, Pawlak DB, Ludwig DS. Childhood obesity: Public health crisis, common sense cure. Lancet 2002;360:473-82.

[3] Ding YA, CHu NF, Wang TW, Lin CC. Anthropometry and lipoproteins-related characteristics of young adult males in Taiwan. Int J Obes Relat Metab Disord 1995;1:392-96.

[4] Chu NF. Prevalence and trends of obesity among school children in Taiwan—the Taiepi Children Heart Study. Int J Obes 2001;25(2):170-6.

[5] Department of Health, The Executive Yuan, ROC. The National Nutritional Guide Book. Taipei, Taiwan: Taiwan Government, 1991:2.

[6] Department of Health, The Executive Yuan, ROC. Public Health in Taiwan Area, Republic of China. Taipei, Taiwan: Taiwan Government, 1995.

[7] Hope P, Big in Taiwan. BBC News. 2000. Available from http://news.bbc.co.uk/1/hi/programmes/crossing_continents/892840.stm

[8] Nogami Y. Eating disorders in Japan: A review of the literature. Psychol Med 1997;51(6):339-46.

[9] Lee AM, Lee S. Disordered eating and its psychosocial correlates among Chinese adolescents in Hong Kong. Int J Eat Disord 1996;20:177-83.

[10] Hill AJ, Oliver S, Rogers PJ. Eating in the adult world: The rise of dieting in childhood and adolescents. Br J Clin Psychol 1992;31:95-105.

[11] Bennink MR, Wang MF, Yamamoto S, Wong Y. Overconcern about thinness in 10- to 14-year-old schoolgirls in Taiwan. J Am Diet Assoc 2000;100(2):234-7.
[12] Wong Y, Huang YC. Obesity concerns, weight satisfaction and characteristics of female dieters: A study on female Taiwanese college students. J Am Coll Nutr 1999;18(2):194-200.
[13] Wong Y, Chen SL, Chan YC, Wang MF, Yamamoto S. Weight satisfaction and dieting practices among college males in Taiwan. J Am Coll Nutr 1999;18(3):223-8.
[14] Huon GF, Mingyi Q, Oliver K, Xiao G. A large scale survey of eating disorder symptamology among female adolescents in the People's Republic of China. Int J Eat Disord 2002;32:192-205.
[15] Wang MC, Ho TF, Anderson JN, Sabry ZI. Preference for thinness in Singapore, a newly industrialized society. Singapore Med J 1999;40:504-9.
[16] Lee S, Lee AM. Disordered eating in three communities of China: A comparative study of female high school students in Hong Kong, Shenzen, and rural Hunan. Int J Eat Disord 2000;27:317-27.
[17] Heatherton TF, Nichols P, Mahamedi AM, Keel P. Body weight dieting, and eating disorder symptoms among college students, 1982 to 1992. Am J Psychiatry 1995;152:1623-9.
[18] Lee S. Reconsidering the status of anorexia nervosa as a Western culture-bound syndrome. Soc Sci Med 1996;42:21-34.
[19] Koh IP, Tian CS. Susceptbility of Singapore Chinese schoolgirls to anorexia nervosa: Part I (psychological factors). Singapore Med J 1994;35:481-5.
[20] Lee S. How abnormal is the desire for slimness? A survey of eating attitudes and behaviour among Chinese undergraduates in Hong Kong. Psychol Med 1993;23:437-51.
[21] Lake AJ, Staiger PK, Glowinski H. Effect of Western culture on women's attitudes to eating and perceptions of body shape. Int J Eat Disord 2000;27:83-9.
[22] Fiengold A. Good-looking people are not what we think. Psych Bull 1992;111:304-11.
[23] Grunbaum JA, Kann L, Kinchen SA, Williams B, Ross JG, Lowry R, Kolbe L. Youth Risk Behavior Surveillance-2001. MMWR 2002:51(SS04):1-64.
[24] Kann L, Kinchen SA, Williams BI, Ross BG, Lowry R, Grunbaum J, Kolbe LJ. Youth risk behavior surveillance-United States. MMWR;49(xx-5):1-95.
[25] Kolbe LJ, Kann L, Collins J. Overview of the youth risk behavior surveillance system. Public Health Rep 1993;108:2-10.
[26] Barlow SE, Dietz WH. Obesity evaluation and treatment: Expert Committee Recommendations. Pediatrics 1998;102(3):E29. (Electronic article).
[27] Lowry R, Galuska DA, Fulton JE, Wechsler H, Kann L. Weight management goals and practices among U.S. high school students: Associations with physical activity, diet, and smoking. J Adolesc Health 2002:31(2):133-4.
[28] Xie B, Liu C, Chou C-P, Xia J, Spruijt-Metz D, Gong J, Li Y, Wang H, Johnson CA. Weight perception and psychological factors in Chinese adolescents. J Adolesc Health 2003:33(3):202-10.
[29] Strauss RS. Self-reported weight status and dieting in a cross-sectional sample of young adolescents. Arch Pediatr Adolesc Med 1999;153:741-7.

[30] Flegal KM, Troiano RP. Changes in the distribution of body mass index of adults and children in the U.S. population. Int J Obes Relat Metab Disord 2000:24(7):807-18.

[31] Centers for Disease Control and Prevention. Body-weight perceptions and selected weight-management goals and practices of high school students-United States, 1990. MMWR 1991;40(43):741,747-50.

[32] Chang VW, Christakis NA. Self-perception of weight appropriateness in the United States. Am J Prev Med 2003;24(4):332-9.

[33] Serdula, MK, Collins ME, Williamson DF, Anda RF, Pamuk E, Byers TE. Weight control practices of U.S. adolescents and adults. Ann Intern Med 1993:82:1251-7.

[34] Kaplan SL, Busner J, Pollack S. Perceived weight, actual weight, and depressive symptoms in a general adolescent sample. Int J Eat Disord 1988;7:107-13.

[35] Rierdan J, Koff E. Weight, weight-related aspects of body image, and depression in early adolescent girls. Adolescence 1997;32:615-24.

In: Obesity and Adolescence: A Public Health Concern
Editors: H.A. Omar, D.E. Greydanus et al.
ISBN: 978-1-60692-821-9

Chapter XV

Overweight Misperception

Kathleen S. Talamayan, Andrew E. Springer*, Steven H. Kelder, Emmanuel C. Gorospe and Karen A. Joye

Centers for Health Promotion and Prevention Research, School of Public Health, University of Texas Health Science Center at Houston, Houston, Texas and School of Public Health, University of Nevada Las Vegas, USA

Abstract

Weight perceptions and weight control behaviors have been documented with underweight and overweight adolescents, yet limited information is available on normal weight adolescents. This chapter investigates the prevalence of overweight misperceptions and weight control behaviors among normal weight adolescents in the United States by sociodemographic and geographic characteristics. We examined data from the 2003 Youth Risk Behavior Survey (YRBS). A total of 9,714 normal weight US high school students were included in this study. Outcome measures included self-reported height and weight measurements, overweight misperceptions, and weight control behaviors. Weighted prevalence estimates and odds ratios were computed. There were 16.2% of normal weight students who perceived themselves as overweight. Females (25.3%) were more likely to perceive themselves as overweight than males (6.7%) ($p < .05$). Misperceptions of overweight were highest among white (18.3%) and Hispanic students (15.2%) and lowest among black students (5.8%). Females (16.8%) outnumbered males (6.8%) in practicing at least one unhealthy weight control behavior (use of diet pills, laxatives, and fasting) in the past 30 days. The percentage of students who practiced at least one weight control behavior was similar by ethnicity. There were no significant differences in overweight misperception and weight control behaviors by grade level, geographic region or metropolitan status. A significant portion of normal weight adolescents misperceive themselves as overweight and are engaging in unhealthy

* Correspondence: Assistant professor Andrew Springer, DrPH, Michael and Susan Dell Center for Advancement of Healthy Living, University of Texas School of Public Health- Austin Regional Campus, 313 E. 12th Street, Suite 220, Austin, Texas 78701 United States. E-mail: andrew.e.springer@uth.tmc.edu

weight control behaviors. These data suggest that obesity prevention programs should address weight misperceptions and the harmful effects of unhealthy weight control methods even among normal weight adolescents.

Introduction

The preference for thinness in the mass media has a strong influence in shaping adolescents' concept of ideal body weight [1,2]. As adolescents have been found to be extremely self-conscious of their bodies [3], social pressures from the mass media may cause even normal weight adolescents to misperceive themselves as overweight. In the US National Health and Nutrition Examination Survey (NHANES III), 42% of adolescents who considered themselves as overweight were actually of normal weight [4]. Based on studies [5,6] reporting the prevalence of unhealthy weight control practices among overweight adolescents, there is potential for normal weight adolescents who misperceive themselves as overweight to also engage in unhealthy weight control behaviors.

Unhealthy weight control behaviors such as fasting, purging, and use of diet pills may adversely affect adolescents' physical and psychosocial development. Unhealthy outcomes include the development of eating disorders [7,8], stress [9], other mental health problems and impairment of cognitive abilities [10,11]. Despite the potential risks associated with unhealthy weight control behaviors, few studies have specifically examined this issue among normal weight adolescents.

This chapter reports the prevalence of overweight misperceptions and weight control behaviors among normal weight adolescents from the 2003 Youth Risk Behavior Survey (YRBS), a nationally representative survey of US high school students. In addition to examining the prevalence of overweight misperceptions and weight control practices by several sociodemographic and geographic characteristics, this paper explores the association between overweight misperception and unhealthy weight control behaviors.

We conducted a secondary analysis of the cross-sectional data from the 2003 Youth Risk Behavior Study (YRBS), a comprehensive school-based adolescent health survey that has been administered biennially in the United States since 1991 by the Centers for Disease Control and Prevention (CDC) with the aim of monitoring priority health risk behaviors among youth. The YRBS is based on a three-stage cluster sample design to produce a nationally representative sample of high school students in grades 9 through 12. Participants completed a self-administered questionnaire that included items on various youth risk behaviors. Participation in the survey was anonymous and voluntary, and local parental permission procedures were followed. The specific sampling design and methods for the YRBS are described in greater detail elsewhere [12].

What did we find?

There were 15,214 respondents from 158 public and private high schools, who participated in the study. The student and school response rate were 83% and 81%, respectively. For the purposes of the present analysis, we selected the 9,714 normal weight students. Normal weight status was based on the CDC Body Mass Index (BMI) percentile categories for age and sex [13]. A weighting factor was applied to each student record to adjust for non-response and for the varying probabilities of selection in order to ensure that the data equaled the total sample size and matched national population proportions.

Body mass index (BMI) was based on self-reported height and weight measurements and was obtained by asking "How tall are you without your shoes on?" in feet, and "How much do you weigh without your shoes on?" in pounds. These values were converted to the metric system to derive the BMI (kilograms/meters^2). Participants were then categorized as underweight, normal, at risk for overweight and overweight. Values were based on the BMI-for-age and sex for pediatric population as per the CDC classifications with normal weight, defined as a BMI between the 5th and <85th percentile.

Weight perception was assessed with the question, "How do you describe your weight?" Adolescents with normal BMI who responded "overweight" and "very overweight" were classified as those with misperception of overweight status. Information on different weight control behaviors was also collected. Trying to lose weight was determined by asking, "Which of the following are you trying to do about your weight?" with responses that included "lose weight" and "gain weight". Exercise was assessed with the question, "During the past 30 days, did you exercise to lose weight or to keep from gaining weight?" Dieting was measured by asking, "During the past 30 days, did you eat less food, fewer calories, or foods low in fat to lose weight or to keep from gaining weight?" Unhealthy weight control behaviors which include fasting, taking diet medicines, and purging were determined with the following questions respectively, "During the past 30 days, did you go without eating for 24 hours or more (also called fasting) to lose weight or to keep from gaining weight?", "During the past 30 days, did you take any diet pills, powders, or liquids without a doctor's advice to lose weight or to keep from gaining weight?", "During the past 30 days, did you vomit or take laxatives to lose weight or to keep from gaining weight?" Fasting was defined as no food intake for more than 24 hours and purging was defined as either vomiting or taking laxatives to lose weight. Having at least one unhealthy weight loss behavior was described as reporting yes to any of the three weight control behaviors. The overweight misperception and weight control behavior variables were all dichotomized with a 'yes' or 'no' response. All outcomes were based on the YRBS questionnaire.

We examined the prevalence and distribution of overweight misperception and weight control behaviors by gender, grade level, race/ethnicity, geographic region, and metropolitan status. For this study, race/ethnicity comprised the following groups: white, black, Hispanics and a combined category of 'other' for those races/ethnicities with small sample size. This variable was based on response to the question "How do you describe yourself?" Geographic region (Northeast, Midwest, South, or West) and metropolitan status ("urban", "suburban", and "rural") were based on the location of the school attended by the student.

Analysis was performed using STATA® version 9.0 statistical program that takes into account the complex sampling design of the YRBS. In describing the prevalence and distribution among the sample, we computed the weighted point prevalence estimates and standard errors of the overweight misperception and weight control behaviors for the sample as a whole and by the various sociodemographic variables described above. Logistic regression was performed to determine the bivariate associations between the principal study variables of interest: overweight misperception and weight control behaviors, with the sociodemographic and geographic variables. In assessing the association between overweight misperception and the weight control behaviors, we used logistic regression to compute the odds ratios while adjusting for gender and race/ethnicity. Differences between prevalence estimates were considered statistically significant at p-value<.05.

In the 2003 YRBS sample, 71.0% of participants were classified as having normal body weight (BMI-for-age: 5th to <85th percentile). Based on this normal weight classification, 9,714 students were included in this study. The sample was equally distributed across gender and grade level and was largely represented by white students (64.3%) and students residing in the suburban area (see table 1).

Of the normal weight respondents, 16.2% misperceived themselves as overweight (seee table 2). Moreover, 35.8% of the students indicated trying to lose weight, including those that did not perceive themselves to be overweight. 11.8% of normal weight students indicated at least one unhealthy weight control behavior. Among the unhealthy weight control behaviors, fasting was the most commonly practiced (11.6%), followed by taking diet medicine (7.4%) and purging (5.2%).

Normal weight adolescents who misperceived themselves as overweight varied by gender and race (see table 2). Females (25.3%) were more likely to misperceive themselves as overweight than males (6.7%). There were more white (18.3%) and Hispanic (15.2%) students who misperceived themselves as overweight compared to black students (5.8%).

The misperception of being overweight tends to increase from the 9th to the 12th grade (see table 2). The number of those trying to lose weight was greater among the higher grade levels. Parallel to this trend was the higher number of 11th and 12th grade students practicing at least one unhealthy weight control behavior compared to the 9th and 10th grade students. This pattern is best seen in the increasing proportion of students who reported taking dieting pills from 9th to 12th grade.

Females persistently outnumbered males in practicing weight control behaviors (see table 2). Females were approximately three times as likely to exercise (OR=2.6, 95% CI: 2.3-2.9) and five times as likely to diet (OR=4.8, 95% CI: 4.0-5.7) than males (data not shown in tables). Unhealthy weight control behaviors (fasting, taking diet medicines and purging) were also more common in females than in males (see table 2). For example, females were approximately three times as likely to report at least one weight control behavior compared to males (OR= 2.8, 95% CI: 2.1-3.7; data not shown in tables).

Table 1. Descriptive characteristics of normal weight[a] U.S. high school students by sociodemographic and geographic characteristics, YRBS 2003

		n	%
Total	Normal Weight	9714	100%
Gender	Males	4716	48.5
	Females	4998	51.5
Grade level	9th	2713	28.0
	10th	2578	26.6
	11th	2268	23.4
	12th	2135	22.0
Race/ethnicity	Blacks	1211	12.5
	Hispanics	1261	13.0
	Whites	6242	64.3
	Others[b]	999	10.3
Geographic region	Northeast	2206	22.7
	Midwest	2535	26.1
	South	3310	34.1
	West	1663	17.1
Metropolitan status	Urban	2492	25.7
	Suburban	5058	52.1
	Rural	2163	22.3

[a] Normal weight based on a Body Mass Index (BMI)-for-age of 5th to <85th percentile.

[b] "Others" include American Indian or Alaskan Native, Asian, Native Hawaiian or Other Pacific Islander, Multiple Hispanic, Multiple non-Hispanic.

White and Hispanic students were twice as likely to engage in physical activity (OR=1.8, 95% CI: 1.4-2.4 and OR= 2.0, 95% CI 1.6-2.6, respectively) and diet (OR= 2.2, 95% CI: 1.7-2.8 and OR 2.5, 95% CI: 2.1-3.0, respectively) as compared to black students (data not shown in tables). These same ethnic groups were also approximately thrice as likely to attempt losing weight (OR= 2.7, 95% CI 2.2-3.3 and OR= 2.5, 95% CI: 2.1-3.0, respectively) and to take diet pills (OR= 2.9, 95% CI: 1.9-4.4 and OR= 3.2, 95% CI: 1.9-5.5, respectively) than black students (data not shown in tables). There was no significant difference in the prevalence of having at least one unhealthy weight control behavior among the ethnic groups.

In addition, there were no significant differences observed in overweight misperception and weight control behaviors by grade level, geographic region or metropolitan status.

The associations between overweight misperception and the different weight control behaviors were determined while controlling for gender and race/ethnicity (see table 3). Among the normal weight students, those who perceived themselves as overweight were three times as likely to engage in each of the unhealthy weight control behaviors examined as those who did not perceive themselves as overweight.

Table 2. Prevalence of overweight misperception and weight control behaviors by sociodemographic and geographic characteristics, YRBS 2003

Characteristic	Perceived themselves as overweight % (CI)	Were trying to lose weight %(CI)	Exercised to lose weight or keep from gaining weight % (CI)	Ate less food, fewer calories, or foods low in fat to lose weight or to keep from gaining weight % (CI)	Went without eating for ≥24 hours to lose weight or to keep from gaining weight % (CI)	Took diet medicines to lose weight or to keep from gaining weight % (CI)	Vomited or took laxatives to lose weight or to keep from gaining weight % (CI)	At least 1 Unhealthy Weight Control Behavior % (CI)
Total	16.2 (±1.5)	35.8 (±2.3)	54.6 (±3.0)	36.8 (±2.0)	11.6 (±1.3)	7.4 (±1.5)	5.2 (±1.3)	11.8 (±2.5)
Gender								
Males	6.7 (±1.0)	15.5 (±2.1)	42.7 (±2.8)	19.2 (±2.3)	6.3 (±1.2)	4.6 (±1.7)	2.6 (±1.1)	6.8 (±1.6)
Females	25.3 (±3.0)	54.8 (±4.0)	65.8 (±3.8)	53.4 (±2.9)	16.6 (±2.0)	10.0 (±1.7)	7.6 (±1.9)	16.8 (±1.9)
Grade level								
9th	15.3 (±3.0)	33.5 (±3.1)	55.6 (±4.2)	34.5 (±2.7)	12.4 (±2.4)	6.6 (±2.3)	4.8 (±1.9)	11.8 (±2.5)
10th	15.7 (±2.1)	36.2 (±3.6)	56.1 (±4.8)	37.7 (±4.5)	12.1 (±2.0)	6.2 (±1.8)	6.2 (±2.0)	10.9 (±1.9)
11th	15.8 (±2.0)	36.0 (±2.9)	53.4 (±3.9)	36.4 (±2.8)	12.3 (±2.3)	7.9 (±2.3)	5.1 (±1.4)	12.0 (±2.0)
12th	18.7 (±2.1)	38.0 (±3.1)	53.0 (±4.5)	39.2 (±3.3)	9.1 (±2.0)	9.2 (±1.6)	4.7 (±1.2)	12.8 (±2.4)
Race								
Blacks	5.8 (±1.1)	19.7 (±2.2)	39.6 (±3.6)	20.9 (±2.5)	9.7 (±1.6)	2.8 (±1.3)	3.6 (±1.3)	10.2 (±1.5)
Hispanics	15.2 (±3.8)	39.6 (±4.2)	54.7 (±4.7)	36.8 (±4.0)	12.5 (±2.2)	7.6 (±3.8)	5.8 (±2.8)	13.6 (±3.0)
Whites	18.3 (±2.0)	37.9 (±3.1)	57.1 (±4.0)	39.8 (±2.6)	11.3 (±1.7)	8.4 (±2.0)	5.2 (±1.6)	11.4 (±1.5)
Others[a]	17.3 (±4.0)	37.1 (±6.0)	57.1 (±7.3)	37.7 (±4.5)	14.5 (±3.3)	6.1 (±2.5)	6.5 (±2.8)	13.8 (±3.4)
Geographic region								
Northeast	16.9 (±1.2)	35.5 (±5.0)	51.7 (±8.8)	38.0 (±2.2)	12.0 (±2.9)	8.9 (±5.0)	7.3 (±4.0)	12.0 (±4.2)
Midwest	17.8 (±4.4)	40.1 (±3.8)	59.4 (±2.8)	42.0 (±4.2)	12.5 (±1.3)	6.9 (±1.6)	4.6 (±1.2)	12.8 (±1.9)
South	14.1 (±1.3)	32.2 (±3.2)	51.3 (±2.9)	31.1 (±2.2)	11.0 (±1.7)	6.2 (±1.4)	4.3 (±1.1)	10.9 (±1.6)
West	17.4 (±3.3)	36.6 (±5.8)	57.8 (±5.8)	39.1 (±4.2)	11.0 (±3.7)	8.6 (±5.0)	5.3 (±4.3)	11.8 (±2.6)
Metropolitan status								
Urban	14.9 (±3.5)	31.5 (±5.0)	50.7 (±5.6)	32.0 (±3.4)	10.7 (±2.2)	6.7 (±3.1)	5.8 (±2.8)	9.7 (±1.9)
Suburban	16.7 (±1.3)	37.6 (±1.9)	57.1 (±2.3)	37.6 (±2.3)	12.1 (±1.8)	6.8 (±1.3)	4.5 (±1.5)	12.4 (±1.6)
Rural	16.8 (±2.5)	36.4 (±7.9)	53.3(±11.1)	40.8 (±3.7)	11.6 (±2.4)	9.6 (±4.3)	6.1 (±3.7)	12.8 (±3.3)

Abbreviations: CI - 95% confidence interval.

[a] "Others" include American Indian or Alaskan Native, Asian, Native Hawaiian or Other Pacific Islander, Multiple Hispanic, Multiple non-Hispanic.

Table 3. Odds ratios of overweight perception and weight control behaviors of U.S. normal weight students, *YRBS 2003*

	Exercised to lose weight or keep from gaining weight		Ate less food, fewer calories, or foods low in fat to lose weight or to keep from gaining weight		Went w/o eating for $\geq$24 hours to lose weight or to keep from gaining weight		Took diet medicines to lose weight or to keep from gaining weight		Vomited or took laxatives to lose weight or to keep from gaining weight		At least 1 Unhealthy Weight Control Behavior	
Perceived themselves as overweight[a]	OR (CI 95%)		OR (CI 95%)		OR (CI 95%)		OR (CI 95%)		OR (CI 95%)		OR (CI 95%)	
Crude OR	4.1	(3.5-4.9)	6.8	(5.6-8.1)	3.8	(3.0-4.7)	4.1	(2.9-5.7)	3.9	(2.6-6.0)	3.3	(2.5-4.3)
Adjusted OR[b]	3.0	(2.5-3.6)	4.6	(3.8-5.7)	3.0	(2.4-3.7)	3.1	(2.3-4.3)	3.0	(2.0-4.5)	2.6	(2.0-3.4)

Abbreviations: OR- odds ratio; CI - confidence interval.

[a] Referent group = students who did not perceive themselves as overweight.

[b] Adjusted for gender and ethnicity.

Discussion

This chapter investigated the prevalence of overweight misperception and weight control practices of normal weight adolescents in the United States. We found that a significant percentage of normal weight high school students (16.2%) misperceived themselves as overweight and that more than a third (35.8%) reported trying to lose weight in spite of their normal BMI. Of particular concern, 11.8% of students reported practicing at least one unhealthy weight control behavior such as purging or fasting in the past 30 days. These findings suggest that normal weight adolescents may be at risk for adverse health effects related to unhealthy weight control behaviors.

Similar to past studies, this study observed several important gender [4,14-17] and ethnic [4,17] differences in overweight misperceptions. Our finding of a higher prevalence of overweight misperceptions among female adolescents may be a result of a greater concern with body image as compared to their male counterparts [15,18,19]. In spite of the large gender difference in the prevalence of overweight misperception and unhealthy weight control behaviors, there is nevertheless a significant number of male students (>6%) who reported overweight misperceptions and engagement in more than one unhealthy weight control behavior.

With regard to ethnic differences in overweight misperceptions, our findings are consistent with the results of the NHANES III and the 1990 North Carolina YRBS report, which found white females to be more inclined to misperceive themselves as overweight [4,20]. This study also found African American adolescents with normal weight to be the least likely to perceive themselves as overweight. Even as children, African Americans are most satisfied with their body weight compared to whites and other racial minorities [21]. Studies have suggested lesser social and cultural pressure for blacks to be thin as compared to their white and Hispanic counterparts [22,23].

Having distorted weight perception may set unrealistic goals and unhealthy weight control behaviors among adolescents [17]. There is some evidence to suggest that body weight misperception may be more influential than actual weight status in enticing adolescents to practice weight control [4,24]. This study supports the hypothesis that students who misperceive themselves as overweight are more likely to engage in various unhealthy weight control behaviors.

Of particular concern was our finding of a substantial prevalence of fasting (11.6%) and diet pill use (7.4%) among our normal weight sample. Unaware of their ill effects, adolescents might consider these behaviors as the fastest and easiest course to lose weight. Fasting has been found in previous research to be highest among younger adolescents [25]. Our results also suggest that fasting is higher among those in the first three years of high school, with a slight decrease by 12th grade. The intake of diet pills, on the other hand, was more prevalent among higher grade levels. As exercise and healthy dieting remained constant throughout the grade levels in this study, the increase in diet pill consumption may reflect an increasing pressure to lose weight through the fastest means possible, especially for older adolescents who may have greater access to diet pills compared to their younger schoolmates. Concern for the use of diet pills is underscored when comparing the prevalence of diet pill use among adolescents in previous studies. In the 1990 YRBS, the use of dieting pills was only 4% among females and 2% among males [22]. In our data, 10% of females and 4.6% of males have used dieting pills. While results from the 1999 YRBS showed higher prevalence of abnormal weight control behavior in the Midwestern and southern states [26], we did not find significant differences in the prevalence of unhealthy weight control practices by geographic region and metropolitan status. The lack of association between the prevalence of weight control behaviors and place of residence found in this study may suggest the popularity of unhealthy weight control across the United States that results from widespread exposure of media among US adolescents.

An important limitation of this study was the determination of the BMI status and classification of normal weight adolescents based on self-reported height and weight. As adolescents have been found to over-report their height and underreport their weight [27], it is possible that some students who were actually overweight were misclassified as normal weight. The potential misclassification of overweight students as normal weight may have led to an overestimate of the prevalence of overweight misperceptions and weight control behaviors among this sample.

In conclusion, a significant portion of normal weight adolescents misperceived themselves as overweight and are practicing at least one unhealthy weight loss behavior. This study's findings also suggest that overweight misperception is associated with unhealthy weight control behaviors. With the increasing prevalence of childhood obesity [28,29], our results recommend the need for a holistic perspective in addressing healthy weight issues among adolescents. Many program implementers working with the childhood obesity issue may be tempted to focus their efforts on strategies for reducing weight among overweight adolescents, with little attention given to the majority of the adolescents who, in spite of their normal weight, may be struggling to maintain or to lose further weight. Childhood obesity prevention programs need to include educational components that address the risks of unhealthy weight control behaviors among adolescents, regardless of BMI status, in addition to the benefits of healthy weight maintenance behaviors.

Acknowledgments

The authors would like to acknowledge Bob Addy, Research Associate at the Centers for Health Promotion and Prevention Research, University of Texas-Houston School of Public Health, and Julia Sanders, Graduate Research Assistant at the Human Nutrition Center, University of Texas-Houston School of Public Health, for their insightful guidance with the analysis of the YRBS data. Preparation of this manuscript was made possible in part by the National Cancer Institute/NIH Grant# 2R25CA57712-11 which supported Dr. Springer's Postdoctoral Fellowship as well as the Cancer Prevention and Control Training Program in the Centers for Health Promotion and Prevention Research, University of Texas-Houston School of Public Health. This chapter is based on an earlier published paper: Talamayan KS, Springer AE, Kelder SH, Gorospe EC, Joye KA. Prevalence of overweight misperception and weight control behaviors among normal weight adolescents in the United States. ScientificWorldJournal 2006;6:365-73.

References

[1] Rodin J. Cultural and psychosocial determinants of weight concerns. Ann Intern Med 1993;119(7 Pt 2):643-5.

[2] Field AE, Camargo CA, Jr., Taylor CB, et al. Relation of peer and media influences to the development of purging behaviors among preadolescent and adolescent girls. Arch Pediatr Adolesc Med 1999;153(11):1184-9.

[3] Phelps L, Johnston L, Jimenes D, et al. Figure preference, body dissatisfaction, and body distortion in adolescence. J Adolesc Res 1993;8:297-311.

[4] Strauss RS. Self-reported weight status and dieting in a cross-sectional sample of young adolescents: National Health and Nutrition Examination Survey III. Arch Pediatr Adolesc Med 1999;153(7):741-7.

[5] Boutelle K, Neumark-Sztainer D, Story M, et al. Weight control behaviors among obese, overweight, and nonoverweight adolescents. J Pediatr Psychol 2002;27(6):531-40.

[6] Neumark-Sztainer D, Story M, Falkner NH, et al. Sociodemographic and personal characteristics of adolescents engaged in weight loss and weight/muscle gain behaviors: who is doing what? Prev Med 1999;28(1):40-50.

[7] Killen JD, Taylor CB, Hayward C, et al. Weight concerns influence the development of eating disorders: a 4-year prospective study. J Consult Clin Psychol 1996;64(5):936-40.

[8] Killen JD, Taylor CB, Hayward C, et al. Pursuit of thinness and onset of eating disorder symptoms in a community sample of adolescent girls: a three-year prospective analysis. Int J Eat Disord 1994;16(3):227-38.

[9] Rosen T, Howel D. Life stress, psychological symptoms and weight reducing behavior in adolescent girls: a prospective analysis. Int J Eat Disord 1990;9:7-26.

[10] Rogers PJ, Green MW. Dieting, dietary restraint and cognitive performance. Br J Clin Psychol 1993;32 (Pt 1):113-6.

[11] Stice E, Cameron RP, Killen JD, et al. Naturalistic weight-reduction efforts prospectively predict growth in relative weight and onset of obesity among female adolescents. J Consult Clin Psychol 1999;67(6):967-74.

[12] Centers for Disease Control and Prevention. National School-based Youth Risk Behavior Survey: Public-use Data Document. 2003. Available from http://www.cdc.gov/HealthyYouth/yrbs/data/2003/yrbs2003codebook.pdf

[13] Centers for Disease Control and Prevention. Body Mass Index: BMI for children and teens. 2005. Available from http://www.cdc.gov/nccdphp/dnpa/bmi/bmi-for-age.htm

[14] Childress AC, Brewerton TD, Hodges EL, et al. The Kids' Eating Disorders Survey (KEDS): a study of middle school students. J Am Acad Child Adolesc Psychiatry 1993;32(4):843-50.

[15] Gustafson-Larson AM, Terry RD. Weight-related behaviors and concerns of fourth-grade children. J Am Diet Assoc 1992;92(7):818-22.

[16] Field AE, Camargo CA, Jr., Taylor CB, et al. Overweight, weight concerns, and bulimic behaviors among girls and boys. J Am Acad Child Adolesc Psychiatry 1999;38(6):754-60.

[17] Felts WM, Parrillo AV, Chenier T, et al. Adolescents' perceptions of relative weight and self-reported weight-loss activities: analysis of 1990 YRBS (Youth Risk behavior Survey) national data. J Adolesc Health 1996;18(1):20-6.

[18] Thelen M, Powell A, Lawrence C, et al. Eating and body image concern among children. J Clinical Psychology 1992;21:41-46.

[19] Feldman W, Feldman E, Goodman JT. Culture versus biology: children's attitudes toward thinness and fatness. Pediatrics 1988;81(2):190-4.

[20] Felts M, Tavasso D, Chenier T, et al. Adolescents' perceptions of relative weight and self-reported weight loss activities. J Sch Health 1992;62(8):372-6.

[21] Welch C, Gross SM, Bronner Y, et al. Discrepancies in body image perception among fourth-grade public school children from urban, suburban, and rural Maryland. J Am Diet Assoc 2004;104(7):1080-5.

[22] Serdula MK, Collins ME, Williamson DF, et al. Weight control practices of US adolescents and adults. Ann Intern Med 1993;119(7 Pt 2):667-71.

[23] Kumanyika SK. Special issues regarding obesity in minority populations. Ann Intern Med 1993;119(7 Pt 2):650-4.

[24] Brener ND, Eaton DK, Lowry R, et al. The association between weight perception and BMI among high school students. Obes Res 2004;12(11):1866-74.

[25] Maloney MJ, McGuire J, Daniels SR, et al. Dieting behavior and eating attitudes in children. Pediatrics 1989;84(3):482-9.

[26] Forman-Hoffman V. High prevalence of abnormal eating and weight control practices among US high-school students. Eat Behav 2004;5(4):325-36.

[27] Brener ND, McManus T, Galuska DA, et al. Reliability and validity of self-reported height and weight among high school students. J Adolesc Health 2003;32(4):281-7.

[28] Hedley AA, Ogden CL, Johnson CL, et al. Prevalence of overweight and obesity among US children, adolescents, and adults, 1999-2002. Jama 2004;291(23):2847-50.

[29] Strauss RS, Pollack HA. Epidemic increase in childhood overweight, 1986-1998. JAMA 2001;286(22):2845-8.

VI. Nutrition, Environment and Special Populations

In: Obesity and Adolescence: A Public Health Concern
Editors: H.A. Omar, D.E. Greydanus et al.
ISBN: 978-1-60692-821-9

Chapter XVI

Obesity and Nutrition

Vinay N. Reddy*

Pediatrics and Human Development, Michigan State University College of Human Medicine, Michigan State University/Kalamazoo Center for Medical Studies, Kalamazoo, Michigan, United States of America

Abstract

The prevalence of obesity has increased to epidemic proportions in the United States in recent years. Obesity in the Western world is a disease of poverty that is seen much more often in minority populations. Obesity-related illnesses, such as type II diabetes, are now seen frequently in adolescents and even in younger children. Caloric intake has increased in adolescents over the last two decades along with changes in dietary composition fueled by advertisements of unhealthy foods by various food producers. Nutritional modification is an essential part of any weight-loss program. This chapter discusses various diet changes that are important to reverse this current trend of increasing obesity in all populations and ages. Highly-restrictive diets should be reserved only for the morbidly obese child or for those with obesity-related problems such as sleep apnea.

Introduction

In recent years the prevalence of obesity has increased steadily in the United States, and the rate of increase has itself increased, especially over the last 25 years [1-5]. Although one might expect obesity to be more prevalent among people of higher socioeconomic status with better nutritional access, the converse is true; indeed, the prevalence of obesity in much of the

* Correspondence: Vinay N Reddy MD, Assistant professor, Pediatrics and Human Development, Michigan State University College of Human Medicine, Michigan State University/Kalamazoo Center for Medical Studies, 1000 Oakland Drive, Kalamazoo, Michigan 49008-1284 United States. Tel: 269-337-6450; Fax: 269-337-6474; E-mail: Reddy@kcms.msu.edu

developed world increases with poverty. In the United States obesity is much more prevalent among American Hispanics (21.8%) and African-Americans (21.5%) than among Caucasians (12.3%), with a prevalence of 26.6% among teenage and preteen African-American females [1,6-8]. Obesity-related illnesses, such as type II diabetes mellitus, previously observed only in later adulthood, are being seen more often in adolescence and sometimes in the preteen years.

Many problems with treatment of obesity arise from obesity risk factors [9]. Health-care professionals and the general publicassume that increases in adolescent's caloric intake, coupled with decreases in their physical activity, are responsible for the increased prevalence of obesity. However, published data from the United States shows that caloric intake among children over the last three decades remained relatively constant from the 1970s until the late 1980s. From then until 2000, caloric intake increased among adolescent females, especially white and black females, with larger increases toward the end of this period [10]. Similarly, the United States Department of Agriculture data shows decreased average caloric intake for the general United States population from the mid-1960s to 1991, followed by an increase in the mid-1990s [11]. These trends do not explain the steady and accelerating increase in prevalence of obesity over the past thirty years, nor do they fit the observed increases in prevalence among ethnic groups, especially Hispanics.

Many experts conclude that decreased physical activity and the resulting fall in caloric consumption have contributed to the recent increase in obesity, and that physical activity has decreased due to the rapid increase in television watching since the 1960s, and more recently to the even more rapid increase in adolescent's use of the internet, both of which are physically sedentary activities. Many studies of risk factors for obesity in adolescents have shown significant associations between obesity and television watching, although some studies did not support this conclusion [11-18]. Increased television watching is associated with increased BMI [19,20], increased food consumption [21] and decreased fruit and vegetable consumption [22]. Other contributing factors for children in urban areas may include use of cars or mass transit rather than walking [17] and inability to play safely outdoors due to neighborhood crime in association with low socioeconomic status [23,24]. Significantly decreased physical activity has been observed among female college freshmen within 5 months after starting college; this gain is accompanied by a significant decrease in caloric intake along with significant increase in body-weight parameters, suggesting suggests that decreased activity was a major contributor to this weight gain [25]. Unfortunately, there is little data available on how children's or adolescent's physical activity and caloric consumption have changed over the years, and there is evidence that decreased physical activity occurs after obesity develops, rather than before [26].

Changes in dietary carbohydrate and fat intake are also blamed for the increased prevalence of obesity. Excessive fat intake by some persons, especially those predisposed to obesity, certainly seems to lead to obesity. Although fat-laden foods -- especially fast foods -- have been strongly linked to the development of obesity in the media, fat consumption by children has decreased over the last 30-35 years [10,27]. Carbohydrate consumption, on the other hand, has increased over the same time period and seems to be related to the emphasis seen in recent years on decreasing dietary fat intake, which has resulted in fat calories being largely replaced by simple carbohydrate calories [28]. Calcium intake has decreased due to the substitution of soft drinks and non-citrus fruit juices for milk, which is perceived to be a source of fat. Many parents believe that fruit juices and fruit drinks are "healthier" than milk because they contain nutrients found in the source fruits. However, the actual nutritional value of fruit juices is quite low, especially for clear juices such as those from apples and grapes which are little more than flavored sugar water in which grape juice is 1/7 sugar by weight [29,30]. Carbohydrate composition of foods is commonly classified using the glycemic index [31], which is in general higher for simple sugars and starches (e.g., potatoes, refined grains, and many fruit juices), lower for whole grains and legumes, and lowest for non-starchy fruits and vegetables. High glycemic-index diets have been associated with obesity [32] and type II diabetes mellitus [33] in adults; these associations may hold in children and adolescents, but this has not yet been confirmed. Also, postprandial hyperinsulinemia is associated with weight gain, and low glycemic-index diets appear to decrease postprandial hyperinsulinemia, while also being associated with weight loss in obese patients [9].

Unfortunately, foods high in fat and/or refined carbohydrates taste good, especially to children and adolescents. They are also less expensive and more convenient than more nutritionally valuable foods, especially in the Western world; this may explain why economically disadvantaged children in the United States are more likely to be obese. Attempts to replace high-fat, high-carbohydrate foods in school lunch programs have been met with protests from children and adolescents served by those programs, who would much rather eat nachos and pizza [6]. The media affects children's dietary choices as well as their activity levels. Saturday-morning children's television is largely financed by brand-name advertising for fast-food chains and food manufacturers, and much of that advertising is for high-fat, high-sugar, and high-salt foods. A similar pattern is seen in food-related advertising on prime-time television, and young children prefer the taste of food in fast-food chain packaging to the identical food in plain wrappers, especially if they have multiple TV sets in their homes and/or if they eat fast food frequently [34]. A 1999 analysis of the percentage of advertising for each food group in the USDA Food Guide Pyramid [35] showed a massive overemphasis on high-calorie foods (fats, oils, sweets, and grain-based foods), with only 12% of food advertising promoting vegetables and fruits [36].

There is an inherited component to obesity as well. Many genetic syndromes are associated with obesity, as are endocrine disorders such as Cushing's disease and hypothyroidism [37,38]. Hypothyroidism does not appear to be a primary cause of massive obesity, although modest weight loss is noted with treatment [39]. However, much of the familial component of obesity seems to be environmental. Obesity in children and adolescents has been associated with both maternal and paternal obesity [18,40-42]. Although this may be partly genetic and, in the case of maternal obesity, partly due to gestational influences, socioeconomic factors shared by parents and children are certainly responsible as well; examples include lack of physical activity and indulgence in fast foods and other high-fat, high-carbohydrate food.

In some countries, although not in Western countries, adolescents have been found to underestimate their body weight significantly, especially when they are overweight or obese [43]. This is in contrast to the overestimation seen in anorexia nervosa and bulimia nervosa, but appears to be related to cultural norms and their effect on self-image. Obesity has also been associated with social factors, including low family income and lower cognitive stimulation at home [44]. This may explain in part racial and ethnic differences in the prevalence of obesity, although some of these differences persist when corrected. A history of neglect and/or abuse, especially sexual abuse, is also associated with obesity [45,46].

Nutritional Treatment

Even a brief look at the media reveals multitudes of weight-loss programs, diets, and medical treatments for obesity. Some of them may actually work, at least for a while, at least in adults, and at least until deleterious effects or lack of long-term relief are seen. The story of damage produced by fenfluramine should be remembered in this regard, as reviewed elsewhere in this issue on obesity. Obese children and adolescents are more difficult to treat. Social and economic considerations, especially family issues, must be addressed, and the entire family must make the required lifestyle changes [47].

The goals of treatment must also be realistic. Many patients expect the same results seen in the before-and-after advertisements for weight-loss programs; however, weight loss of that extent is often not possible without medication and/or surgery. However, moderate weight loss -- 5-10% of weight at presentation, for example -- can produce significant improvement in blood pressure, glucose, and lipids [48]. It may be most practical, and beneficial especially to the growing child or teenager to maintain weight at a particular range rather than to seek actual weight loss. Also, early treatment is of benefit even in young children, both to avoid childhood complications (e.g., sleep apnea, orthopedic disease) as well as adult complications (e.g., type 2 diabetes, coronary vascular disease) and to avoid or lessen the psychosocial consequences of obesity. Dietary modification, combined with increased and regular physical activity, is a cornerstone of therapy for obesity. These interventions work best when they take place simultaneously [49].

Diet changes should be made by the entire family and emphasize increasing consumption of healthy foods that include vegetables, whole fruits, and whole grains while avoiding high-fat, high-simple-carbohydrate foods such as juices, sweetened drinks, fats (especially saturated fats), and refined carbohydrates (sweets, baked goods containing white flour and/or simple sugars). Many dietary modification plans are based on the USDA Food Guide Pyramid [35], which is easier to follow for most children and families than counting calories with every meal. Table 1 lists simple and realistic strategies for diet modification [50].

One program, the "Traffic Light Diet" [52] uses simple categories (Red Light [avoid], Yellow Light [approach-with-caution], and Green Light [at-all-you-want]; it also provides a list of foods in each of the major food groups (grains, fruits/vegetables, dairy, and meat, with a fifth miscellaneous category). This program teaches children and families to make healthy food choices. When used in combination with exercise and behavioral modification, this diet program has produced long-term weight loss in children [53].

Table 1. Simple and realistic strategies for diet modification [50]

- • Reducing consumption of specific high-calorie foods, such as candy or potato chips, without entirely eliminating them from the diet.
- • Replacing high-calorie snacks such as cookies or baked goods with low-calorie alternatives such as fruits.
- • Reducing portion sizes when preparing meals, and when eating out.
- • Eating out less often, and choosing low-calorie foods such as vegetables instead of high-calorie foods such as French fries.
- • Limiting drinks containing large amounts of sugar, including fruit juices (even 100% juices are high in simple sugars) and soft drinks.
- • Eating meals as a family as frequently as possible (this helps children and their parents support each other in implementing the above strategies, and has been shown to be of benefit in adolescents51 as well as in younger children).

Regular meals, especially breakfast, also seem to be important in prevention of obesity. Cross-sectional studies have shown an inverse relationship between regularly eating breakfast and development of obesity. One recent prospective study shows a direct association between breakfast frequency and carbohydrate as well as fiber intake; it also noted an inverse and dose-related relationship between breakfast frequency and BMI, although these relationships have not yet been shown to be causal [54].

Severely obese patients, such as the morbidly obese or those with acute obesity-related problems such as sleep apnea, may need more restricted diets such as those high in protein (i.e., 1.5 to 2.5 g/kg/day) and very low in calories (i.e., 600-900 kcal/day) with extremely limited carbohydrate as well as fat intake and a minimum water intake of 1.5 liters per day. These diets are usually deficient in essential vitamins and in some minerals, which must be provided by appropriate supplements. Close monitoring by the physician and nutritionist is essential when using these diets to ensure compliance by the patient and family as well as to avoid, detect, and treat potential medical complications [55-57].

Exercise is important, but cannot by itself reduce weight [58]. Since ability to exercise decreases with increased BMI, regular exercise must begin before morbid obesity renders the patient immobile [59]. There are many approaches possible to increasing physical activity and reducing a sedentary lifestyle; examples include increased activity at school during lunch and recess, walking or bicycling to school, enrollment in summer schools or summer camps [60] and reducing television viewing [13,21,61]. Psychotherapy may also be helpful in selected cases [62] and inpatient treatment may be especially useful when family support for treatment is lacking. A combination of dietary changes, organized and supervised exercise, and cognitive-behavioral therapy in a 10-month (one school year) inpatient program resulted weight loss at discharge that was sustained 14 months after discharge [63]. If diet modification and increased exercise do not yield weight stabilization or weight loss, further investigation should address the extent and severity of obesity co-morbidities. Pharmacologic treatment may be considered at this stage as an adjunct to continued diet and exercise, as reviewed elsewhere in this issue on obesity.

Conclusions

The prevalence of obesity has increased to epidemic proportions in the United States in recent years. Factors behind this problem include some increase in caloric intake stimulated by the good taste of high-fat and high-carbohydrate foods along with strong advertising for these unhealthy foods by their producers. Nutritional modification is an essential part of any weight-loss program. Diet changes, which should be made by the patient's entire family for best results, include adding more vegetables, whole fruits, and whole grains to the diet while avoiding high-fat and high-simple-carbohydrate foods such as juices, sweetened drinks, fats (especially saturated fats), and refined carbohydrates. Reducing consumption of specific high-calorie foods such as candy and potato chips, replacing high-calorie snacks with low-calorie ones, limiting high-sugar drinks, eating smaller portions, eating more often at home, and eating meals as a family are simple and realistic strategies for reducing caloric intake. Eating regular meals, especially breakfast, may also help avoid obesity. Highly-restrictive diets should be reserved only for the morbidly obese child or teenager and for those with obesity-related problems such as sleep apnea.

References

[1] Troiano R, Flegal K, Kuczmanski R, Campbell S, Johnson C. Overweight prevalence and trends for children and adolescents: The National Health and Nutrition Examination Surveys, 1963 to 1991. Arch Pediatr Adolesc Med 1995;149:1085-91.

[2] Visscher T, Seidell J. The Public Health Impact of Obesity. Annu Rev Public Health 2001;22:355-75.

[3] Wald N, Willett W. Reversing the obesity epidemic. Lancet 2004;364:140.

[4] LeBlanc C. The Growing Epidemic of Child and Youth Obesity - Another Twist? Can J Pub Health 2003;94(5):329-30.

[5] Stubbs C, Lee A. The obesity epidemic: both energy intake and physical activity contribute. Med J Austral 2004;181(9):489-91.

[6] Weil E. Heavy Questions. The New York Times Magazine 2005 02 Jan 2005:34-39.

[7] Kimm S, Glynn N, Kriska A, Fitzgerald S, Aaron D, Similo S, et al. Racial divergence in adiposity during adolescence: The NHLBI Growth and Health Study. Pediatrics 2001;107:E34.

[8] Ogden C, Flegal K, Carroll M, Johnson C. Prevalence and trends in overweight among US children and adolescents, 1999-2000. JAMA 2002;288:1728-32.

[9] Slyper A. The Pediatric Obesity Epidemic: Causes and Controversies. J Clin Endocrinol Metab 2004;89:2540-7.

[10] Troiano R, Briefel R, Carroll M, Bialostosky K. Energy and fat intakes of children and adolescents in the United States: data from the National Health and Nutrition Examination surveys. Am J Clin Nutr 2000;725(5 Suppl):1343S-53.

[11] Kennedy E, Bowman S, Powell R. Dietary fat intake in the US population. J Am Coll Nutr 1999;18:207-12.

[12] Tucker L. The relationship of television viewing to physical fitness and obesity. Adolescence 1986;21:797-806.
[13] Robinson T, Hammer L, Killen J, Kraemer H, Wilson D, Hayward C, et al. Does television watching increase obesity and reduce physical activity? Cross-sectional and longitudinal analyses among adolescent girls. Pediatrics 1993;91:273-80.
[14] Gortmaker S, Must A, Sobol A, Peterson K, Colditz G, Dietz W. Television viewing as a cause of increasing obesity among children in the United States, 1986-1990. Arch Pediatr Adolesc Med 1996;150:356-62.
[15] Dietz W, Gortmaker S. Do we fatten our children at the TV set? Obesity and television in children and adolescents. Pediatrics 1985;75:807-12.
[16] Krassas G, Tzotzas T, Tsatmetis C, Konstantinidis T. Determinants of body mass index in Greek children and adolescents. J Pediatr Endocrinol Metab 2001;14(Suppl 5):1327-33.
[17] Giles-Corti B, Macintyre S, Clarkson J, Pikora T, Donovan R. Environmental and lifestyle factors associated with overweight and obesity in Perth, Australia. Am J Health Promot 2003;18:93-102.
[18] Al-Isa A. Dietary and socio-economic factors associated with obesity among Kuwaiti college men. Br J Nutr 1999;82:369-74.
[19] Kaur H, Choi W, Mayo M, Harris K. Duration of Television Watching is Associated with Increased Body Mass Index. J Pediatr 2003;143:506-11.
[20] Hancox R, Milne B, Poulton R. Association between child and adolescent television viewing and adult health: a longitudinal birth cohort study. Lancet 2004;364:257-62.
[21] Matheson DM, Killen JD, Wang Y, Varady A, Robinson TN. Children's food consumption during television viewing. Am J Clin Nutr 2004;79(6):1088-94.
[22] Boynton-Jarrett R, Thomas T, Peterson K, Wiecha J, Sobol A, Gortmaker S. Impact of television viewing patterns on fruit and vegetable consumption among adolescents. Pediatrics 2003;112:1321-6.
[23] Gordon-Larsen P, MacMurray R, Popkin B. Determinants of Adolescent Physical Activity and Inactivity Patterns. Pediatrics 2000;105:e83-e90.
[24] Wilson D, Kirtland K, Ainsworth B, Addy C. Socioeconomic status and perception of access and safety for physical activity. Ann Behav Med 2004;28:20-8.
[25] Butler S, Black D, Blue C, Gretebeck R. Change in diet, physical activity, and body weight in female college freshmen. Am J Health Behav 2004;28(1):24-32.
[26] Kimm S, Glynn N, Kriska A, Barton B, Kronsberg S, Daniels S, et al. Decline in physical activity in black girls and white girls during adolescence. N Engl J Med 2002;347:709-15.
[27] Wright J, Wang C, Kennedy-Stephenson J, Ervin R. Dietary intake of ten key nutrients for public health, United States 1999-2000. Hyattsville, MD: Nat Center Health Stat, 2003, Report 334.
[28] Cavadini C, Siega-Riz A, Popkin B. US adolescent food intake trends from 1965 to 1996. Arch Dis Child 2000;83:18-24.
[29] United States Department of Agriculture Nutrient Data Laboratory.
[30] Wagner PM. Grapes into wine. New York: Alfred A Knopf, 1976: 105.

[31] Ludwig D, Eckel R. The glycemic index at 20 y. Am J Clin Nutr 2002;76(suppl):264S-5.

[32] Brand-Miller J, Holt S, Pawlak D, McMillan J. Glycemic index and obesity. Am J Clin Nutr 2002;76(suppl):281S-5.

[33] Willett W, Manson J, Liu S. Glycemic index, glycemic load, and risk of type 2 diabetes. Am J Clin Nutr 2002;76(suppl):274S-80.

[34] Robinson TN, Borzekowski DLG, Matheson DL, Kraemer HC. Effects of fast food branding on young children's taste preferences. Arch Pediatr Adolesc Med 2007;161(8):792-7.

[35] United States Departments of Agriculture and Health and Human Services. Nutrition and your health: Dietary guidelines for Americans, 4th ed. Washington, DC: US Dept Agriculture, 2000.

[36] Byrd-Bredbenner C, Grasso D. A comparative analysis of television food advertisements and current dietary recommendations. Am J Health Studies 1999;15:169-80.

[37] Snyder E, Walts B, Perusse L, Chagnon Y, Weisnagel S, Rankinen T, et al. The Human Obesity Gene Map: The 2003 Update. Obes Res 2004;12(3):369-439.

[38] Jones K. Smith's recognizable patterns of human malformation, 5th ed. Philadelphia, PA: WB Saunders, 1997.

[39] Styne D, Schoenfled-Warden N. Obesity. In: Rudolph C, Rudolph A, eds. Rudolph's pediatrics, 21 ed. New York: McGraw Hill, 2003:2136-42.

[40] Ramos de Marins V, Almeida R, Pereira R, de Azevedo Barros M. The relationship between parental nutritional status and overweight children/adolescents in Rio de Janeiro, Brazil. Public Health 2004;118(1):43-9.

[41] Savva S, Kourides Y, Epiphanou-Savva M, Tonaritis M, Kafatos A. Short-term predictors of overweight in early adolescence. Int J Obes Relat Metab Disord 2004;28(3):451-8.

[42] Power C, Parsons T. Nutritional and other influences in childhood as predictors of adult obesity. Proc Nutr Soc 2000;59:267-72.

[43] Al-Sendi A, Shetty P, Musaiger A. Body weight perception among Bahrain adolescents. Child Care Health Dev 2004;30(4):369-76.

[44] Strauss RS, Knight J. Influence of the home environment on the development of obesity in children. Pediatrics 1999;103(6):e85.

[45] Lissau I, Sorenson T. Parental neglect during childhood and increased risk of obesity in young adulthood. Lancet 1994;343(8893):324-7.

[46] Zametkin AJMD, Zoon CKBS, Klein HWBS, Munson SBA. Psychiatric Aspects of Child and Adolescent Obesity: A Review of the Past 10 Years. J Am Acad Child Adolesc Psychiatry 2004;43(2):134-50.

[47] Strauss R. Childhood obesity. Ped Clin North Am 2002;49(1):175-201.

[48] Goldstein D. Beneficial health effects of modest weight loss. Int J Obes Relat Metab Disord 1992;16(6):397-415.

[49] Fulton J, McGuire M, Casperson C, Dietz W. Interventions for weight loss and weight gain prevention among youth: Current issues. Sports Med 2001;31(3):153-65.

[50] Mullen MC, Shield J, eds. Childhood and adolescent overweight: The health professional's guide to identification, treatment and prevention. Chicago, IL: Am Diet Assoc, 2004.

[51] Neumark-Sztainer D, Eisenberg ME, Fulkerson JA, Story M, Larson NI. Family meals and disordered eating in adolescents: Longitudinal findings from project EAT. Arch Pediatr Adolesc Med 2008;162(1):17-22.

[52] Epstein L. Family-based behavioural intervention for obese children. Int J Obes Relat Metab Disord 1996;20(Suppl 1):S14-S21.

[53] Epstein LH, Valoski A, Wing RR, McCurley J. Ten-year outcomes of behavioral family-based treatment for childhood obesity. Health Psychol 1994;13(5):373-83.

[54] Timlin MT, Pereira M, Story M, Neumark-Sztainer D. Breakfast eating and weight change in a 5-Year prospective analysis of adolescents: Project EAT (Eating Among Teens). Pediatrics 2008;121(3):e638-45.

[55] Hirsch J, Hudgins L, Leibel R, Rosenbaum M. Diet composition and energy balance in humans. Am J Clin Nutr 1998;67(3):551S-5.

[56] St. Jeor ST, Howard BV, Prewitt TE, Bovee V, Bazzarre T, Eckel RH. Dietary protein and weight reduction: A statement for healthcare professionals from the nutrition committee of the council on nutrition, physical activity, and metabolism of the American Heart Association. Circulation 2001;104(15):1869-74.

[57] Willi S, Oexmann M, Wright N, Collop N, Key L. The effects of a high-protein, low-fat, ketogenic diet in adolescents with morbid obesity composition, blood chemistries, and sleep abnormalities. Pediatrics 1998;101:61-6.

[58] Saris W. Exercise with or without dietary restriction and obesity treatment. Int J Obes Relat Metab Disord 1995;19(Suppl 4):S113-6.

[59] Speiser PW, Rudolf MCJ, Anhalt H, Camacho-Hubner C, Chiarelli F, Eliakim A, et al. Childhood obesity. J Clin Endocrinol Metab 2005;90(3):1871-87.

[60] Jago R, Baranowski T. Non-curricular approaches for increasing physical activity in youth: a review. Prev Med 2004;39(1):157-63.

[61] Robinson TN. Reducing children's television viewing to prevent obesity: A randomized controlled trial. JAMA 1999;282(16):1561-7.

[62] Eliakim A, Kaven G, Berger I, Friedland O, Wolach B, Nemet D. The effect of a combined intervention on body mass index and fitness in obese children and adolescents - a clinical experience. Eur J Pediatr 2002;161:449-54.

[63] Braet C, Tanghe A, Decaluwe V, Moens E, Rosseel Y. Inpatient treatment for children with obesity: Weight loss, psychological well-being and eating behavior. J Pediatr Psychol 2004;29(7):519-29.

In: Obesity and Adolescence: A Public Health Concern
Editors: H.A. Omar, D.E. Greydanus et al.
ISBN: 978-1-60692-821-9

Chapter XVII

Obesity Prevention, Environment and School Transportation

Chanam Lee* and Xuemei Zhu
Department of Landscape Architecture and Urban Planning, College of Architecture, Texas A&M University, College Station, Texas, United States of America

Abstract

Obesity rates among children around the world have reached an epidemic level. Having an option to walk or bike to school is important for mobility, health and equity purposes. However, fewer students are walking or biking to school today than a generation ago, and fewer students live within a walkable distance to schools. This chapter highlights the existing evidence from multiple disciplines on health and equity issues related to school transportation. It then assesses the literature dealing with the built environmental correlates of walking or biking to school. Travel distance and safety were found to be the strongest predictors of walking or biking to school. Studies suggested that about one-half to one mile (0.8-1.6 km) between home and school was generally considered walkable. Other factors such as roadway conditions, sidewalk continuity, bike lane availability, signals, lighting, and neighborhood design appeared important but with some inconsistencies in the findings. Many commonly reported environmental barriers were related to transportation infrastructure, such as high-volume and high-speed roadways, unsafe street crossings, and railroads. Compared with distance, safety and transportation infrastructure, neighborhood characteristics such as density, land use, and overall street patterns appeared less significantly associated with school transportation. Our review revealed evidence supporting the link between school transportation and the built environment. It also discovered many remaining questions for future research, such as interactions and causalities between personal and environmental factors, environmental

* Correspondence: Chanam Lee, PhD, Department of Landscape Architecture and Urban Planning, College of Architecture, Texas A&M University, W014D Williams Administration Building, College Station, TX 77843-3137 USA. Tel: 1-979-845-7056; Fax; 1-979-862-1784; E-mail: chanam@tamu.edu

influences from multiple spatial scales, and differences between objective and perceived measures.

Introduction

This chapter discusses health and equity issues related to school transportation and the environment. The focus is on the roles of built environments in promoting or deterring physically active commuting to school. Increased automobile dependency and sedentary lifestyle have contributed to many public health problems such as obesity and diabetes. Obesity rates have reached an epidemic level across all age, race, gender and income groups. Childhood obesity is of significant concern because of its lifelong consequences involving much comorbidity. Walking or biking to school can help incorporate routine physical activity into children's daily life and therefore fight against obesity. However, fewer students are walking or biking to school today than a generation ago, due to many personal and environmental barriers. Leading environmental deterrants include dangers from traffic and crime, long distances between homes and schools, and poor infrastructure conditions. In addition to the health benefits, creating a supportive environment for walking and biking is also important for mobility and equity purposes. Walking and biking are more important and more common travel modes for lower income populations than for higher income groups. However, lower income people often bear greater risks while walking or biking, because their neighborhoods tend to have more traffic crashes and crimes, and more automobile-emitted pollutants.

In this chapter we review the existing evidence from multiple disciplines concerning the personal and environmental correlates of school transportation. It emphasizes the public health implications of walking or biking to school as healthy physical activities and as ways to establish lifelong habits of active living. After summarizing the current state of knowledge on the topic, it concludes with discussions about future research needs to fill in the remaining gaps.

School Transportation and Health

Physical Activity and Health

Without reversing the current trend of unhealthy lifestyles and health disparity, the advances in modern medicine may no longer be sufficient to add quality and length to human lives. Physical activity holds particular significance as the most powerful tool to prevent and manage chronic diseases such as obesity, asthma, hypertension, type 2 diabetes, cardiovascular diseases, and depression [1] and to reduce healthcare costs [2]. Benefits of physical activity among children and adolescents are even greater with additional developmental and health benefits, such as stress management and improved academic performance [3-5]. Play activities are important for children's social developments [6,7]. According to the Surgeon General's Report on Physical Activity and Health [1], even moderate-intensity daily activities such as walking for 30 minutes or jogging for 15 to 20 minutes can be beneficial to health for people of all ages. This report recommends at least 30 minutes of physical activity on five or more days per week.

Despite the many proven health benefits, more than half of US adults are not sufficiently active to meet this recommendation and 26% are not active at all [1]. Physical activity levels and the opportunities for children to be active have continued to decrease over the past several decades. This decline is due to increased parental safety concerns related to traffic and crime, reduced physical education classes offered at schools, greater dependency on automobiles for commuting to schools, and shift in the forms of play from active to sedentary. An observation study found that children from low-income families spent about 58% of their free playtime in sedentary behaviors [8]. About 14% of young people in the US engage in no regular physical activity [9]. Enrollment in physical education classes among high school students has reduced from 42% in 1991 to 25% in 1995 [9]. Among children aged 9 to 13 years, only 38.5% engaged in organized sports but 77.4% reported performing some free-time physical activity in a week [10]. Physical activities decrease dramatically during the teen years [11,12]. Looking specifically at school transportation, children who walk or bike to school reduced from 42% in 1969 to 16% in 2001 [13]. During the same period, students living within one mile from schools, generally considered a walkable distance, decreased from 34% to 21% [13]. This prevalence of physical inactivity and sedentary lifestyle has contributed to the recent obesity epidemic. Childhood obesity has tripled over the past two decades and adult obesity has doubled since 1980, reaching over 30% [13].

Physically active commuting to school alone may not be sufficient to bring about the health benefits related to physical activity. However, physical activity habits are formed early in childhood, and walking and biking are the most attractive, accessible, and feasible forms of physical activity. Walking was found to be the most preferred type of physical activity among primarily Mexican American 7th grade students from San Antonio, Texas, followed by roller-skating/blading and running [14]. Walking is the most preferred physical activity among adults as well [15,16]. In addition, a study of 9-year-old Danish children found that walking to or from school was a good indicator of overall physical activity among children [17]. Another US study among the 5th-grade students found that walking to or from school was associated with 24 additional minutes of moderate to vigorous physical activity per day [18].

Utilitarian transportation behaviors such as walking and biking are especially important, because they are sustainable, lifestyle activities. They serve dual purposes as transportation modes and healthy exercises [19]. As travel modes, they are affordable, environmentally clean, and efficient and reliable in covering short distances [20]. As part of lifestyle intervention programs, they are more likely to induce long-term lifestyle changes, to be effective for currently sedentary people, and to be more cost effective than structured interventions [21-23]. Further, if even a small proportion of automobile trips can be replaced by nonmotorized modes, additional environmental benefits will be significant through reduced air pollution and reduced land consumption [24]. As outdoor activities, walking and biking can potentially bring added health benefits through the exposure to pleasant natural settings, which is shown to facilitate recovery from daily stresses [25, 26]. However, one may question if walking is rigorous enough to actually lower the risks of developing chronic diseases. Although the scientific evidence is not as extensive as that available for overall physical activity, empirical studies have shown that walking alone without other physical activities can and does bring health benefits such as improved cardiovascular, respiratory, and metabolic fitness [27-29]. Sesso and colleagues found that walking more than 10 city blocks everyday resulted in a 33% reduction in cardiovascular disease risks [30].

Physical Activity, Health and Built Environments

Multiple factors influence people's decision to engage in physical activity, including personal, social, and physical environmental factors. Adding to the strong empirical knowledge on the roles of personal and social correlates, a recent and growing body of studies now confirms the significance of the physical environment. As the prevalence of physical inactivity has reached an epidemic proportion, environmental approaches that target large populations at a time and target lifestyle changes are gaining increasing support [31,32]. Previous studies have shown that the designs and uses of built environments (e.g., sidewalks, street network patterns, shops, recreational facilities, and other destinations) and the related environmental characteristics (e.g., safety, lighting, traffic, and aesthetics) are associated with physical activity, walking, and other transportation behaviors [33-41]. A study conducted in Seattle, Washington, showed that if neighborhood environments are supportive, people can meet the recommended amount of physical activity by neighborhood walking alone [40]. In addition, studies suggest that built environments can influence diet behaviors. People living closer to a supermarket are likely to eat more fruits and vegetables. Availability and cost of food, especially healthy food, vary by the neighborhood's socioeconomic status. The poor, especially those living in inner-city areas, pay more for their food and have fewer grocery stores nearby [42]. A study of Chicago schools showed that three to four times more fast food restaurants were located within 1.5 kilometers (0.93 miles) from schools than what would be expected without considering the school locations [43]. This increased accessibility may trigger increased consumption of unhealthy, energy-dense fast food by school-aged children.

The health implications of the built environment have become increasingly important in this highly urbanized society where the majority of the population's everyday experiences are dominated by human-built elements. Cumulative scientific evidence now lets us believe that the built environment does and can make people sick. It does so by exposing people to toxins and hazards. For example, proximity to high-volume streets has been shown to have a role on asthma diagnosis and hospitalization [44]. Recent trends in land use and infrastructure developments appear to foster unhealthy lifestyles such as poor diet and sedentary behaviors, as discussed earlier. Unfortunately, however, the exact mechanism through which the built environment interacts with human behaviors and health is not clearly understood.

Built environments are the physical settings for youth activities and development. Urban development patterns in the US since World War II have been dominated by automobile-oriented infrastructure with divided land uses. Urban landscapes have been shaped to make it easier for people to adopt unhealthy lifestyles than healthy ones. Young people are especially vulnerable to their surrounding environments, because they do not have control over the types of environment in which they live, learn, or play. Children have limited mobility due to their limited physical capacity and their lack of access to private automobiles. Therefore, the magnitude of impact by the given and proximal environments on children is much greater compared to that on adults with greater physical capacity and mobility options.

Equity in School Transportation

Elimination of health disparity is one of the two overarching goals in Healthy People 2010 [45]. The burden of chronic diseases is not equally distributed among different subpopulations. Among the many alarming facts, up to 80% of Hispanic populations are overweight or obese and they are twice as likely to have diabetes than non-Hispanic whites [46]. Type 2 diabetes is the most common comorbidity of obesity among children, estimated to result in the reduction of 15 to 27 years in life expectancy [47], and undiagnosed cases are much more prevalent among minorities than among whites [48]. Over 38% of Hispanics with diagnosed diabetes do not have any healthcare coverage, compared with only 12.4% for whites and 19.8% for African Americans [48]. Hispanics and African Americans, as well as those living in rural and underserved areas, tend to have much higher risks for being overweight or obese and have limited access to healthcare services [49]. The current cost of obesity, in Texas for example, is about $500 per person per year and is expected to double by 2040. Compared with those of normal weight, obese people spend 36% more for their healthcare and 77% more for their medication [50]. The economic burdens of obesity, diabetes, and other health problems are greater among those with lower socioeconomic status.

Physical activity levels differ across different population groups. Minorities, females, low-income groups, and rural residents report the highest rates of inactivity, and these differences emerge in early childhood [51,52]. About 50% of Hispanic and 47% of black adolescent females engage in regular vigorous physical activity, compared to 60% among white counterparts [53]. Females are generally less active than males. A study reported that only 36.3% of non-Hispanic black females and 42.3% of Hispanic females engaged in regular physical activity, compared to 49.7% among non-Hispanic whites [54]. Gender differences are also shown in environmental influences on outdoor physical activity. While distance to the closest open play area was important for boys, violent crime was a key consideration for girls [14]. In addition, rural residents are more sedentary according to leisure-time physical activity than urban residents, and they face more personal barriers to physical activity [52]. Rural children or adolescents walk or cycle less than their urban counterparts [55] and are more likely to be obese or overweight [56]. Another key factor is income, which is often strongly correlated with ethnicity and education. Residents of low-income neighborhoods were 36% less likely to be vigorously active than were those from high-income areas [35]. Children from lower income families were more likely to be inactive and overweight [35,57]. Lower income neighborhoods were generally perceived less walkable, and students from lower-income schools consumed more baked foods, chips, sodas, and candies, compared to those from higher income neighborhoods [58]. They also spent more time watching television and sitting in front of the computer [58]. Another study conducted in Cincinnati, Ohio, reported that poverty rate among young children was positively associated with proximity to fast food restaurants [59].

While health problems, especially those related to physical inactivity, are more common among minority and low-income populations, their access to physical activity resources tends to be more limited [60]. Even if these resources are available, they often suffer from poor quality and maintenance, crime and gang activities, and pollution [61-63]. It should be noted that the issues of disparity are related to multiple, interrelated dimensions, including socioeconomic and environmental dimensions. For example, while children in inner-city or lower income communities may rely more on freely available public parks and streets for their outdoor play activities [64], the availability and the quality of such facilities in these communities are usually far worse than those available in higher-income, suburban neighborhoods. Consequently, inner-city children are shown to report lower levels of physical activity [57] and higher rates of obesity. Further, children from low-income and minority communities are more likely to suffer from poor pedestrian infrastructure conditions and safety problems [65], but may be forced to walk because they are deprived of other mobility options. Lower income parents are more likely to report unpleasant walking conditions and to perceive dangers from crime, drug dealers, and violence [66]. Schools with high percentage of low-income or minority students were exposed to more traffic, which can increase exposure to polluted air and traffic dangers [67].

In general, empirical studies on the environmental or spatial disparities related to health and physical activity behaviors are limited [68]. Most existing studies focus on simple comparisons of prevalence rates among different income, age, gender, or ethnic groups. Further, the different attitude and perceptions toward walking and physical activity across different subgroups should be considered. Bostock states that while utilitarian physical activity such as walking is encouraged for everyone as healthful activity, the reality of people's daily living may tell a different story [69]. For instance, for mothers with young children from low-income families who have no other means to run daily errands, walking will come with the added pressure and labor demand, performed in deprived, unsafe, and polluted environments. In cases like this, the mental stress and physical fatigue, as well as increased risks for respiratory diseases, may outweigh the benefits of walking as healthy exercise.

Correlates of Walking and Biking to School

A limited but growing body of literature has explored the multilevel correlates of walking and biking to school behaviors, including personal, social, and physical environmental factors (see table 1). Although it is too early to draw conclusions on exactly what variables play what roles, some important patterns are discovered from the literature. In general, smaller and more compact neighborhood schools located centrally in neighborhoods that have safe and connected street system appear supportive of students' walking and biking to school. Kouri's work found that older schools (built before 1983), which were primarily small neighborhood schools, had four times more students walking to school, compared to newer schools [71]. The related issue of school siting emerged as a key factor predicting the travel distance and mode choice [70]. Contradictory to what is shown to be desirable for walking and biking, current trend in school developments, however, shows a pattern toward larger schools farther away from the students' homes. These schools are often located near high-volume arterials and highways, making it unsafe or even impossible to walk or bike to school.

Personal correlates of walking or biking to school are many. Overall, boys are more likely to walk or bike to school than are girls [72-75]. Younger elementary school children walked more than older elementary school students in two US studies [73,74]. However, another Australian study reported a reverse association [75] and a few other studies reported insignificant results [72,76,77]. It appears that Hispanic and African American children and children with lower socioeconomic status walk more [72,78,79], but, again, insignificant results have also been reported [73,74, 77]. Parents' education levels were insignificant in four studies [72-74,76]. The child's level of independence, the parents' perceived benefits of active commuting, and having the father as the responsible parent had a positive correlation with walking or biking to school [75]. In contrast, convenience of driving was a negative factor [74]. Other factors such as parents' marital status [73,75] and car ownership [75,77,78,80] have yielded inconsistent results.

A growing number of studies have shed light on the environmental attributes that may encourage or deter children to walk or bike to school (see table 1). These variables cover the environmental attributes at both the larger neighborhood level and the detailed microscale level. First of all, distance and safety are definitely two of the most important environmental correlates of walking or biking to school. In a national survey by the Centers for Disease Control and Prevention (CDC), parents reported long distances, traffic dangers, and crime as the topmost barriers to walking to school [81]. Empirical studies have also confirmed the importance of both objective and perceived measures of distance and safety. For walkable distances, studies report about one-half to one mile (0.8-1.6 km) between home and school to be the maximum threshold for walking to school [74,75,77,82], although this threshold will likely vary depending on the children's personal characteristics and the environmental conditions. Safety concerns were related to traffic and crime, and the parents' perceptions played especially significant roles [74-76]. While the actual crash rates have declined over the years, the perceived fear of traffic crashes has not. The CDC survey found that about one third of the parents reported traffic danger to be a barrier to walking to school [81]. Along the same line, fear of abduction seems to encourage automobile use for school transportation [83,84].

Sidewalk and other street characteristics have significant impacts on walking or biking to school, although insignificant results have also been reported (see table 1). These factors include sidewalk and bike lane availability, sidewalk continuity, traffic signals, street crossings, slope, and lighting [73,78,80,82,85,86]. While the majority of the previous studies are cross-sectional, a small number of longitudinal studies identified certain environmental interventions to be effective, including sidewalk gap closures at locations with moderate or heavy pre-existing walking/biking traffic and the replacement of four-way stops with traffic signals [85,86].

Compared with the roles of distance, safety, and infrastructure conditions, the influence of neighborhood characteristics such as density, land use, and street patterns appeared somewhat weaker with less consistent results [77-80]. Neighborhood locations in rural areas were found to be negatively correlated with active school travel, consistent with findings from the physical activity literature [73]. Table 1 shows that the research on built environmental correlates on walking or biking to school behaviors is a work in progress, with inconsistent results and missing variables. Also lacking are systematic comparisons between objective and perceptual measures and investigation into the interrelations between different environmental factors as well as between environmental and personal factors.

Table 1. Built environmental correlates of walking or biking to school

Class	Variable	Measure Type[a]	Association[b]	Source
Travel Distance	Travel time (distance)	O, PP	(−)	[74, 75, 77, 78, 80-82, 87]
	Route directness	O	(×)	[77]
	Route directness for 5-6 year old	O	(×)	[82]
	Route directness for 9-12 year old	O	(−)	[82]
Safety	Neighborhood safety for child to	PP	(×)	[74]
	walk/bike to/from school alone	PP	(−)	[88]
	Neighborhood safety for playing	CP	(×)	[73]
	Safety concerns	PP	(−)	[76]
	Safety concerns about strangers	PP, CP	(×)	[82]
	Crime	PP	(−)	[81]
	Traffic dangers	PP, CP	(×)	[82]
		PP	(−)	[75, 81]
School	School size (enrollment)	O	(−)	[79]
		O	(×)	[78, 80, 87]
	Age of school (built before 1983]	O	(+)	[89]
	School locations (urban vs. suburban)	O	(×)	[18]
School Environment	Population density	O	(+)	[79]
	(Residents + jobs) density	O	(×)	[78, 80, 87]
	Land-use mix	O	(×)	[78, 80, 87, 88]
	Abandoned buildings in surroundings	O	(+)	[88]
	Windows facing streets in surroundings	O	(×)	[88]
Roadway Conditions	Intervention: replacing 4-way stops with traffic signals	O	(+)	[85, 86]
	Intersection density	O	(+)	[77]
		O	(×)	[79]
	Dead end density	O	(−)	[77]
	Street width	O	(+)	[88]
	Block length	O	(×)	[88]
	Speed humps	O	(×)	[88]
	Street lighting	O	(−)	[88]
	No light/crossings	PP	(−)	[82]
	Street tree coverage	O	(×)	[78, 87]

Class	Variable	Measure Type[a]	Association[b]	Source
Non-Motorized Facility	Interventions: sidewalk gap closures	O	(+)	[85, 86]
	Interventions: new sidewalks and sidewalk gap closure	O	(+)	[85, 86]
	Interventions: crossing improvement	O	(×)	[85, 86]
	Interventions: development of bicycle facility in areas with low pre-existing bicycle travel	O	(×)	[86]
	Sidewalk coverage	O	(×)	[88]
		O	(+)	[78, 80, 87]
	Bike lane or paved shoulder coverage	O	(×)	[78, 80, 87]
Neighborhood	Neighborhood locations in central cities, suburbs, or small cities/towns vs. rural areas	PP	(+)	[73]
	Neighborhood locations in urban vs. suburban areas	O	(×)	[88]
	Neighborhood aesthetics	PP	(+)	[76]
	Access to local stores (within 20-min walk)	PP	(+)	[76]
	Access to biking/walking facilities	PP	(+)	[76]
	Walkability in high-income neighborhood	O	(+)	[76]
	Walkability in low-income neighborhood	O	(×)	[76]
Barriers	High-speed road barriers (> 30 mph)	PP	(–)	[88]
	Major road barriers	O	(×)	[77]
	Busy road barriers	O	(–)	[82]
	Railroad track barriers	O	(–)	[77]
	Steep road barriers for 5-6 year old	O	(–)	[82]
	Steep road barriers for 9-12 year old	O	(×)	[82]
	Need to cross several roads	PP	(×)	[82]
	Limited public transport	PP	(×)	[82]
	Not having many other children around	PP	(–)	[82]
Others	Multi-level interventions including engineering improvement	O	(+)	[90]

[a] O, objective measures; PP, parents' perceptions; CP, children's perceptions

[b] (+), positive association; (–), negative association; (×), no association with walking or biking to school

Discussion

This chapter discussed several important public health and social equity issues related to school transportation and the roles of the built environment. Existing literature was reviewed identifying specific environmental correlates of walking or biking to school behaviors and confirming the importance of the built environment in promoting or detering these behaviors. It should be noted that this paper did not review exhaustively all published literature on this topic, and focused on selected empirical studies published in peer-reviewed journals. The scope of the reviews and discussions in this paper was to cover the broad categories of themes emerged from the literature. Despite these limitations, several important findings are emerged from the literature reviewed in this paper and major gaps in the current knowledge on this topic are identified.

First, school siting is the foremost important factor in assessing walkability because it determines the distance that students have to travel and therefore the mode choice. It is clearly shown that beyond certain distance thresholds (between one half to one mile), walking is not considered a viable travel option. Parallel to the strategies to promote locating or keeping schools near residential neighborhoods and urban centers, policies such as minimum acreage requirements and financial incentives for new school constructions require re-examination.

Second, along with distance, safety is another key factor in children's school transportation. A national survey reported that traffic-related dangers were the second most common barriers reported by parents of 5- to 18-year-old children, followed by distance [81]. Although other previous studies reported some inconsistency in the roles of safety [76,82, 88], safety still demands full attention in both research and promotion efforts. The "perception" of safety, rather than the factual crime or crash data, and the "perception" of physical barriers, such as high-volume and high-speed roadways and unsafe street crossings, seem crucial. Findings suggest that several improvements in the built environment may contribute to increase safety perceptions, including traffic-calming devices, signalized crossings, continuous sidewalks, and increased surveillance in areas around schools and along the major home-to-school routes. It is encouraging that most of these interventions are considered feasible. However, comprehensive cost-benefit analyses of these options, considering both the short-term and the long-term costs and benefits, seem necessary to guide future research and intervention efforts.

Third, school transportation has potentially significant equity implications. We know that people of lower socioeconomic status walk more for transportation purposes, but they do so in poorly maintained and unsafe environments. Green and colleagues found that schools with higher percentage of minority and low-income students are exposed to more traffic and air pollution when they walk to school [67]. Many advocates are promoting walking and walkable communities, as a way to incorporate healthy physical activities into people's daily routines and to reduce reliance on automobiles. However, walking for children and for lower income populations may not be perceived positively as a healthful activity but rather as a socially stigmatized activity for persons of lower socioeconomic status who do not own a car [69]. This is especially true when they are forced, rather than they choose, to walk. For certain populations, walking can add significantly to the already intensive labor demand of their job or other daily burdens. Cumulative findings suggest that the environments where people do walk are less safe and less walkable than the environments where people do not walk. Future research and promotion efforts should consider social equity aspects related to walking or biking to school behaviors.

Fourth, this review identified multi-level factors associated with walking or biking to school, confirming that school transportation is not an independent individual choice but is decided by multiple household-related and environmental characteristics. Among the non-environmental factors, parental characteristics were found to be the key determinants of children's school transportation. Future promotion efforts can be more effective if they target parents as well as children. Also importantly, more research is needed to understand the complicated interactions among the environmental, policy, and personal (children and family) factors that influence children's school transportation. Further, the literature showed that the necessary conditions required for children to be able to walk or bike to school vary depending on the characteristics the students and their parents. A study by Kerr et al. showed that the objectively measured walkability of a neighborhood was important in high-income neighborhoods but not in low-income neighborhoods [76]. Future efforts targeting active commuting to school should consider the different needs of and concerns for the specific target students and parents.

Several additional gaps in the previous literature are identified from this review. More work is needed to understand diverse environmental settings (e.g., urban, suburban, and rural settings) and the differences in the roles of specific environmental features in school transportation behaviors. Further, what and how different environmental conditions influence school travels across different groups of children (e.g., by age, gender, ethnicity, and income) are still unclear. From the methodological perspective, many school transportation-environment research remains descriptive or observational. Longitudinal experimental research necessary to investigate causal relationships is rare in this area of research, because of the technical difficulty and ethical concerns involving children. Boarnet further suggests that children represent an important population for studying environment-physical activity relationships because they do not select where to live, and therefore the problem of self-selection bias is resolved or reduced [91]. Although truly experimental research is not feasible, quasi-experimental studies can be designed, which can add valuable insights into the currently fragmented picture in understanding school transportation behaviors.

Conclusions

Boarnet's studies are two of the few such studies that we found, and more longitudinal studies are needed, perhaps taking advantage of the natural experiments (intervention programs) that are being increasingly planned [85, 86]. Finally, future research should also consider the additional roles of streets as venues for play activities for children, especially those who do not have parks or private yards to play in.

Despite the growing number of empirical studies on this topic, this area of research is still in its early stage of development with many questions waiting to be answered. The "what" questions relating to correlates are beginning to be revealed, but the "why" and "how" questions about school travel choices remain largely unanswered.

References

[1] Centers for Disease Control and Prevention Physical activity and health: A report of the Surgeon General. Atlanta, GA: CDC, 1996.

[2] Swinburn B, Egger G, Raza F. Dissecting obesogenic environments: The development and application of a framework for identifying and prioritizing environmental interventions for obesity. Prev Med 1999;29:563-70.

[3] Taylor WC, Sallis JF. Determinants of physical activity in children. In: Simopolous AP, Pavlou KN, eds. Nutrition and fitness: Metabolic and behavioral aspects in health and disease. World Rev Food Nutr 1997;82:159-67.

[4] Ellefsen KA. Physical activity as a moderator of life stress in elementary school children. Dissertation Abstr Int Section A: Humanities Soc Sci 1998;59: 0417.

[5] Cheatum BA, Hammond AA. Physical activities for improving children's learning and behavior: A guide to sensory motor development. Champaign, IL: Human Kinetics, 2000.

[6] Moore RC. Streets as playgrounds. New York, NY: Van Nostrand Reinhold, 1987.

[7] Loukaitou-Sideris A. Children in Los Angeles parks: A study of equity, quality and children satisfaction with neighborhood parks. Cleveland, OH: Assoc Coll Schools Planning, 2001.

[8] Sallis JF, Patterson TL, McKenzie TL, Nader PR. Family variables and physical-activity in preschool-children. J Dev Behav Pediatrics 1988;9: 57-61.

[9] Centers for Disease Control and Prevention. Kids walk-to-school then and now: Barriers and solutions. Atlanta, GA: CDC, 2007.

[10] Duke J, Huhman M, Heitzler C. Physical activity levels among children aged 9-13 years, United States, 2002. MMWR 2003;52: 785-8.

[11] Sallis JF, Prochaska JJ, Taylor WC. A review of correlates of physical activity of children and adolescents. Med Sci Sports Exercise 2000;32: 963-75.

[12] Telama R, Yang XL. Decline of physical activity from youth to young adulthood in Finland. Med Sci Sports Exercise 2000;32:1617-22.

[13] Centers for Disease Control and Prevention. Kids walk-to-school: A guide to promote walking to school. Atlanta, GA: CDC, 2007.

[14] Gomez JE, Johnson BA, Selva M, Sallis JF. Violent crime and outdoor physical activity among inner-city youth. Prev Med 2004;39: 876-81.

[15] Bull FC, Milligan R, Rosenberg M, MacGowan H. Physical activity levels of western Australian adults 1000. Perth: Health Dept Western Aust, 2000.

[16] Lee C, Moudon AV. Physical activity and environment research in the health field: Implications for urban and transportation planning practice and research. J Plan Literature 2004;19:147-81.

[17] Cooper AR, Andersen LB, Wedderkopp N, Page AS, Froberg K. Physical activity levels of children who walk, cycle, or are driven to school. Am J Prev Med 2005;29: 179-84.
[18] Sirard JR, Riner WF, McIver KL, Pate RR. Physical activity and active commuting to elementary school. Med Sci Sports Exercise 2005;37:2062-9.
[19] Pucher J, Dijkstra L. Promoting safe walking and cycling to improve public health: Lessons from the Netherlands and Germany. Am J Public Health 2003;93:1509-16.
[20] Litman TA. Economic values of walkability. Transport Res Record 2003:1828.
[21] Owen N, Bauman A. The descriptive epidemiology of a sedentary life-style in adult Australians. Int J Epidemiol 1992;21:305-10.
[22] Dunn AL, Marcus BH, Kampert JB, Garcia ME, Kohl HW, Blair SN. Comparison of lifestyle and structured interventions to increase physical activity and cardiorespiratory fitness - A randomized trial. JAMA 1999;281:327-34.
[23] Sevick MA, Dunn MS, Morrow BH, Marcus GJ, Chen SN. Cost-effectiveness of lifestyle and structured exercise interventions in sedentary adults: Results of project ACTIVE. Am J Prev Med 2000;19:1-8.
[24] Frank LD, Sallis JF, Conway TL, Chapman JE, Sealens BE, Willians B. Many pathways from land use to health: Associations between neighborhood walkability and active transportation, body mass index, and air quality. J Am Plan Assoc 2006;72:75-87.
[25] Ulrich RS. Visual landscape and psychological well being. Landscape Res 1979;4: 17-23.
[26] Kaplan R, Kaplan S. The experience of nature: A psychological perspective. Cambridge, MA: Cambridge Univ Press, 1989.
[27] Pollock ML, Wilmore JH, Fox III SM. Health and fitness through physical activity. New York: Wiley, 1978.
[28] LaCroix AZ, Leveille SG, Hecht JA, Grothaus LC, Wagner EH. Does walking decrease the risk of cardiovascular disease hospitalizations and death in older adults? J Am Geriatr Soc 1996;44: 120.
[29] Oja P, Vuori I, Paronen O. Daily walking and cycling to work: Their utility as health-enhancing physical activity. Patient Educ Counseling 1998;33(Suppl 1): S87-94.
[30] Sesso HD, Paffenbarger RS, Ha T, Lee IM. Physical activity and cardiovascular disease risk in middle-aged and older women. Am J Epidemiol 1999;150:408-16.
[31] Sallis JF, Kraft K, Linton LS. How the environment shapes physical activity. A transdisciplinary research agenda. Am J Prev Med 2002;22:208.
[32] World Health Organization. A physically active life through everyday transport: With special focus on children and older people with examples and approaches from Europe. Copenhagen: WHO, 2002.
[33] Brownson RC, Housemann RA, Brown DR, Jackson-Thompson J, King AC, et al. Promoting physical activity in rural communities: Walking trail access, use, and effects. Am J Prev Med 2000;18:235-41.
[34] Cervero R, Ewing R. Travel and the built environment. A synthesis. Transport Res Record 2001:1780.

[35] Giles-Corti B, Donovan RJ. Socioeconomic status differences in recreational physical activity levels and real and perceived access to a supportive physical environment. Prev Med 2002;35:601-11.

[36] Handy SL, Boarnet MG, Ewing R, Killingsworth RE. How the built environment affects physical activity: Views from urban planning. Am J Prev Med 2002;23:64-73.

[37] Cervero R, Duncan M. Walking, bicycling and urban landscapes: Evidence from the San Francisco Bay Area. Am J Public Health 2003;93:1478-83.

[38] Humpel N, Owen N, Iverson D, Leslie E, Bauman A. Perceived environment attributes, residential location, and walking for particular purposes. Am J Prev Med 2004;26:119-25.

[39] Frank LD, Schmid TL, Sallis JF, Chapman J, Sealens BE. Linking objectively measured physical activity with objectively measured urban form: Findings from SMARTRAQ. Am J Prev Med 2005;28:117-25.

[40] Lee C, Moudon AV. Correlates of walking for transportation or recreation purposes. J Phys Activity Health 2006;3:S77-98.

[41] Moudon AV, Lee C, Cheadle AD, Garvin C, Johnson DB, et al. Attributes of environments supporting walking. Am J Health Promot 2007;21:448-59.

[42] Helling A, Sawicki D. Race and residential accessibility to shopping and services," Housing Policy Debate 2003;14: 69-101.

[43] Austin SB, Melly SJ, Sanchez BN, Patel A, Buka S, Gortmaker SL. Clustering of fast-food restaurants around schools: A novel application of spatial statistics to the study of food environments. Am J Public Health 2005;95:1575-81.

[44] Edwards J, Walters S, Griffiths RK. Hospital admissions for asthma in preschool-children. Relationship to major roads in Birmingham, United-Kingdom. Arch Environmental Health 1994;49:223-7.

[45] US Department of Health and Human Services. Healthy people 2010: Understanding and improving health, Washington, DC: US Gov Printing Office, 2000.

[46] Cowie C, Rust K, Byrd-Holt D, Eberhardt M, Flegal K, et al. Prevalence of diabetes and impaired fasting glucose in adults in the US Population: National Health and Nutrition Examination Survey 1999-2002. Diabetes Care 2006;29:1263-8.

[47] Panzram G. Mortality and survival in type 2 (non-insulin dependent) diabetes mellitus. Diabetologia 1987;30:123-31.

[48] Texas Diabetes Council. The changing face of diabetes: A plan to prevent and control diabetes in Texas 2006-2007. Austin, TX: Texas Dept State Health Serv, Texas Diabetes Council, 2007.

[49] Tai-Seale T, Chandler C. Nutrition and overweight concerns in rural areas: A literature review. Rural Healthy People 2010: A companion document to healthy people 2010. College Station, TX: Texas A&M Univ System Health Sci Center, School Rural Public Health, Southwest Rural Health Research Center, 2003.

[50] Statewide Obesity Taskforce. Strategic plan for the prevention of obesity in Texas. Austin, TX: Texas Dept Health Bureau Nutr Serv, 2003.

[51] Crespo CJ, Smit E, Andersen RE, Carter-Pokras O, Ainsworth BE. Race/ethnicity, social class and their relation to physical inactivity during leisure time: results from

the Third National Health and Nutrition Examination Survey, 1988-1994. Am J Prev Med 2000;18: 46-53.

[52] Wilcox S, Castro C, King AC, Housemann R, Brownson RC. Determinants of leisure time physical activity in rural compared with urban older and ethnically diverse women in the United States. J Epidemiol Community Health 2000;54: 667-72.

[53] Gordon-Larsen P, McMurray RG, Popkin BM. Adolescent physical activity and inactivity vary by ethnicity: The National Longitudinal Study of Adolescent Health," J Pediatrics 1999;135:301-6.

[54] Kruger J, Yore M, Solera M, Moeti R. Prevalence of fruit and vegetable consumption and physical activity by race/ethnicity United States, 2005. JAMA 2007;297:2072-4.

[55] Sjolie AN, Thuen F. School journeys and leisure activities in rural and urban adolescents in Norway. Health Promot Int 2002;17:21-30.

[56] Lewis RD, Meyer MC, Lehman SC, Trowbridge FL, Bason JJ, et al.. Prevalence and degree of childhood and adolescent overweight in rural, urban, and suburban Georgia. J Sch Health 2006;76:126-32.

[57] Lee RE, Cubbin C. Neighborhood context and youth cardiovascular health behaviors. Am J Public Health 2002;92: 428-36.

[58] Merchant AT, Dehghan M, Behnke-Cook D, Anand SS. Diet, physical activity, and adiposity in children in poor and rich neighborhoods: A cross-sectional comparison. Nutr J 2007;6:1.

[59] Burdette HL, Whitaker RC. Neighborhood playgrounds, fast food restaurants, and crime: relationships to overweight in low-income preschool children. Prev Med 2004;38:57-63.

[60] Estabrooks PA, Lee RE, Gyurcsik NC. Resources for physical activity participation: does availability and accessibility differ by neighborhood socioeconomic status? Ann Behav Med 2003;25:100-4.

[61] Shakoor BH, Chalmers D. Co-victimization of African-American children who witness violence. Effects on cognitive, emotional, and behavioral-development. J Natl Med Assoc 1991;83:233-8.

[62] Bullard RD. Environmental justice: It's more than waste facility siting. Soc Sci Quart 1996;77:493-9.

[63] Rasmussen A, Aber MS, Bhana A. Adolescent coping and neighborhood violence: Perceptions, exposure, and urban youths' efforts to deal with danger. Am J Community Psychol 2004;33:61-75.

[64] Loukaitou-Sideris A. Urban form and social context: Cultural differentiation in the uses of urban parks. Plan Educ Res 1995;14:89-102.

[65] Zhu X, Lee C. Walkability and safety around elementary schools: Economic and ethnic disparities. Am J Prev Med 2008;34(4):282-90.

[66] Gielen AC, DeFrancesco S, Bishai D, Mahoney P, Ho S, Guyer B. Child pedestrians: the role of parental beliefs and practices in promoting safe walking in urban neighborhoods. J Urban Health Bul NY Acad Med 2004;81:545-55.

[67] Green RS, Smorodinsky S, Kim JJ, McLaughlin R, Ostro B. Proximity of California public schools to busy roads. Environ Health Perspect 2004;112:61-6.

[68] Northridge ME, Stover GN, Rosenthal JE, Sherard D. Environmental equity and health: Understanding complexity and moving forward. Am J Public Health 2003;93: 209-14.

[69] Bostock L. Pathways of disadvantage? Walking as a mode of transport among low-income mothers. Health Soc Care Community 2001;9:11-8.

[70] Ewing R, Forinash CV, Schroeer W. Neighborhood schools and sidewalk connections: What are the impacts on travel mode choice and vehicle emissions? Transport Res News 2005;237:4-10.

[71] Kouri C. Wait for the bus: How Lowcountry school site selection and design deter walking to school and contribute to urban sprawl. Durham, NC: South Carolina Coastal Conservation League, Duke Univ Terry Sanford Inst Public Policy, 1999.

[72] Evenson KR, Huston SL, McMillen BJ, Bors P, Ward DS. Statewide prevalence and correlates of walking and bicycling to school. Arch Pediatr Adolesc Med 2003;157: 887-92.

[73] Fulton JE, Shisler JL, Yore MM, Caspersen CJ. Active transportation to school: Findings from a national survey. Res Quart Exerc Sport 2005;76:352-7.

[74] McMillan T, Day K, Boarnet M, Alfonzo M, Anderson C. Johnny walks to school. Does Jane? Sex differences in children's active travel to school. Children Youth Environ 2006;16:75-89.

[75] Merom D, Tudor-Locke C, Bauman A, Rissel C. Active commuting to school among NSW primary school children: implications for public health. Health Place 2006;12: 678-87.

[76] Kerr J, Rosenberg D, Sallis JF, Saelens BE, Frank LD, Conway TL. Active commuting to school: Associations with environment and parental concerns. Med Sci Sports Exerc 2006;38:787-94.

[77] Schlossberg M, Greene J, Phillips PP, Johnson B, Parker B. School trips. Effects of urban form and distance on travel mode. J Am Plan Assoc 2006;72:337-46.

[78] Ewing R, Schroeer W, Greene W. School location and student travel. Analysis of factors affecting mode choice. Transport Res Record 2004;1895:55-63.

[79] Braza M, Shoemaker W, Seeley A. Neighborhood design and rates of walking and biking to elementary school in 34 California communities. Am J Health Promot 2004;19:128-36.

[80] Environmental Protection Agency. Travel and environmental implications of school sitting. Washington, DC: US Environ Protect Agency, 2003.

[81] Martin S, Carlson S. Barriers to children walking to or from school - United States, 2004. JAMA 2005;294:2160-2.

[82] Timperio A, Ball K, Salmon J, Roberts R, Giles-Corti B, et al. Personal, family, social, and environmental correlates of active commuting to school. Am J Prev Med 2006;30:45-51.

[83] Eichelberger MR, Gotschall CS, Feely HB, Harstad P, Bowman LM. Parental attitudes and knowledge of child safety. A National Survey. Am J Dis Child 1990;144:714-20.

[84] DiGuiseppi C, Roberts I, Li L, Allen D. Determinants of car travel on daily journeys to school: cross sectional survey of primary school children. BMJ 1998;316:1426-8.

[85] Boarnet MG, Anderson CL, Day K, McMillan T, Alfonzo M. Evaluation of the California safe routes to school legislation. Urban form changes and children's active transportation to school. Am J Prev Med 2005;28:134-40.
[86] Boarnet MG, Day K, Anderson C, McMillan T, Alfonzo M. California's safe routes to school program. Impacts on walking, bicycling, and pedestrian safety. J Am Plan Assoc 2005;71:301-17.
[87] Ewing R, Forinash CV, Schroeer W. Neighborhood schools and sidewalk connections: What are the impacts on travel mode choice and vehicle emissions? Transport Res News 2005;237:4-10.
[88] McMillan TE. Walking and urban form: Modeling and testing parental decisions about children's travel. Irvine, CA: Dept Urban Regional Plan, Univ of California, 2003.
[89] Kouri C. Wait for the bus: How Lowcountry school site selection and design deter walking to school and contribute to urban sprawl. Durham, NC: South Carolina Coastal Conservation League, Duke Univ Terry Sanford Inst Public Policy, 1999.
[90] Staunton CE, Hubsmith D, Kallins W. Promoting safe walking and biking to school: The Marin County success story. Am J Public Health 2003;93:1431-4.
[91] Boarnet MG. The built environment and physical activity: Empirical methods and data resources. Washington, DC: Transport Board and Inst Med, 2004.

In: Obesity and Adolescence: A Public Health Concern
Editors: H.A. Omar, D.E. Greydanus et al.
ISBN: 978-1-60692-821-9

Chapter XVIII

Obesity and Persons with Down Syndrome

Joav Merrick[1,2,*], Isack Kandel[1,3], Mohammed Morad[1,4], Jason Ahn[1,5] and Brian Seth Fuchs[1,5]

[1]National Institute of Child Health and Human Development, Office of the Medical Director, Division for Mental Retardation, Ministry of Social Affairs, Jerusalem, Israel, [2]Kentucky Children's Hospital, University of Kentucky, Lexington, United States of America, [3]Faculty of Social Sciences, Department of Behavioral Sciences, Ariel University Center of Samaria, Ariel, Israel, [4]Department of Family Medicine, Faculty of Health Sciences, Ben Gurion University of the Negev, Beer-Sheva, Israel and [5]Harvard Medical School, Boston, United States of America

Abstract

Obesity in childhood has particular concern, because if it continues into adulthood, the result will be increased morbidity and decreased life expectancy. An increase in obesity in the general population in the developed world has been documented in recent years. This trend is also seen in persons with intellectual disability and in particular in persons with Down syndrome (DS). Persons with DS are prone to obesity already at an early age and several studies have shown a high prevalence in this population compared to persons with intellectual disability without DS and the general population. Persons with DS have a low resting metabolic rate and low dietary intake of individual nutrients and therefore exercise and vitamin-mineral supplement diet must be instituted in this population to prevent or minimize obesity and its adverse consequences.

* Correspondence: Professor Joav Merrick, MD, MMedSci, DMSc, Medical Director, Division for Mental Retardation, Box 1260, IL-91012 Jerusalem, Israel. E-mail: jmerrick@zahav.net.il

Introduction

Obesity in childhood and adolescence presents a challenging and sometimes frustrating problem in clinical practice. Obesity is of particular concern, because of the health risk associated with it, such as hypertension, hyperlipidemia, hypertriglyceridemia, diabetes mellitus, coronary heart disease, pulmonary and renal problems, surgical risks and degenerative joint disease.

The prevalence of overweight among children and adolescents in the United States has increased between 1980 and 2004 [1]. Height and weight measurements were obtained from 8,165 children and adolescents as part of the 2003-2004 and 2005-2006 National Health and Nutrition Examination Survey (NHANES)[1]. During 2003-2006, 11.3% (95% confidence interval [CI], 9.7%-12.9%) of children and adolescents 2-19 years were at or above the 97th percentile of the 2000 BMI-for-age growth charts, 16.3% (95% CI, 14.5%-18.1%) were at or above the 95th percentile, and 31.9% (95% CI, 29.4%-34.4%) were at or above the 85th percentile.

Studies of Obesity in Persons with Intellectual Disability

Polednak and Auliffe in 1976 studied [2] 161 adults in an institution for people with intellectual disability (ID) in Canada (aged 18-73 years, 108 males, 53 females) and found that 20.4% of the males and 17.0% of the females were obese. The frequency of obesity was higher, but not statistically significant, in moderate ID than mild or severe ID. Burkart et al in 1985 [3] reviewed the literature and found that obesity was a prevalent problem in the population of persons with ID with a higher incidence among females than males.

A study from Northern Finland [4] in 1991 calculated the BMI at the age of 20 for all the 132 survivors (83%) out of the 159 persons born in that region with ID in 1966. Reliable information for 112 cases (84.8%) did not deviate significantly from the average Finnish population at age 20-29 years. 41.5% with mild ID (IQ 35-70) and 28.6% with severe ID (IQ less than 35) were of ideal weight (BMI 20-24), while 9.8% of all the persons studies were moderately obese (BMI greater than 30) and 7.1% severely obese (BMI greater than or equal to 32). 91% of the severe obese cases lived with their parents and did not participate in any occupational therapy or work. 29.5 % of the persons studied were underweight (BMI less than 20) and most of these cases were with severe ID.

Takeuchi [5] studied 20,031 pupils and students at special schools in Japan. The degree of obesity was computed as actual weight devided standard weight times 100. Standard weight was the average weight for the child's sex, age and height. 11.1% of males and 14.5% of females were obese and 2.5 % of males and 3.1% of females were severely obese.

Frey and Rimmer [6] studied 210 adults with ID residing in a residential setting in United States and one in Germany. Mean age was 31.7 years. Skinfold measurements were used to estimate percent body fat (PBF) and height and weight were used to compute BMI. PBF was significantly higher among females and persons in institutional settings had significantly lower BPF and BMI levels than persons in the family setting. PBF and BMI levels were significantly higher in persons from the United States than Germany.

Another study from Rimmer et al [7] studied 364 adults (mean age 36.8 years) from four residential settings (state institution, private community facility (ICF/MR), private group home and living with family) in Illinois. The rates of obesity were higher among females (58.8% versus 27.5%), persons with severe ID had the lowest overall rates of obesity (29.4% versus 53.2 for moderate and 46.5% for mild) and the institutional group had the lowest incidence of obesity (16.5%, 50.0% for ICF/MR, 40.9 % for group home and 55.3% for natural family). A total of 27.5% of males and 58.5% of females were obese, higher than the national data for the general population in the United States.

In a study from Israel [8]of persons with ID aged 40 years and older living in residential care centers (2,282 persons) we found that the mean BMI was 25.7 and 35% classied as overweight. 45.7% with mild ID, 45.1% with moderate, 27.1% with severe and 15% with profound ID had a BMI over 27.

A recent large study of of 1,119 adults with ID aged 20 years and older [9] from the United Kingdom Leicestershire Learning Disability Register, who participated in a programme of universal health checks and home interviews with their carers, looked at weight and hight and compared the observed and expected prevalences of body mass index categories in the ID and general populations using indirect standardisation for age. They found [9] in those aged 25 years and older, that the standardised morbidity ratio (SMR) for obesity was 0.80 (95% CI 0.64-1.00) in men and 1.48 (95% CI 1.23-1.77) in women. The SMR for underweight was 8.44 (95% CI 6.52-10.82) in men and 2.35 (95% CI 1.72-3.19) in women. Among those aged 20 years and older, crude prevalences were 20.7% for obesity, 28.0% for overweight, 32.7% for normal weight and 18.6% for underweight. Obesity was associated with living independently or with family, ability to feed/drink unaided, being female, hypertension, Down syndrome and the absence of cerebral palsy.

From the above studies it seems that a disproportionate high number of persons with ID display obesity and especially females. It also seems that living arrangements and environment plays an important role in obesity rates for this population.

Studies of Obesity in Persons with Down Syndrome

A study Children's Hospital in Philadelphia [10] on 730 children with Down syndrome (DS) showed a tendency to overweight beginning in late infancy and throughout the remainder of the growing years. The percentage of children with overweight increased to 50 % of the girls by the third year of life and 50 % of the boys by early childhood. The percentage of children, who were overweight fluctuated to 18 years, but the percentage above the 85th percentile of weight per height always was greater than 30 %.

A study from Australia [11] determined the resting metabolic rate of children with DS living at home (11 males, 7 females aged 10-14 years) and found a depressed rate compared to normal values for children of similar age. These findings seems to support the theory of "metabolic sluggishness" as a contributing factor to the etiology of obesity in children with

DS and therefore a nutritional energy-controlled diet with daily physical activity could work against obesity in DS.

Bell and Bhate [12] from Northumberland in the United Kingdom studied 183 adult persons (58 with DS) with ID living in the community. They found that 70.58% of males and 95.83% of females with DS and 49.29 % males and 62.96 % females with non-DS retardation were overweight and obese compared to 40% of males and 32% of females from the general population.

A study from the University of Illinois at Chicago [13] with 283 adults with Down syndorme (146 males, 137 females, aged 15-69 years) living with family or group home found that 45% of males and 56% of females were overweight with BMI levels higher in the family setting than at the group homes.

A Japanese study from 2000 [14] with 325 school children with Down syndrome aged 6-18 years showed obesity for the children with DS compared to the average Japanese child (34.3% and 7.47% respectively). Obesity started to increase in the obese group around age 7 year and the obese group tended to have greater intake of sweets, juice and total foods in their preschool days, but unexpectedly had been physically more active in their primary school days.

A detailed method was used to identify all adults with ID in Leicestershire, United Kingdom [15], which included medical examination and measurement of height and weight. For each person with Down syndrome, an individual matched for gender, age and accommodation type was identified. Data was obtained for 247 matched pairs and it was found that women with Down syndrome had lower mean height and weight, but greater mean BMI than the matched pairs. Men with Down syndrome had a lower mean height and weight, but there was no statistical difference in BMI compared to the matched pairs. Using World Health Organization categories of BMI, women with Down syndrome were more likely to be overweight or obese than their matched pairs (odds ratio=2.17). Men with Down syndrome were more likely to be in the overweight category than their matched pairs, but were less likely to be obese (odds ratio=0.85).

Looking at the physical activity of children with DS researchers from Wake Forest University School of Medicine in Winston Salem, NC, United States [16] studied 28 children with DS compared with their siblings ($n = 30$), between 3-10-years (mean +/- SD 7.1 +/- 2.1 years). Physical activity was measured over seven days. The children with DS were younger (6.6 vs. 7.1 years) and heavier (BMI 18.4 vs. 16.7) than their siblings ($p < 0.05$). Children with DS accumulated less vigorous-intensity activity than their siblings (49.5 vs. 68.6 minutes per day; $p = 0.04$) and for shorter bouts (2.5 vs. 5.1 minutes per bout; $p < 0.01$), but spent similar time in moderate physical activity and low-intensity physical activity. Physical activity should therefore be encouraged in this population from an early stage in life [16,17].

Conclusions

Obesity is a major public health problem in the population of persons with intellectual disability and especially in the persons with Down syndrome. Obesity limits the capacity of the child and adolescent with Down syndrome to participate in recreational and sports activities and obesity also have social adverse consequences. The management of obesity in children with DS is complicated due to their low resting metabolic rate and low dietary intake of individual nutrients, but exercise and a vitamin-mineral supplement diet should be efforts in the right direction to minimize obesity and its adverse effects.

References

[1] Ogden CL, Carroll MD, Flegal KM. High body mass index for age among US children and adolescents, 2003-2006. JAMA 2008;299(20):2401-5.

[2] Polednak AP, Auliffe J. Obesity in an institutionalised adult mentally retarded population. J Ment Defic Res 1976;20(1):9-15.

[3] Burkart JE, Fox RA, Rotatori AF. Obesity of mentally retarded individuals: prevalence, characteristics and intervention. Am J Ment Defic 1985;90(3):303-12.

[4] Simila S, Niskanen P. Underweight and overweight cases among the mentally retarded. J Ment Defic Res 1991;35(2):160-4.

[5] Takeuchi E. Incidence of obesity among school children with mental retardation in Japan. Am J Ment Retardation 1994;99(3):283-8.

[6] Frey B, Rimmer JH. Comparison of body composition between German and American adults with mental retardation. Med Sci Sports Exerc 1995;27(10):1439-43.

[7] Rimmer JH, Braddock D, Fujiura G. Prevalence of obesity in adults with mental retardation: Implications for health promotion and disease prevention. Ment Retardation 1995;31(2):105-10.

[8] Merrick J, Davidson PW, Morad M, Janicki MP, Wexler O, Henderson CM. Older adults with intellectual disability in residential care centers in Israel: health status and service utilization. Am J Ment Retard 2004;109(5):413-20.

[9] Bhaumik S, Watson JM, Thorp CF, Tyrer F, McGrother CW. Body mass index in adults with intellectual disability: distribution, associations and service implications: a population-based prevalence study. J Intellect Disabil Res 2008;52(Pt 4):287-98.

[10] Cronk C, Crocker AC, Pueschel SM, Shea AM, Zackai E, Pickens G, Reed RB. Growth charts for children with Down syndrome: 1 month to 18 years of age. Pediatrics 1988;81(1):102-10.

[11] Chad K, Jobling A, Frail H. Metabolic rate: A factor in developing obesity in children with Down syndrome ? Am J Ment Retardation 1990;95(2):228-35.

[12] Bell AJ, Bhate MS. Prevalence of overweight and obesity in Down syndrome and other mentally handicapped adults living in the community. J Intellect Disabil Res 1992:36(4):359-64.

[13] Rubin SS, Rimmer JH, Chicoine B, Braddock D, McGuire DE. Overweight prevalence in persons with Down syndrome. Ment Retardation 1998;36(3):175-81.

[14] Kawana H, Nonaka K, Takaki H, Tezuka F, Takano T. [Obesity and life style of Japanese school children with Down syndrome]. Nippon Koshu Eisei Zasshi 2000;47(1):87-94. [Japanese]

[15] Melville CA, Cooper SA, McGrother CW, Thorp CF, Collacott R. Obesity in adults with Down syndrome: a case-control study. J Intellect Disabil Res 2005;49(Pt 2):125-33.
[16] Whitt-Glover MC, O'Neill KL, Stettler N. Physical activity patterns in children with and without Down syndrome. Pediatr Rehabil 2006;9(2):158-64.
[17] Sayers Menear K. Parents' perceptions of health and physical activity needs of children with Down syndrome. Downs Syndr Res Pract 2007;12(1):60-8.

VII. International Aspects

In: Obesity and Adolescence: A Public Health Concern
Editors: H.A. Omar, D.E. Greydanus et al.
ISBN: 978-1-60692-821-9

Chapter XIX

Obesity: A Public Health Concern in Australia

Elizabeth Denney-Wilson, and Louise A. Baur*
Discipline of Paediatrics and Child Health, University of Sydney,
Sydney NSW 2006 Australia

Abstract

Adolescent obesity is a major public health problem in Australia, and in many other parts of the world. Recent data suggest that as many as one quarter of young people in Australia are either overweight or obese, and that the majority of obese young people have one or more risk factors for chronic disease. Efforts to reduce the health and economic burden of obesity must focus on both management of affected individuals and prevention of further cases. This chapter reviews some of the research currently underway in Australia, and includes recent data on both the prevalence of obesity and the associated complications, from large surveys and smaller cohorts. State and Federal governments have developed policies aimed at obesity prevention, but these are yet to be fully evaluated. Two large-scale community-based interventions are underway, one of which has reported positive preliminary findings. A number of smaller research programs are examining macro and individual level causation of obesity and include unique research examining the way adolescents perceive their environment. Other research includes the development and evaluation of service delivery models specifically targeting adolescents. A greater emphasis on environmental determinants and management of adolescent obesity is needed in future programs.

* Correspondence: Professor Louise A Baur, Clinical School, The Children's Hospital at Westmead, Locked Bag 4001, Westmead NSW 2145, Australia. Tel: 612-98453393; Fax: 612-98453389; E-mail: Louiseb3@chw.edu.au

Introduction

Despite a reputation as an active, sport-loving nation, Australians, including adolescents, have not escaped the obesity epidemic sweeping the world. Currently, more than 25% of adolescent boys and almost 20% of adolescent girls are either overweight or obese [1], with the prevalence of overweight having doubled, and that of obesity trebled, over the past twenty years [2,3]. This chapter summarises the current situation in Australia, in terms of epidemiology, causes, morbidity, clinical management and recent policy and research developments that include provision of funds for large scale community-based interventions. A number of challenges are evident: firstly, to develop strategies for prevention to reverse the current trends in obesity; and secondly, to provide clinical management appropriate for obese adolescents.

Measurement of Overweight

Body mass index (BMI; weight/height2) is a simple, cost-effective measure of body fatness for children, adolescents and adults [4]. Among adults, a person with a BMI of 25.00-29.99 kg/m2 is considered overweight, while those with a BMI >30.00 kg/m2 are classified as obese; cut-points that relate to the point at which health risks rise steeply, at least in adult European populations [5]. However, among adolescents there is insufficient evidence to provide an absolute definition of health-related overweight. BMI also varies dramatically with age and sex during development, rising in the first year, falling during preschool years, before then rising once more into adolescence. Therefore, the standard adult BMI cut-points cannot be used to define overweight or obesity in childhood or adolescence.

In 2000, the International Obesity Taskforce (IOTF) published a table of age- and sex - specific BMI cut-points for people aged <18 years which were based upon a compilation of nationally representative cross¬-sectional growth studies from a number of countries, and which relate to the adult cut-points of 25 kg/m2 and 30 kg/m2 [6]. An Australian expert committee has recommended that for epidemiological studies in children and adolescents, the BMI cut-points identified by the IOTF [6] be used to categorize individuals as being overweight, obese or not overweight or obese [7].

Epidemiology

The most recent national prevalence data on overweight and obesity in the Australian adolescent population were collected in 1995, however more recent data collections have occurred in NSW, Queensland and Western Australia. Other States have collected data on younger age groups [8], and yet other data are available from smaller studies.

In NSW, Australia's most populous State, the NSW Schools Physical Activity and Nutrition Survey (SPANS 2004) collected data on measured height, weight and waist circumference among over 5,000 students aged 5-16 years in early 2004 [9]. Table 1 shows the prevalence of overweight and obesity among adolescent boys and girls in school years 6, 8 and 10 with mean ages of 11.3, 13.3 and 15.3 years respectively [10]. The prevalence of both overweight and obesity was higher among boys than girls, with the exception of overweight prevalence in year 8 girls. Analysis of the trend in obesity prevalence from 1997-2004 among year 8 and 10 students found that the rate of increase is much higher in boys than girls: 0.94% per year compared with 0.27% per year [1]. While BMI increased among all socioeconomic status (SES) categories in the SPANS study, there is evidence of an inverse association between SES and BMI [10], although the difference between socioeconomic groups is not as great as that reported in the United States [11]. Earlier research has also found an inverse association between SES and BMI, waist circumference and waist-hip ratio [12] and SES and BMI and weight control practices [13] in Australian adolescents.

It is not just BMI that is increasing; Garnett et al measured 342 boys and girls based in western Sydney at age 7-8 and again five years later, and found that waist circumference had increased at a greater rate than BMI [14]. Waist circumference provides an indication of central adiposity (or abdominal fat), which is associated with adverse risk factors for cardiovascular disease and diabetes [15].

Causes of Overweight

Put simply, excess body fat accumulation primarily occurs when energy intake is greater than energy expenditure, but this must be examined within the context of changing food, family and physical activity environments. While genetic and biological factors make a major contribution to an individual's susceptibility to the development of obesity, unless the "correct" environmental conditions exist, an individual's genetic predisposition for obesity may not be fully expressed. The dramatic increase in obesity prevalence in recent decades highlights the central role of environmental change on the development of obesity. Some of these recent trends, as they affect adolescents, are highlighted below.

Table 1. Prevalence of overweight and obesity in boys and girls from the 2004 NSW Schools Physical Activity and Nutrition Survey [10]

	Boys			Girls		
	Year 6 (n= 483)	Year 8 (n=408)	Year 10 (n=555)	Year 6 (n= 496)	Year 8 (n=393)	Year 10 (n=415)
BMI Category*						
Not Overweight	68.4	73.7	73.5	76.6	76.2	81.2
Overweight	22.2	18.2	19.6	15.7	19.1	14.7
Obese	9.4	8.2	7.0	7.7	4.7	4.2

• BMI defined according to International Obesity Taskforce criteria [6]

Food Habits

Comparison of data from two National Nutrition Surveys conducted in 1985 and 1995 found that energy intake had increased by 12-15% in the adolescent age-group over the ten year period [16], and that more than 50% of total energy intake came from carbohydrate. Sugars (including fruit sugars) were the major source of carbohydrate [17].

Several studies suggested that soft drink consumption may contribute to excess energy intake and obesity in young people [18,19]. Soft drink and "fast food" are examples of energy dense food and beverages that are heavily marketed to adolescents [18,20,21]. Recent data from SPANS 2004 indicate that over one-half of boys and one-third of girls drink more than one cup of soft drink each day and 7-12% of boys drink more than one litre each day [10]. Not surprisingly, increasing consumption is associated with excess weight gain [18,22].

Soft drinks are very popular with adolescents who are at a life-stage where they experience increased autonomy, both in terms of availability of meals outside the home and discretionary income [23,24]. Taste preferences, parental (especially maternal) modelling, convenience, food availability (in the home, in school canteens and elsewhere) and relative cost may all play a role in influencing purchasing and consumption patterns [25-27].

Physical Activity

The way that adolescents or their parents perceive their environment may impact on their activity levels and weight status. In a study of adolescents aged 13 years in western Sydney, adolescents were more likely to walk or cycle if their parents perceived the area as being safe and as having good places for physical activity, or if the young people had friends living nearby or found the neighbourhood easy to get around [28]. Timperio and her colleagues found that 10-12 year olds in metropolitan Melbourne who perceived their environment as "safe" were more likely to walk and cycle in their area [29]. Further, the children of parents who were concerned about road safety were significantly more likely to be overweight or obese [30]. Thus, such factors as neighbourhood cohesion, safety and quality may be important predictors of adolescents' level of active transport and resilience to the development of obesity. In Australia, both walking and cycling to school have declined dramatically between 1985 and 2001 [31], and fewer than 20% of high school students reported walking and fewer than 3% of students regularly cycled to school in SPANS 2004 [10]. Okely and colleagues, however, compared self-reported physical activity among adolescents from 1985-2004 and found that the prevalence of participation in moderate to vigorous physical activity significantly increased in both boys and girls aged 13-16 years [10]. The authors acknowledge the potential weakness of self-report data [32].

Table 2. Prevalence of chronic disease risk factors in Year 10 boys and girls from the 2004 NSW Schools Physical Activity and Nutrition Survey [10]

	Boys			Girls		
	Year 6 (n= 483)	Year 8 (n=408)	Year 10 (n=555)	Year 6 (n= 496)	Year 8 (n=393)	Year 10 (n=415)
BMI Category*						
Not Overweight	68.4	73.7	73.5	76.6	76.2	81.2
Overweight	22.2	18.2	19.6	15.7	19.1	14.7
Obese	9.4	8.2	7.0	7.7	4.7	4.2

Sedentary Behaviors

Increases in sedentary behaviours, and in particular small screen recreation, are implicated in the increasing prevalence of obesity among adolescents. Hardy et al [33] found that Australian adolescents spend between 34 and 45 hours each week involved in such sedentary pastimes as small screen recreation, homework and other educational pursuits, travel and cultural and social activities. Another study [14] from western Sydney found that those children who watch more than two hours of television per day at age eight years were significantly more likely to be overweight or obese by early adolescence.

Consequences

Overweight and obese adolescents in Australia are afflicted with co-morbidities common to adolescents throughout the world. Recent data from the SPANS study indicate a very high prevalence of risk factors for cardiovascular disease, non-alcoholic fatty liver disease (NAFLD) and type 2 diabetes among the overweight and obese students [10] (see Table 2). Obese boys and girls were significantly more likely to have multiple risk factors [34].

Policy

The Australian Federal Government has developed a healthy weight strategy (Healthy Weight 2008) focussed upon young people and families that describes prevention strategies in multiple settings including food supply, marketing, primary care and schools. The program was launched in 2004, has been only partially implemented and has not been formally evaluated; the impact on adolescents cannot be estimated. State governments, with responsibility for government schools, have implemented healthy school canteen policies that include bans on soft drinks within the school environment. An evaluation of the NSW School Canteen strategy indicated that more than 98% of school canteen managers had adopted all or some of the program in the first year of implementation [35]. Other environmental strategies that may potentially enhance the adolescent's food and physical activity environment, including bans on food marketing, pricing structures that favour healthy food and availability of safe active transport options, have not been addressed in the Australian context.

Community-Based Interventions

Two large scale community-based obesity prevention trials are underway: one in the Barwon-South Western region of Victoria [36] and the other in the Hunter-New England region of New South Wales [37]. Both trials have received substantial funding from their respective State governments and represent an opportunity to develop multiple strategies for obesity prevention in a wide range of settings, and include school media and policy dimensions. Early results from the Barwon intervention indicate a high level of parental awareness and recall of the intervention messages [38].

Clinical Management

Programs and policies aimed at preventing the development of obesity in young people are important, but so too is the provision of effective clinical services for the assessment and management of affected individuals. In 2003, the Australian National Health and Medical Research Council published its clinical practice guidelines for the management of overweight and obesity in children and adolescents [39]. Unfortunately, this evidence-based set of recommendations which was aimed at general practitioners was not accompanied by an education or dissemination programme so awareness and use of the guidelines remains limited [40].

The conventional components of weight management include dietary modification, increased physical activity, decreased sedentary activity, behaviour modification and family involvement [39,41]. However evidence for most of these is based on studies dealing with pre-adolescent children and their parents, the majority of such studies occurring either in schools or tertiary clinical settings and few specifically focussing on adolescents [42]. Indeed, there is only extremely limited evidence to guide effective weight management interventions in the adolescent age group, especially at an intensity that would be sustainable in health care settings such as in Australia. In Australia, several randomized clinical trials (RCT) in adolescent obesity have commenced, or are recently completed. They differ in their focus on patients or clients with different levels of severity of obesity and in the intensity and type of intervention offered. For example, the Loozit® trial, underway in Sydney [43], is a group-based weight management program for overweight or obese adolescents developed for delivery in a variety of primary care or community settings by a range of health professionals with outcomes to be measured at two years. In Melbourne, a 12 session cognitive behavioural therapy intervention achieved significant differences in body fat between the intervention and control groups that were maintained over 6-months of follow-up [44]. The first RCT of bariatric surgery in severely obese older adolescents is currently underway in Melbourne –

this is a trial of what is essentially a quaternary level of intervention [45]. Results of these and other studies, when available, will help inform the development of clinical service delivery in the area of adolescent obesity management.

Future Directions

Although innovative research is being undertaken throughout Australia, prevention and treatment of adolescent obesity needs further commitment to prevent an overwhelming burden on the public health system in the future. In particular, the development of health service delivery models that acknowledge the unique needs of adolescents, and provide appropriate care for affected young people, be they mildly or severely obese.

Efforts toward prevention must focus on better understanding the determinants and causes of obesity in adolescents in an effort to develop evidence-based prevention strategies. This would include not just individual level causes such as food and activity behaviours but environmental determinants such as urban planning, transport infrastructure, food sale policies and the effects of advertising on young people. Finally, ongoing monitoring of the prevalence of obesity as well as determinants is vital in order that the immediate effect of the epidemic and its impact on young adults be quantified.

References

[1] Booth ML, Dobbins TA, Denney-Wilson E, Hardy LL, Okely AD. Trends in the prevalence of overweight and obesity among Australian children and adolescents 1985 -1997-2004. Accepted by Obesity 2007.

[2] Booth ML, Chey T, Wake M, Norton K, Hesketh K, Dollman J, et al. Change in the prevalence of overweight and obesity among young Australians, 1969-1997. Am J Clin Nutr 2003;77(1):29-36.

[3] Magarey AM, Daniels LA, Boulton TJ. Prevalence of overweight and obesity in Australian children and adolescents: reassessment of 1985 and 1995 data against new standard international definitions. [comment] [erratum appears in Med J Aust 2001;175 (7):392]. Med J Aust 2001;174(11): 561-4.

[4] Bellizzi MC, Dietz WH. Workshop on childhood obesity: summary of the discussion. Am J Clin Nutr 1999;70(1): 173S-5S.

[5] WHO. Obesity: Preventing and managing the global epidemic. Report of a WHO consultation on obesity. Geneva: WHO,1998.

[6] Cole TJ, Bellizzi MC, Flegal KM, Dietz WH. Establishing a standard definition for child overweight and obesity worldwide: international survey. [comment]. BMJ 2000;320 (7244): 1240-3.

[7] Denney-Wilson E, Booth ML, Baur LA. Development of the Australian standard definition of child/adolescent overweight and obesity. Nutr Diet 2003; 60(2): 74-77.

[8] Vaska VL, Volkmer R. Increasing prevalence of obesity in South Australian 4-year olds: 1995-2002. J Paediatr Child Health 2004;40:353-5.

[9] Booth ML, Denney-Wilson E, Okely AD, Hardy LL. Methods of the NSW Schools Physical Activity and Nutrition Survey (SPANS). J Sci Med Sport 2005;8(3):284-93.

[10] Booth ML, Okely A.D, Denney-Wilson E, Hardy LL, Yang B, Dobbins TA. NSW Schools Physical Activity and Nutrition Survey (SPANS 2004)- Full Report. Sydney: NSW Dept Health,2006.

[11] Gordon-Larsen P, Adair LS, Popkin BM. The relationship of ethnicity, socioeconomic factors, and overweight in US adolescents. Obes Res 2003; 11(1):121-9.

[12] Booth ML, Macaskill P, Lazarus R, Baur LA. Sociodemographic distribution of measures of body fatness among children and adolescents in New South Wales, Australia. Int J Obes Relat Metab Disord 1999; 23(5): 456-62.

[13] O'Dea JA, Caputi P. Association between socioeconomic status, weight, age and gender, and the body image and weight control practices of 6- to 19-year-old children and adolescents. Health Educ Res 2001;16(5):521-32.

[14] Garnett SP, Cowell CT, Baur LA, Shrewsbury VA, Chan A, Crawford D et al. Increasing central adiposity: the Nepean longitudinal study of young people aged 7-8 to 12-13 y. Int J Obes 2005;29(11):1353-60.

[15] Field AE, Colditz GA. Overweight, central adiposity, and cardiovascular disease risk patterns in children. [comment]. J Pediatrics 1999;135 (4):409-10.

[16] Cook T, Coles-Rutishauser I, Seeig M. Comparible data on food and nutrient intake and physical measurements from the 1983, 1985 and 1995 National Surveys. Canberra: Commonwealth Dept Health Ageing, 2001.

[17] Gill T, Story E, Webb K. Report on the weight status of NSW: 2003. Sydney: NSW Health, 2003.

[18] Ludwig DS, Peterson KE, Gortmaker SL. Relation between consumption of sugar-sweetened drinks and childhood obesity: a prospective, observational analysis. Lancet 2001;357(9255):505-8.

[19] Tam CS, Garnett SP, Cowell CT, Campbell K, Cabrera G, Baur LA. Soft drink consumption and excess weight gain in Australian school students: results from the Nepean study. Int J Obes 2006;30(7):1091-3.

[20] Prentice AM, Jebb SA. Fast foods, energy density and obesity: a possible mechanistic link. Obes Rev 2003;4(4): 187-94.

[21] Zuppa JA, Morton H, Metha K. Television food advertising: Counterproductive to children's health? A content analysis using the Australian Guide to Healthy Eating. Nutr Diet 2003;60(2):78-84.

[22] Kassem NO, Lee JW, Modeste NN, Johnston PK. Understanding soft drink consumption among female adolescents using the Theory of Planned Behavior. Health Educ Res 2003;18(3): 278-91.

[23] French SA, Story M, Neumark-Sztainer D, Fulkerson JA, Hannan P. Fast food restaurant use among adolescents: associations with nutri¬ent intake, food choices and beha¬vioral and psychosocial variables. Int J Obes Relat Metab Disord 2001;25(12): 1823-33.

[24] Johnson F, Wardle J, Griffith J. The Adolescent Food Habits Checklist: reliability and validity of a measure of healthy eating behaviour in adolescents. Eur J Clin Nutr 2002;56(7):644-9.

[25] Neumark-Sztainer D, Story M, Perry C, Casey MA. Factors influencing food choices of adolescents: findings from focus-group discussions with adolescents. J Am Diet Assoc 1999; 99(8): 929-37.

[26] Grimm GC, Harnack L, Story M. Factors associated with soft drink consumption in school-aged children. J Am Diet Assoc 2004;104 (8):1244-9.

[27] Campbell K, Crawford D, Salmon J, Carver A, Garnett SP, Boulton J et al. Associations between the home food environment and obesity-promoting eating behaviours in adolescence. Accepted by Obesity 2007.

[28] Carver A, Salmon J, Campbell K, Baur LA, Garnett SP, Crawford D. How do perceptions of local neighborhood relate to adolescents' walking and cycling? Am J Health Promot 2005; 20:139-47.

[29] Timperio A, Crawford D, Telford A, Salmon J. Perceptions about the local neighborhood and walking and cycling among children. Prev Med 2004; 38(1):39-47.

[30] Timperio A, Salmon J, Telford A, Crawford D. Perceptions of local neighbourhood environments and their relationship to childhood overweight and obesity. Int J Obes 2005;29(2): 170-5.

[31] Salmon J, Timperio A, Cleland V, Venn A. Trends in children's physical activity and weight status in high and low socio-economic status areas of Melbourne, Victoria, 1985-2001. Aust NZ J Public Health 2005;29(4):337-42.

[32] Okely AD, Booth ML, Denney-Wilson E, Hardy LL, Yang B, Dobbins TA. Secular trends in the self-reported physical activity among adolescents in NSW, Australia from 1985-1997-2004. Sydney: 10th Int Congr Obes, 2006:97.

[33] Hardy LL, Dobbins T, Booth ML, Denney-Wilson E, Okely AD. Sedentary behaviours among Australian adol¬escents. Aust NZ J Public Health 2006; 30(6):534-40.

[34] Denney-Wilson E, Booth ML, Okely AD, Hardy LL, Dobbins T, Baur LA. Clustering of metabolic risk factors in obese adolescents: the NSW Schools Physical Activity and Nutrition Survey (SPANS 2004). Obes Rev 2006;7:193.

[35] NSW Health. NSW Healthy School Canteen Strategy Evaluation Report 2005. http://www.health.nsw.gov.au/ pubs/2006/canteens_evaluation.html 2006 [cited 7 A.D. Feb 7].

[36] Deakin University. WHO Collaborating Centre for Obesity Prevention and Related Research and Training. http://www.deakineduau/ hmnbs/who-obesity/ 2007 [cited 7 A.D. Feb 13].

[37] HNE Health. Hunter New England Child Obesity Prevention Program. www.hnehealthnsw.gov.au.2007 [cited 7 A.D. Feb 23].

[38] Bell AC, Brennan M, Cutter R, Sanigorski A, Simmons A, Kremer P et al. Colac's Be Active Eat Well program outcomes. Obes Rev 2006;7: 27-8.

[39] NHMRC. Clinical practice guidelines for the management of overweight and obesity in children and adolescents. Canberra: NHMRC,2003.

[40] Spurrier NJ, Magarey AM, Wong C. Recognition and management of childhood overweight and obesity by clinicians. J Paediatr Child Health 2006;42(7-8),411-8.

[41] Lobstein T, Baur LA, Uauy R. Childhood obesity: a crisis in public health. Obes Rev 2004;5(4):245.

[42] Summerbell CD, Ashton V, Campbell K, Edmunds L, Kelly S, Waters E. Interventions for treating obesity in children (Cochrane Review). Cochrane Database Syst Rev 2003;(3).

[43] O'Connor J. The Loozit pilot study of adolescent weight management, and rationale for a randomised controlled trial: what do young people want? Sydney: Proceed Youth Health Conf, 2006:42.

[44] Brennan L, Wilks R, Walkley J, Fraser S, Greenway K. Efficacy of cognitive behaviour therapy in the treatment of overweight and obese adolescents. ObesRev2006;7:88-9.

[45] Monash University. Centre for Obesity Research and Education. Current Research. Monash University 2007; Available from: http:// www.core.monash.org/current-research-studies.html [cited 7 A.D. Feb 23].

In: Obesity and Adolescence: A Public Health Concern
Editors: H.A. Omar, D.E. Greydanus et al.
ISBN: 978-1-60692-821-9

Chapter XX

Food Choice of Children in Bangkok

Chulanee Thianthai*
Department of Sociology and Anthropology, Chulalongkorn University, Bangkok, Thailand

Abstract

Research has focused on adolescent's food choice with the hope of finding key factors preventing obesity. We aimed to specifically spot relevant key factors that influence Bangkok children, aged 9-11 years old, their food buying preferences and behaviors in schools. Nutritional anthropological research methodology namely, participant observation, in-depth interviews, and buying and eating behaviors-related observation questionnaires were carried out among 27 participating elementary schools in Central Bangkok. This research aimed to discover detailed factors associated with individuality, sociality, environmental, and external influence over children's food choices. First, individuality factors associated to children's food choices involved the amount of daily allowance, children's food preferences, students' perception towards food ability in correlation with the frequency of school breaks, and children's rationale of food prices (reasonable/affordable range). Second, sociality factors concerned how individual(s) have shaped children's knowledge of food, food-related beliefs, and individual(s) that accompany/are present at the moment when children are buying foods. Third, environmental factors discovered were the location, distance, and quality of where food is being sold, shelving/how food is being displayed, and the availability of food knowledge the school displayed/provided for their students. Last, external factors identified the variety of mass media channels, which triggered children to desire new food items, were tested and shown no influence over children's food choice on school days. In conclusion, the insights gained can enlighten ways in which in-depth understanding of children's food choice and behaviors can be obtained in order to create a more efficient and culturally suited future obesity prevention plan.

* Correspondence: Assistant Professor Dr. Chulanee Thianthai, Department of Sociology and Anthropology, Faculty of Political Science, Chulalongkorn University, Patumwan, Bangkok 10330, Thailand. Tel: (662) 218-7292; Fax: (662) 218-7300; E-mail: chulanee00@hotmail.com or chulane.t@chula.ac.th

Introduction

Today's health scientists are focusing on the importance of children's nutritional-related habits, because of the increasing rate of child obesity. It has been proven that children's nutritional eating habits will have a strong influence over their adult years [1]. Children, especially those who live in urban areas, are being bombarded by unhealthy food alternatives, such as high calorie, sugary, and fattening foods. Not only do these unhealthy food alternatives not provide the essential nutrients a child needs, but the sense of fulfillment from eating these types of foods also reduces the child's appetite to want other nutrient enriched foods, particularly vegetables and fruits. Many studies have been conducted to stress how children's unhealthy eating habits can cause obesity, diabetic type 2, high blood pressure, dental disease, and heart failure [2-4]. However, many societies believe that a part of these unhealthy eating habits have been built up due to the support of mass media influence [5,6].

Recent literatures have found that there are multiple factors that contribute to children's food choice and eating behaviors. These factors were such as family influence, given health information, availability and accessibility, exposure to new food types, food environment, socioeconomic status, and cultural beliefs [7-9]. Not only do these factors shape children's food choice and eating behaviors, but they are also factors that will instigate modifications in those choices and behaviors [7]. However, not all of these factors may apply to certain populations. Moreover, due to variation in children's food choice and eating behaviors from society to society, researchers should not limit their examination to only the above factors. Therefore, in order to gain realistic insights on obesity prevalence, researchers should focus on a particular societal circumstance.

Using Thai society as an example, the World Health Organization has showed that in just over a period of two years, the prevalence of obesity among Thai children aged 5-to-12 years old had risen from 12.2% to 15-16% [10]. Another recent research has proven that children who live in Bangkok have a higher risk of being obese than those who live in the rural areas [11]. In supporting the latter research result, another research found that 1 out of 4 Thai children who attended well-known schools within Central Bangkok district were obese [12]. In order to efficiently create a health program that specifically targets on reducing the obesity rate among children who live in urban areas, like Bangkok, one needs to gain cultural insight dimension and have an in-depth understanding of why and how urban children's food choice appear to be that way. Thus, this research proposes to identify the main influential factors affecting Bangkok children and young adolescents' food choice on their school days through illustrative insights.

Our Research

The fieldwork data was obtained from intensive fieldwork in Bangkok from mid 2006 to 2007. Bangkok, known as Krung Thep, the capital of Thailand, was selected to be the most appropriate setting for this research. Bangkok is known for having the best educational institutions, which attracts students from different regions in Thailand, enabling the researcher to receive students with various socio-economic backgrounds. In addition, students in Bangkok were the group that has been bombarded with a greater variety of food through mass media influence. Having Bangkok students as the target population also permits the researcher to examine whether or not their food choices during their school hours involved Western and international variety of foods and to what extent.

Through permission from 27 public elementary schools located in Central Bangkok, the researcher was able to observe and participate in food buying and selling-related activities of elementary school children, aged 9-11 years old, during their school hours on school days. This age group was selected, because they just started their own decision making in spending their allowance on food and they are among the most at risk group for obesity. Moreover, this study was able to capture the majority of children's food choice behaviors because it covers five days out of the week when they must make their own decisions.

The data collection started with the process of mapping out and defining the boundary of Central Bangkok. The research team then visited over 50 public elementary schools in Central Bangkok and explained the research objectives. Out of 50 elementary schools, 27 were willing to participate in this research. The researchers then visited these schools and observed the children, while buying and eating during the school hours (08:00-16:00). Observation records were kept and found it to be interesting in the form of field notes. After several months of utilizing systematic observation, the researchers moved on to participate in children's food related activities at school. For example, they assisted school teachers and food vendors to sell food and beverages during the school hours, helped teachers make food-related posters to hang in the cafeterias, and facilitated the children to form lines for buying food. Through the methodology of participant observation, the researchers were able to gain essential firsthand experience needed for building a realistic buying and eating behaviors-related observation questionnaire. The questionnaire was composed of three parts: 1) school information and drawing of physical site where foods were sold in schools; 2) demographic questions of who were being observed, at what time, and where and 3) sets of closed-end and opened-end questions needed for further in-depth interviews with students. At least 20 students per school, who portrayed the characteristics being articulated and showing regularity in buying foods and beverages during school hours were selected for in-depth interviews.

Observation and participation in children food buying and selling-related activities were limited to when they buy foods of any type or form within the school courtyard during school hours. The activities related to food buying inside and outside of the schools after school hours were excluded. Their food choices that we observed were mainly the types of foods that they bought other than what their school provided for their lunch.

The researcher used the data gained from participant observation field notes and the first and second parts of the questionnaire to examine and highlight the pattern of children's food choice in each school. The data obtained through the third part of the closed-ended questions were calculated with the help of Statistical Package for the Social Sciences (SPSS) and the output was shown in percentages, whereas the data drawn from open-ended questions were used to cross-check with the data gained from participant observation and to further clarify what has been the children's perspective.

What did we find?

The following are findings that revealed detailed factors associated with the four areas of examination: individual, social, environmental and external factors believed to have influence over food choice patterns.

Individual Factors

Individuality involved factors that were mainly created by the children themselves, which contributed to their food choice behaviors. Individual factors were the amount of children's daily allowance, children's food preference, children's perception towards food availability in correlation with the frequency of school breaks, and children's rationale of food prices (reasonable/affordable range) factors.

The amount of money Bangkok children received per day to spend on buying food and beverages on school days was on average $0.60 cents (equivalent to 20 Baht). With this amount of money, children can only afford certain quality and quantify of food. For example, in this study the average number of food items bought per day was 1-2.

Food preference was being tested in terms of what were Bangkok children's most favorite food items (listed in order): Fried food (i.e. fried chicken wings, french fries, fried sausages, and fried wontons), ice cream, chips/snacks in small packages, food items that represent meals (i.e. a one dish meal such as rice and curry or noodles), various kinds of milk products, and types of flour related foods (wafer, bread, cookies, and sandwich). From the observation and in-depth interviews, this research found that children were highly fond of sweet-tasting beverages such as soda pops and Thai ice tea and ice coco drinks and smoothies. Also through the in-depth interviews, the study has found that milk was categorized not as a beverage, but rather seen as a food item.

Children's perception towards food availability in correlation with the frequency of school breaks revealed that lunch time was the peak time for them to buy food and beverages in schools. Almost every child in this study bought food and beverages after they ate their school-provided meals. From the in-depth interviews, the research has found that Bangkok children defined food-buying-and-eating activities as their leisure time.

Children's rationale of what is the reasonable food price was $0.20-0.30 cents (equivalent to 5-10 baht) per item. Every food item at this price range was in the small size packaging.

Social Factors

Sociality concerns other individual(s)/source(s) that have shaped and contributed to children's food choices and eating patterns. Examples of these individuals were parents, teachers, friends, food and beverages sellers. Thus, the social category we found in this study covered individual(s)/source(s) that had influenced food knowledge, food-related beliefs, and individual(s) that accompanied or was present at the moment when children were buying foods.

Individual(s)/source(s) that had influenced these Bangkok children's food knowledge and food-related beliefs (ranked in order) were their elementary school teachers, parents and television commercials. Although television commercials were mentioned as one of the sources that influenced food choice, it had only shaped their perception of what was good and nutritious food, but had no impact on their food buying decisions.

Individual(s) that Bangkok children wanted to accompany or be present with when they buy food was their friends. Friends usually accompany friends to buy food in a group of 1-2 friend(s) at a time. However, this study revealed that there were no influence related to the choice of food and beverages they buy at this age.

Environmental Factors

Environment is being defined as factors that were created by physical things that surrounded children on school days. Thus, environmental factors found involved the location, distance, and quality of where food was sold, food display, ice cream commercial food pricing posters displayed above the ice cream freezers, and the availability of food knowledge the school displayed/provided for their students.

The location where food was sold in schools usually came in the form of student union shops, food stands located inside school cafeterias and outdoor food stands within the school gate and food vending machines. This study found that the location and distance were correlated to the decision-making of children when they want to buy food, that is children often go to buy foods at the closest location to their classrooms. Listed in order that shows this correlation between the closest distance and where food were most bought by these children were food stands in school cafeterias, student union shops, outdoor food stands and food vending machines.

Regarding the quality of where food is being sold we found that in schools with only elementary level, only one venue was provided for selling foods during break time. In contrast, in schools that have both elementary and high school level, children would have more variety in choosing places to buy food. From the in-depth interviews, the ideal quality food place was defined as a place that sells a variety of foods. Moreover, the food sold there should be fresh, clean and delicious.

The ice cream commercial food pricing posters displayed above the ice cream freezer had an influence on food choice only to a certain extent, that is to help them know the price and make their decision if they can afford it or not and provide them with easier access to quickly grab the right kind of ice cream in the freezer by memorizing the packaging.

In every school we visited, the food sold most were often displayed and shelved at a distance that is easy for the children to grab and gain access to (leveling to student's reachable height or placed towards the front of the table where food is sold). When we collected our data, the most popular food was fried foods and small package chips/snacks, located as easy access.

The types of food knowledge these elementary schools displayed/provided for their students came in the form of posters that provided nutritional food facts and hygienic facts relating to proper hand washing before eating, broadcasting on school radio, and leaflets/handouts in the school library. The most popular food knowledge displayed was the five food group posters. Rarely have the researchers witnessed a link between the children's food choice and information from these media.

External Factors

External category included influences outside of the school arena. Externality largely was identified as the variety of mass media channels (what children read in books and magazines and/or watch on television commercials), which triggered them to desire new food items.

The study showed that there were little influential factors dominated by what children read in books and magazines or watch on television commercials that cause them to desire new food items. This is maybe due to the fact that the variety of foods sold in schools were limited and the way in which they can buy the types of food they really like through what they read/see on commercials can be more apparent on the weekends. Through the in-depth interviews we found that at this age, children would mainly buy food on their school days based on the delicious taste of the food, the color of the food, the attractive packaging and the free stuff that came with the food.

Conclusions

In conclusion, the insights gained provided in-depth details of Bangkok children's food choices on school days. As we can see, participant observation of buying and eating behaviors, questionnaires, and in-depth interviews served as amazing tools that can provide insight into what really has an influence over our children. These factors are not isolated from one another, but rather associated to one another in shaping Bangkok children's decision-making and food habits. Building upon this information would help in constructing a more efficient future obesity prevention plan in schools. For example, if a greater variety of food stalls that provide reasonable prices (not exceeding their daily allowance), fresh, delicious, clean, and healthy foods are needed to be located near children's classrooms and at places they can easily access. This change can alter and improve their decision-making and behaviors with regard to food. Meanwhile, there is an urgent need to reduce the consumption of fried foods and sweet beverages that are not nutritious in Bangkok elementary schools. The reduction can be made through limiting the amount of these types of foods as well as making it more difficult to buy these foods in schools. The types of food knowledge these elementary schools displayed near food shops or broadcast during the lunch time (which is the peak time when children would buy foods) should also cover information on negative health consequences resulting from eating high fattening and high calorie foods, namely fried foods and sweet beverages. Displaying food facts and harmful consequences relating to their current food buying behaviors would have a stronger impact on their food selections.

It is refreshing to learn that mass media and negative peer influences have very little influence over these children's food choices on school days. We suggest that there is room for healthy foods to make its way into Bangkok elementary schools. Moreover, the data gained from this research can also act as a foundation to create healthy food alternatives for elementary school children in Bangkok. Such research methodologies can easily be applicable in other cultures to improve the study of child obesity.

Acknowledgments

The author wishes to thank the students, teachers, and participating schools, the Thailand Research Fund (TRF) Grant and Commission of Higher Education for making this study possible, Dr. Chitr Sitthi-Amorn in contributing valuable comments, and Raksaya Aunsnunta for her constructive editing skills.

References

[1] Healthy eating in childhood persists into older age. Nurs Standard 2006;20:17.
[2] Unhealthy foods bulk of school vending machine choices. Nation's Health 2004;June-July:7.
[3] Deborah JA. Approaches to the study of children, food and sweet eating: a review of the literature. Early Child Dev Care 2005;175: 407-17.
[4] Holffer J. Child obesity can lead to heart problems. New York Amsterdam News 2005;November: 38.
[5] Lewis MK, Hill AJ. Food advertising on British children's television: a content analysis and experimental study with nine-year olds. Int J Obes 1998;22:206-14.
[6] Krisberg K. Food marketing toward youth contributing to unhealthy choices. Nation Health 2006;January/February:19.
[7] Cooke, L. The development and modification of children's eating habits. Nutrition Bull 2004;29(1):31-5.
[8] Huon GF, Wardle J. Improving children's eating patterns: intervention programs and underlying principles. Aust J Nutr Dietetics 1999;56(3):156-65.
[9] Green J, Waters E, Haikerwal A, O'Neill C, Raman S, Booths ML, Gibbons K. Social, cultural and environmental influences on child activity and eating in Australian migrant communities. Child Care Health Dev 2003;29(6):441-8.
[10] Obesity and overweight. Accessed 2008 Jun 08.URL: http://www.who.int/dietphysicalactivity/publications/facts/obesity/en/
[11] Chaiamnuan P. A personal documentary report on how to prevent and cure obesity in Thai population. Bangkok: Natl Defense Coll Thailand, 2002.
[12] Neannui P. Tooth decay: A little problem that is not little. In: Brain Bank for Health. Bangkok: Office Natl Economic Soc Dev Board, 2004:242-8.

In: Obesity and Adolescence: A Public Health Concern
Editors: H.A. Omar, D.E. Greydanus et al.
ISBN: 978-1-60692-821-9

Chapter XXI

Obesity, Adolescence and Israel

Brian Seth Fuchs[1,2], Mohammed Morad[1,3], Isack Kandel[1,4], Jason Ahn[1,2] and Joav Merrick[1,5,*]

[1]National Institute of Child Health and Human Development, Office of the Medical Director, Division for Mental Retardation, Ministry of Social Affairs, Jerusalem, Israel, [2]Harvard Medical School, Boston, United States of America, [3]Department of Family Medicine, Faculty of Health Sciences, Ben Gurion University of the Negev, Beer-Sheva, Israel, [4]Faculty of Social Sciences, Department of Behavioral Sciences, Ariel University Center of Samaria, Ariel, Israel and [5]Kentucky Children's Hospital, University of Kentucky, Lexington, United States of America

Abstract

Childhood and adolescent obesity are risk factors for poor health later in life as well as decreased life expectancy. This short communication reviews literature on obesity in Israel and examines several recent studies, which have clearly demonstrated rising rates of childhood and adolescent obesity similar in magnitude to those trends observed in other Westernized nations. It is incumbent upon relevant authorities within Israel to reverse these trends so as to prevent the long-term adverse health consequences associated with childhood and adolescent obesity. We recommend initiating a national educational campaign to promote exercise and healthy eating. This campaign would target children and adolescents and would rely upon evidence based guidelines for diet and exercise.

* Correspondence: Professor Joav Merrick, MD, MMedSci, DMSc, Medical Director, Division for Mental Retardation, Box 1260, IL-91012 Jerusalem, Israel. E-mail: jmerrick@zahav.net.il

Introduction

Obesity is recognized as an important risk factor for many chronic diseases, such as cardiovascular disease, diabetes and cancer. Children who are overweight are at an even greater risk of developing such diseases, because of their extended exposure to the harmful effects of excessive weight; and there is often an accelerated onset of chronic disease within this population. In addition, children who are overweight are more likely to suffer from impaired physical, psychological, and social development. In this short communication we examine recent research on obesity among Israeli children and adolescents.

Research Findings from Israel

We conducted a Medline search from 2000 for papers relevant to this review (search entry was adolescence and overweight and Israel).

Because Israel has large number of army recruits each year who are given physical exams, researchers were able to conduct a population-based study of Israeli Jewish males prior to army enrollment [1]. This study provided valuable information for two body mass index (BMI) reference points: a national reference (NR), and an ethnic-specific reference (ER). This study included 109,570 Jewish males 17 years of age. Weight, height and blood pressure values were recorded, and BMI was calculated. The 85th percentile of BMI was used as a lower limit for defining overweight status for NR and ER. Hypertension prevalence among recruits was used as a biomarker to confirm the reliability of the ER when discrepancies in classification between the two references were found. Compared to the NR, three ethnic groups had a BMI distribution shifted to the left (light sub-population) and five had a BMI distribution shifted to the right (heavy sub-population). In the light sub-population, 7% of the recruits who were classified as normal weight by the NR were considered overweight by the ER and had a hypertension rate similar to that of those defined as overweight by both references (3.1 per 1,000). In the heavy sub-population, 4% of the subjects who were classified as overweight by NR and normal by ER had hypertension rates similar to that of those defined as normal weight by both references (2.7 per 1,000), and significantly lower than that of those classified as overweight by both references (10.8 per 1,000).

Type 2 diabetes has been increasing even among children and adolescents during the past decade. A case report [2] of a boy (14 years) and two girls (16.5 and 17 years) and a larger study [3] of 22 children and adolescents linked extreme obesity (BMI 39-47) with acanthosis nigricans, elevated diastolic blood pressure, hirsutism, menstrual disorders and insulin resistance as part of this metabolic syndrome.

One study of a weight management program included 177 obese children (6-16 years); this longitudinal, non-randomised study compared three and six month combined dietary-behavioural-exercise interventions with matched control. The researchers demonstrated that body weight and BMI were reduced ($P<0.05$) and physical endurance was improved ($P<0.0005$) by the three month intervention. Obese children who were given six months of intervention were able to successfully maintain their weight loss and further improved their physical endurance time. In contrast, the obese children who did not participate in the structured intervention gained weight and increased their BMI. Gender, pubertal status, and the degree of obesity had no influence on BMI changes, but children of normal weight parents demonstrated significantly greater weight loss than children of obese parents [4].

An innovative long-term follow-up (seven years) study, which focused on educating the parents of 50 obese children rather than only the children, evidenced a larger treatment effect compared with the conventional approach of treating only children.

Inadequate dietary habits can result in iron deficiency, as shown in a study of 321 children and adolescents who were treated in Israel between 1999 and 2001 [6]. Iron deficiency was common in this sample of overweight and obese children, and the prevalence of this deficiency was significantly greater among obese children compared with their normal-weight counterparts. This result was confirmed by another study [7] which demonstrated an elevated risk of vitamin B12 deficiency in obese children.

One recent study investigated the correlation between early postnatal weight gain and obesity in Arab adolescents [8]. Growth records were examined from the first 24 months of life. Eighty eight obese and 214 non-obese 12 year-old Arab children were evaluated in this study. Height and weight at birth were comparable for the obese and non-obese adolescents, while the rate of breastfeeding was significantly lower in the obese group ($p < 0.01$), suggesting that breastfeeding had a protective effect. The evidence also indicated that obese adolescents had a small but significant weight gain at four ($p = 0.002$) and 12 ($p = 0.01$) months of age relative to their non-obese counterparts. Furthermore, weight gain during the first two months of life and feeding pattern were independent predictors of BMI at the age of 12.

Israel Compared To Europe and the United States

Israel participated in a cross-sectional, nationally representative school-based survey in 1997-1998 (991 Israeli students participated out of a total of 29,242 boys and girls, 13 to 15 years) by means of identical data collection methods [9]. The following countries participated in this study: Austria, Czech Republic, Denmark, Flemish Belgium, Finland, France, Germany, Greece, Lithuania, Ireland, Israel, Portugal, Slovakia, Sweden and the United States.

The United States evidenced the highest prevalence of overweight children and Lithuania the lowest. In the United States 12.6% of 13-year-old boys were overweight, 10.8% of 13-year-old girls, 13.9% of 15-year-old boys, and 15.1% of 15-year-old girls. In contrast, in Israel 3.5% of 13-year-old boys were overweight, 4.8% of 13-year-old girls, 6.8% of 15-year-old boys, and 6.2% of 15-year-old girls [9]. Relative rankings among countries were similar if BMI at or above the 85th percentile were used for comparisons. Although the differences were less dramatic if weight at the 85th percentile was used as a definition of obesity, this approach evidenced the highest prevalence of overweight children in the United States, Ireland, Greece and Portugal [9].

Recent Studies of Army Conscripts

A recent study included 76,732 adolescents, 32,402 (42.2%) females and 44,330 (57.8%) males aged 17 years at the draft examination [10].

Among 17-year-old Israeli conscripts 4.1% of males were obese, and 3.3% of females were obese. The prevalence of individuals categorized as borderline overweight was 12.4% for males and 11.4% for females. Prevalence of hypertension and type 2 diabetes was greater in males than females (P<0.001, 0.015), but for both sexes rates of hypertension and type 2 diabetes were significantly higher among conscripts with BMI>30 kg/m2. Females with BMI>30 kg/m2 were found to be less likely to have completed 10 years of education, but there was no similar difference found among male conscripts.

This study found a relatively low prevalence of obesity, but a high prevalence of individuals who were categorized as borderline overweight; Obesity was positively correlated with hypertension and type 2 diabetes and negatively correlated with level of educational attainment.

Another cross-sectional population-based study conducted from 1996 to 2002 on 560,588 Israeli army recruits 16.5 to 19 years of age determined the prevalence of hypertension and obesity and assessed the relationships between prehypertension, body mass index (BMI), sex and age. These researchers demonstrated that mean systolic BP (SBP) and diastolic BP (DBP) were significantly higher in male subjects than female subjects; 56.8% of males and 35.8% of females were categorized as prehypertensive. There was also a statistically significant positive association between mean SBP and DBP, age and BMI. Moreover, the prevalence of prehypertension was significantly higher in obese subjects; 10.9% of males were overweight and 3.3% were obese, while 11.1% of females were overweight and 3.2% were obese [11].

Health Related Quality of Life

Health-related quality of life (HRQOL) has also been studied in 182 children and adolescents from community pediatric clinics and a hospital-based obesity clinic [12].

Compared with normal weight children, obese children reported significantly lower HRQOL in physical, social and school domains (P<0.01). Dividing the HRQOL results into BMI quartiles demonstrated that scores for emotional and school domains were similar between moderately obese children and normal weight children. Only children in the 4th quartile, with severe obesity, evidenced significantly lower scores. Parents of obese children perceived their children's HRQOL scores to be lower than what was reported by the children themselves.

Conclusions

Recent studies have clearly demonstrated rising rates of childhood and adolescent obesity similar in magnitude to those trends observed in other Westernized nations. It is incumbent upon relevant authorities within Israel to reverse these trends so as to prevent the long-term adverse health consequences associated with childhood and adolescent obesity. We recommend initiating a national educational campaign to promote exercise and healthy eating. This campaign would target children and adolescents and would rely upon evidence based guidelines for diet and exercise.

References

[1] Lusky A, Lubin F, Barell V, Kaplan G, Layani V, Lev B, Wiener M. Body mass index in 17-year-old Israeli males of different ethnic backgrounds; national or ethnic-specific references? Int J Obes Relat Metab Disord 2000;24(1):88-92.

[2] Pinhas-Hamiel O, Koren I, Vardi P. [Type 2 diabetes among adolescents in Israel]. Harefuah 2000;138(3):186-9, 271. [Hebrew]

[3] Kerem N, Guttmann H, Hochberg Z. The autosomal dominant trait of obesity, acanthosis nigricans, hypertension, ischemic heart disease and diabetes type 2. Horm Res 2001;55(6):298-304.

[4] Eliakim A, Kaven G, Berger I, Friedland O, Wolach B, Nemet D. The effect of a combined intervention on body mass index and fitness in obese children and adolescents - a clinical experience. Eur J Pediatr 2002;161(8):449-54.

[5] Golan M, Crow S. Targeting parents exclusively in the treatment of childhood obesity: long-term results. Obes Res 2004;12(2):357-61.

[6] Pinhas-Hamiel O, Newfield RS, Koren I, Agmon A, Lilos P, Phillip M. Greater prevalence of iron deficiency in overweight and obese children and adolescents. Int J Obes Relat Metab Disord 2003;27(3):416-8.

[7] Pinhas-Hamiel O, Doron-Panush N, Reichman B, Nitzan-Kaluski D, Shalitin S, Geva-Lerner L.Obese children and adolescents: a risk group for low vitamin B12 concentration.Arch Pediatr Adolesc Med. 2006 Sep;160(9):933-6.

[8] Shehadeh N, Weitzer-Kish H, Shamir R, Shihab S, Weiss R. Impact of early postnatal weight gain and feeding patterns on body mass index in adolescence. J Pediatr Endocrinol Metab 2008;21(1):9-15.

[9] Lissau I, Overpeck MD, Ruan WJ, Due P, Holstein BE, Hediger ML. Health Behaviour in School-aged Children Obesity Working Group.Body mass index and overweight in adolescents in 13 European countries, Israel, and the United States. Arch Pediatr Adolesc Med 2004;158(1):27-33.

[10] Bar Dayan Y, Elishkevits K, Grotto I, Goldstein L, Goldberg A, Shvarts S, Levin A, Ohana N, Onn E, Levi Y, Bar Dayan Y. The prevalence of obesity and associated morbidity among 17-year-old Israeli conscripts. Public Health 2005;119(5):385-9.

[11] Israeli E, Schochat T, Korzets Z, Tekes-Manova D, Bernheim J, Golan E. Prehypertension and obesity in adolescents: a population study. Am J Hypertens 2006;19(7):708-12.

[12] Pinhas-Hamiel O, Singer S, Pilpel N, Fradkin A, Modan D, Reichman B. Health-related quality of life among children and adolescents: associations with obesity. Int J Obes (Lond) 2006;30(2):267-72.

In: Obesity and Adolescence: A Public Health Concern
Editors: H.A. Omar, D.E. Greydanus et al.
ISBN: 978-1-60692-821-9

Chapter XXII

Self-Image, Adolescence and Italy

Roberta Guarino, Alberto Pellai, Luca Bassoli, Mario Cozzi, Maria Angela Di Sanzo, Daniela Campra and Andrea Guala*

SOC di Pediatria, Ospedale SS Pietro e Paolo, Borgosesia, ASL 11, Regione Piemonte, Istituto di Igiene e Medicina Preventiva, IRCCS Ospedale Maggiore, Milano and Centro di Riabilitazione, Psicomotricità, ASL 1 Tortora, Regione Basilicata, Italy

Abstract

This chapter describes the prevalence rate of overweight and thinness in a population of adolescents living in two different areas of Italy and explores the body self-image perception and unhealthy eating behaviours and strategies to lose weight. A questionnaire was administered to a sample of 2,121 teenage students (1,084 males, 1,037 females). We found that adolescent females and males build and perceive their body images in very different ways. Most of the overall sample perceived their weight as normal, while a relevant 31.6% defined themselves as overweight and another 4.4% as heavily overweight. Analysis based on BMI (calculated through self-referred weight and height) showed that only 9.2% of our sample could be considered overweight and 1.7% obese. Most of female students (485 out of 1,037) were trying to lose weight, demonstrating that strategies to lose weight were undertaken also by girls perceiving themsleves as normal in relation to body weight. 46.8% girls were using strategies to lose weight compared with 21.9% boys. These strategies included very problematic behaviours like self-induced vomiting (3.3% F vs 1.7% M) and dieting pills (2.8% F vs 1.5% M) undertaken along with more usual thinning strategies like dieting and exercising. Girls were more prone than boys to exercise as a way to lose weight (41% vs 31.7%). We found a deep gap between actual weight and perceived body-image and weight. We believe primary prevention and health education programs aimed at

* Correspondence: Andrea Guala, MD, SOC di Pediatria, Ospedale "SS Pietro e Paolo", Piazzale Lora n. 1, 13011 Borgosesia, ASL 11- Regione Piemonte, Italy. Tel: 0163/203111; Fax: 0163/203267. E-mail: pediatria.borgosesia@asl11.piemonte.it

improving teen body-image should be adopted as a strategy to reduce the eating disorder epidemics spreading among young people.

Introduction

The number of teen-agers who perceive themselves as overweight and adopt unhealthy strategies to loose weight is constantly increasing, as clearly put in evidence by some recent epidemiological surveys carried out in Italy [1,2]. Too often, teenage slimming is obtained through problematic eating habits, over-exercising, purging and vomiting. These risk behaviors often brings teenagers to reach a unsuitable body weight or even dangerous for their health [1,3]. Data from the US Centers for Disease Control and Prevention (CDC) indicated that the number of American teen-agers trying to loose weight has been constantly increasing over the past ten years and the percentage of young girls under dietary restraint has grown from 43.5% to 59.5%, while the percentage of boys from 15.5% up to 26% [2,3].

The problem seems to be specifically related to the current cultural attitude, which attach thinness as a valuable aesthetic canon capable of ensuring a successful life [4]. The ideal bodily self-image of the adolescent derives in fact from identification with someone else's body due to mass media influence and from the cultural environment that glorify beauty and physical shape. For example, photos shown in fashion magazines have a deep impact on girls' body size and weight perception, as can be seen from interview of 548 female teenagers (10-17 years), which showed that 69% reported to be influenced in their ideal self-bodily image and 47% reported to wish to loose weight [5].

A number of young girls subject their bodies to heavy thinning efforts in a particular time of growth, when their body specifically requires enriching and strengthening with a negative impact on their pubertal functional levels (organic, psychological and social). Excessive weight concern and indiscriminate dietary restraint might have a potential negative impact on mental and physical health and easily compromise learning ability. A poor nutritional status may have negative effects on cognitive faculties and bad influence on scholastic performances and social acceptance. A reduced calorific intake of some nutritional principles leads in fact to memory diminution, reduced concentration power and irritability increase. A scarcely balanced diet in students finally translates into inactivity, indifference and reduced capacity of interrelating with the environment [6]. A deliberate and prolonged dietary restraint might develop in lack of iron provoking weariness, shorter attention span, lessened capacities in physical and mental activities, weaker resistance to infections as well as a delay in growth and sexual maturity. American surveys reported that 2-4% of teen-aged girls have evidence of iron deficiency)[7].

Weight concern might also affect the adoption of other at-risk behaviors. It is in fact noticed that cigarette smoking onset prevalence is higher among those adolescents on a diet or excessively worried about their weight compared with adolescents satisfied with their body shape and weight. Female students of high schools, white girls and smoke-addicts, reported to use cigarette smoking to keep their weight and appetite under control [8].

The present study was carried out to describe the prevalence rate of unhealthy and risk behaviors in teen Italian students living in two country areas. The research aimed also at revealing how teens value their actual body-image and weight in relation to their BMI (calculated through self-referred weight and height).

Our Research

The survey was carried out in two mountain areas, with similar socio-demographic characteristics, respectively located in the North of Piedmont (Valsesia, Northern Italy) and in Basilicata (Lagonegro, Southern Italy). The survey's tool was an anonymous self-reported questionnaire filled out by all adolescents attending high schools (from I to V-year courses). The research was carried out in the same month in both areas. The sample's age ranged between 14-29 years, but the final sample was obtained after eliminating students 20 years or older (since they represented only 1.5% of the total sample).

Participants filled in their questionnaire at school, during a morning class. Time available to complete the survey was half an hour. The survey tool was the Italian version of the YRBSS (Youth Risk Behavior Survey System) used since 1989 by the US Centers for Disease Control and Prevention (CDC) to monitor at-risk behaviors among teen agers[9]. The YRBSS is currently employed in US surveys with high school students to monitor preventive interventions[10,11,12]. More specifically, the YRBSS is used to analyse eight at-risk behaviours that play an important role in determining the health profile and social aspects of the teen population. Our research used only some sections of the global YRBSS questionnaire, in particular those dealing with body weight, body self-image and strategy to lose or control weight with a total of 12 multiple-choice questions. Besides all students were asked to report their sex, age, weight and height. BMI (Body Mass Index) was calculated by putting in relation weight (expressed in kilograms) with squared height in meters (BMI = Kg/m2). The phenotype classification by BMI size ranges was corrected by age and by Italian data[13,14]: underweight (M <16 at 14 y, <18 at 19 y; F <16,5 at 14y, <17,5 at 19y), average weight (M 16-24 at 14 y, 18-24,9 at 19y; F 16,5-24,9 at 14y, 17,5-24,9 at 19y), overweight (M 24,1-29,5 at 14y, 25-29,9 at 19y; F 25 – 29.9), obesity (M 29,6 and more at 14y, 30 and more at 19y; F 30 and more).

What did we find?

The secondary schools participating in the study were seven in Valsesia with a total number of 1,950 collected questionnaires, and four in Lagonegro with a total number of 937 collected questionnaires. Of the 2,887 questionnaires, 2,158 (75% response rate, 1,350 from Valsesia and 808 from Lagonegro) were available for data analysis. 25% of the returned questionnaires were considered invalid due to blank or unanswered questions. Distribution by age and gender is provided in table 1. On all the items of the two geographical samples, statistical analysis was performed using the Chi Square Test, but no statistical significance (p< 0,05) was found to differentiate some characteristics of the two subsamples. For this reason, this paper presents results obtained through analysis of a unique database, containing both Valsesia's and Lagonegro's data.

Table 1. Participants age and gender

Age (years)	14	15	16	17	18	19	Total
Female	113 10.9%	220 21.3%	196 18.8%	204 19.7%	235 22.7%	69 6.6%	1037 48.9%
Male	159 14.7%	292 26.9%	242 22.3%	186 17.1%	138 12.8%	67 6.2%	1084 51.1%
Total	272 12.8%	512 24.1%	438 20.7%	390 18.4%	373 17.6%	136 6.4%	2121

Table 2 indicate the participants' actual weight, on the basis of BMI stratifications (underweight, average weight, overweight and obese), calculated on the basis of their self-reported measure, for age class. Body weight perception was assessed through the question "How would you define your weight?" The given choices were the following: extremely underweight, a little underweight, average, a little overweight, obese. Table 3 reports self-perceived body weight, stratified by BMI. In our sample, on the basis of BMI values, 194 students can be considered actually "overweight" (9.1%) and 37 "obese" (1.7%). Perception of being overweight and obese interests a much larger group: infact, 670 (31.6%) consider himself as "overweight" and 93 (4.4%) as "obese". The perception of being overweight/obese (36%) resulted associated with actions or attitudes aimed at reducing body weight (34,1%) (table 4).

Table 2. Participant actual body size by BMI classes (underweight, average weight, overweight and obese), corrected for age and italian data [8-9]

Age (years)	Numbers	Underweight	Average	Overweight	Obese
14	272	170	75	24	3
15	512	300	174	35	3
16	438	238	146	41	13
17	390	178	161	42	9
18	373	199	134	35	5
19	136	58	57	17	4
Total	2121	1143 53.9%	747 35.3%	194 9.1%	37 1.7%

Table 3. Perception of own body self-image in relation with BMI, adjusted for age and Italian standard [8-9]

Percezione	N. (%)	M	F	BMI	M	F
Underweight	34 (1,6%)	25	9	1143 (53,9%)	488	655
Underweight	275 (13%)	192	83			
Normal weight	1040 (49%)	573	467	747 (35,2%)	422	325
Overweight	670 (31,6%)	252	418	194 (9,2%)	144	50
Obese	93 (4,4%)	37	56	37 (1,7%)	30	7
No answer	9 (0,4%)	5	4	-----	----	----
Total	2121	1084	1037	2121	1084	1037

Most female respondents reported that they were currently trying to lose weight, while the percentage of males who reported to follow some weight-losing strategy were consistently lower, the ratio between females and males being nearly 2:1. Female responders trying to put on weight were only one third of the corresponding percentage of males. The percentages of female and male respondents trying to maintain the same weight were not statistically different. Sport activities were the most employed weight-controlling strategy, followed by slimming diets in general, self-induced vomiting and use of slimming tablets or remedies. The slimming or weight-controlling strategies and their frequencies by gender are presented in table 5. Some students combine more than one strategy to lose weight in a unhealthy way: infact among those who declared the practice of self-induced vomiting (n=53, 34F, 19M), 15 used also slimming tablets or remedies (9F, 6M).

Table 4. Desire to lose/maintain/increase weight among 2,121 teens

	M 1,084	%	F 1,037	%	Total 2,121	%
I'm trying to lose weight	238	21,9%	485	46,8%	723	34,1%
Keeping my weight	695	64,2%	510	49,2%	1205	56,8%
Trying to improve weight	151	13,9%	42	4%	193	9,1%

Table 5. Slimming strategies adopted by teens dissatisfied with their weight

	F	%	M	%	Numbers	%
Sporting activities	425	41	344	31,7	769	36,2
Slimming diet	260	25	78	7.2	338	15,9
Self-induced vomit	34	3,3	19	1.7	53	2,5
Medecine - remedies	29	2,8	16	1.5	45	2,1

Numbers refer to strategies and not to individuals, considering that some subjects adopt more than one strategy.

Actual BMI was not related with strategies employed to lose weight. Among those who practiced self-induced vomiting (n=53) only four were obese and six overweight, while eight could even be considered underweight, on the basis of their BMI. Among those using dieting pills (n= 45), two were obese, six overweight and nine underweight.

Strategy employed to lose weight were homogeneously distributed in all age classes. Only in a class group of a school in Valsesia, an anomalous situation has been put in evidence: in this class, a relevant group of six students (5F, 1M) aged 16 years, were employing both self-induced vomiting and slimming pills use to lose weight.

Discussion

This survey showed how different Italian teen boys and girls rate and perceive their body self image, as clearly pointed out by the 2:1 ratio between females and males with overweight/obese body perception. Though most students in our sample perceived themselves with "normal weight", still the percentages of those perceving themselves as "a little overweight" (31.6%) or "extremely overweight" (4.4%) appeared quite relevant.

The adoption of weight-losing strategies was reported by almost half of the female sample enrolled in this survey (485 out of 1,037; 46,8%), though almost everybody was ranked as normal through their BMI. Of the female participants who perceived themselves to be "overweight" (418 out of the 1,037 interviewed girls; 40.3%) only 51 were actually overweight (4.9%) according to their BMI. As far as male participants were concerned, those who perceived themselves to be "overweight" were 252 (23.2% of the 1,084 interviewed boys) vs. 143 (13.2%) really ranking in the overweight BMI category. These data show that girls were more likely to have a distorted body self image, which is in accordance with the findings of others [1,15-17]. Regarding weight-losing strategies, we found data consistent with those reported for American teen-agers [3].

The percentage of teen-age girls reporting self-induced vomiting after eating was 3,3%, thus indicating the presence of at least one student for each high school class suffering from consistent eating disturbances, which might easily develop into clear and serious eating disorders [1,7,15,17]. The number of females adopting weight-losing strategies was also higher than males. In addition, the same subjects often reported to follow more than one slimming strategy to lose weight.

Due to these findings the research staff planned and implemented a prevention plan, aimed at reaching the most vulnerable classes, attended by clusters of at-risk adolescents, and discussing the problem of attitudes predisposing to eating disorders. This program took place in Valsesia and brought professionals (a psychologist and nutritionist) into five of the seven III-year classes participating in the current study, for a total of 187 teen-aged students (75% of them were males and 25% females).

The educational intervention consisted of two meetings of one hour each, planned and held with the purpose to clearly explain to the students the harmful effects of unsuitable thinning strategies, as well as to point out actions to prevent eating disorders.

Conclusions

The problem extent, as step by step defined by the current study findings, is certainly wide, although not directly evident, and needs proper attention both at school and within the family. Every education effort in preventing, recognizing and treating the problem of disturbed eating attitudes must be encouraged.

Specifically, school health educators and school health service personnel might be of great help in providing the students with the possibility of dealing with the matter at the class level, in encouraging adolescents to recognize their uneasiness and openly communicate it, to teach them a critical way of "reading" the mass media messages, to address them with basic nutrition information, to explain the risks of a restricted caloric intake as well as the benefits of a well-balanced diet meeting energy needs for growth and development.

School is certainly the privileged environment to recognize the problem for early diagnosis and easy resolution, but it is above all the most suited place to provide adolescents with sound foundations for their adult being and self-esteem building, so that they might become aware of their potentialities as well as of the pressure constantly exerted on them by the prevailing culture. Besides, we firmly believe that any specific preventive actions to be held in the school context, must be extended to the population of primary and lower secondary schools. Although the incidence of eating disturbances reaches its highest peak in puberty, certain attitudes towards food as well as the way of perceiving one's body self-image are consolidated at an earlier age [15]. The current survey was based on self-reported weight and height assessments, which can be seen as a limitation, which might translate in a lower level of accuracy, but this way we avoided long procedures of height and weight measurements with consequent saving of money, time and human resources. In addition, the self-reported method, extensively employed in numerous scientific studies published in the literature was non-invasive [19,20], since it prevented responders with specific weight problems (seriously overweight or underweight) from being subjected to measurements at school. Another limitation is that adolescents suffering from eating disorders tend to deny their condition, which results in under-reporting of abnormal eating patterns [21].

References

[1] Pellai A, Brizzi L, Curci R, Sancini S, Saporetti G, Speich S et al. Valutazione del rischio di disturbi del comportamento alimentare negli adolescenti del Nord Italia. Risultati di uno studio multicentrico. Min Ped 2002;54:139-45.

[2] CDC. Body weight perceptions and selected weight-management goals and practices of high school students, United States 1990. MMWR 1991;40:747-50.

[3] CDC. Youth Risk Behaviour Surveillance, United States 1999. MMWR 2000;49:1-96.

[4] Attie I, Brooks-Gunn J. The development of eating regulation across the life span. In: Cicchetti D, Cohen DJ. Developmental psychopathology. New York, Wiley, 1995:332-68.

[5] Field AE, Cheung L, Wolf AM, Herzog DB, Gortmaker SL, Colditz GA. Exposure to the mass media and wieght concerns among girls, Pediatrics 1999;103:e36.
[6] Tufts University School of Nutrition Science and Policy. Statement on the link between nutrition and cognitive development in children. Boston: Center Hunger Poverty Nutr Policy, 1998.
[7] CDC. Guidelines for school health programs to promote lifelong healthy eating. MMWR 1996;45;RR9.
[8] Tomeo CA, Field AE, Berkey CS, Colditz GA, Fraiser AL. Weight concerns, weight control behaviours, and smoking initiation. Pediatrics 1999;104:918-24.
[9] Pellai A, Marzorati P."Educazione alla salute". Milano: Franco Angeli, 2001.
[10] Kann L, Kinchen SA, William BI, Ross JG, Lowry R, Grunbaum JA et al. Youth Risk Behavior Surveillance. United States, 1999. MMWR CDC Surveill Summ 2000;49:1-32.
[11] Grumbaum JA, Kann L, Kinchen SA, Williams BI, Ross JG., Lowry R et al. Youth Risk Behavior Surveillance. United States, 2001. MMWR CDC Surveill Summ 2002;51:1-62.
[12] Sussman MP, Jones SE, Wilson TW, Kann L. The Youth Risk Behavior Surveillance System: updating policy and program applications. J Sch Health 2002;72:13-7.
[13] Cole TJ, Bellizzi MC, Flegal KM, Dietz WH. Establishing a standard definition for child overweight and obesity worldwide: international survey. BMJ 2000;320:1240-3.
[14] Cacciari E, Milani S, Balsamo A, Dammacco F, De Luca F, Chiarelli F, et al. Italian cross-sectional growth charts for height, weight and BMI (6-20 y). Eur J Clin Nutr 2002;56:171-80.
[15] Saporetti G, Sancini S, Bassoli L, Castelli B, Pellai A. Analisi del rischio per i disturbi del comportamento alimentare in una scuola media superiore: una ricerca basata sull'Eating Attitudes Test 26. Min Ped 2004;56:83-90.
[16] Bryant-Waugh R, Lask B. Childhood-onset eating disorders. In: Brownell KD, Faiburn CG, eds. Eating disorders and obesity: a comprehensive handbook. New York: Guilford, 1995.
[17] Nelson WL, Hughes HM, Katz B, Searight HR. Anorexic eating attitudes and behaviors of male and female college students. Adolescence 1999;34:621-33.
[18] Mellin LM. Responding to desordered eating in children and adolescents. Nutr News 1988; 51:5-7.
[19] Goodman E, Hinden BR, Khandelwal S. Accuracy of teen and parental reports of obesity and body mass index. Pediatrics 2000;106:52-8.
[20] Taylor CB, Sharpe T, Shisslak C, Bryson S, Estes LS, Gray N, McKnight KM, Crago M, Kraemer HC, Killen JD. Factors associated with weight concerns in adolescent girls. Int J Eat Disord 1998;24:31-42.
[21] Johnson-Sabine E, Wood K, Patton G, Mann A, Wakeling A. Abnormal eating attitudes in London schoolgirls – A prospective epidemiological study: factors associated with abnormal response on screening questionnaires. Psychol Med 1988;18:615-22.

VIII. Treatment Aspects

In: Obesity and Adolescence: A Public Health Concern
Editors: H.A. Omar, D.E. Greydanus et al.
ISBN: 978-1-60692-821-9

Chapter XXIII

Adolescent Obesity and Bariatric Surgery

Tara B. Mancl and Alan A. Saber*

Minimally Invasive Surgery, Bariatric Surgery and Surgery Program, Michigan State University College of Human Medicine, MSU/Kalamazoo Center for Medical Studies, Kalamazoo, Michigan, United States of America

Abstract

Obesity is the most prevalent metabolic disorder in the United States with adolescents and children being the fastest growing segment of the population affected by this disorder. The initial management of obesity entails modification of diet and exercise as well as a trial of medications. Unfortunately, this usually has unsatisfactory results; as a result, bariatric surgery has been used in the adult population and seems to offer improved long term results. Because the results have been quite favorable in the adult population, specialists are also looking at bariatric surgery for the adolescent population. This appears to be a safe approach in conjunction with diet and exercise and it offers improved long term results. This article discusses the use of bariatric surgery in obese adolescents.

* Corrrespondence: Alan A Saber, MD, FACS, Associate Professor of Surgery, Michigan State University College of Human Medicine, Chief, Minimally Invasive Surgery & Bariatric Surgery, Surgery Program, MSU/Kalamazoo Center for Medical Studies, 1000 Oakland Drive, Kalamazoo MI 49008-1284 United States. Tel: 269-337-6230; Fax: 269-337-6441; E-mail: Aasabe@kcms.msu.edu

Introduction

Obesity is the most prevalent metabolic disorder in the United States, with children and adolescents being the fastest growing affected segment of the population [1]. The prevalence of obesity has steadily trended upward over the past three decades; approximately two-thirds of adults in the United States are overweight and one-third are obese [2]. This trend is paralleled in the child and adolescent population with an estimated 25% of children being overweight or obese, a percentage which has doubled over the last 30 years [3]. Up to 77% of obese children grow up to be obese adults [1]. There are also differences noted in incidence of obesity among different racial and ethnic groups; the percentage of childhood obesity tends to be higher in the Hispanic and African American communities [4,5]. The epidemic of childhood obesity is not limited to the United States; for example, childhood obesity is also increasing in China, among other countries [6]. Definition, risk factors, consequences, and non-surgical management of obesity in adolescents are reviewed elsewhere in this journal issue. This discussion focuses on bariatric surgery.

Bariatric surgery has proven to be effective in adults with morbid obesity in both the improvement of long term weight management as well as improvement or resolution of medical comorbid conditions [7]. Given these results, bariatric surgery is becoming increasingly popular in the obese adolescent population. The number of bariatric procedures in adolescents increased five-fold between 1997 and 2003 [8]. In 2003, approximately 1,000 adolescents underwent bariatric surgery; this, however, represents a small percentage of the total number of bariatric procedures that are performed [9]. The long term follow-up of adolescent patients undergoing bariatric surgery is limited, and thus, this is an area in which additional research is necessary [10,11].

Bariatric Surgery

The literature regarding bariatric surgery in adolescents is sparse. (see table 1). Most studies have a sample size of 50 patients or less and there are limited retrospective studies prior to 2000 [9]. In 1991, the NIH developed criteria for weight loss surgery in adults; however, the upper and lower limits of age remain an area of controversy and currently guidelines do not exist for the age group of under age eighteen. In adults, a patient with a BMI >40 without medical comorbidities, or BMI > 35 with comorbidities, who has failed multiple nonsurgical efforts, meets the guidelines for operative intervention [9]. A recent task force has been created by the American Pediatric Surgery Association to look at this issue in children and to address whether these patients, given already increased rates of rebellion and noncompliance, will have similar outcomes to adults [8]. Early studies show that bariatric surgery in adolescents appears to have acceptable results and appears to be the only successful long lasting method for reliable weight loss in severely obese adolescents [12].

A unique feature to consider in adolescents is the attainment of linear growth and physiologic maturity. For adolescents who have reached a majority of their linear growth, there is little reason to suspect that bariatric surgery will adversely affect growth. Girls achieve this usually by age 13, and boys usually achieve this by age 15 years. Girls usually have reached physiologic maturity approximately two years after menarche. Measures to detect physiologic maturity include bone age with nomograms to help determine the appropriate age for bariatric surgery [13].

The rationale for bariatric surgery in adolescents is to prevent or alter the adverse health consequences. The current indications for bariatric surgery as endorsed by the American Pediatric Surgical Association, include: failure of at least six months of organized, medically supervised weight loss attempts, and attained physiologic maturity; severe obesity (BMI >40) with comorbidities or BMI >50; commitment to psychologic and medical evaluation; avoidance of pregnancy for 1 year postoperatively; capability of adhering to nutrition guidelines; and demonstration of adequate decisional capacity and supportive family environment [9].

Contraindications to bariatric surgery include substance abuse, psychiatric diagnosis that would make adherence to postoperative diet and medications difficult, medical causes of obesity, unwillingness to comprehend surgical procedures as well as medical consequences, and refusal to participate in lifelong medical surveillance [9]. Offering bariatric surgery based on severe obesity with resultant comorbidities, however, may lead to higher complication rates and less weight loss. The American Society of Bariatric Surgery does not support a strict BMI cutoff of 40 for obese adolescents and promotes bariatric surgery earlier without the need for pre-existing comorbidities and currently supports the same criteria used for morbidly obese adults [11].

The two most common procedures performed in the adolescent population are adjustable gastric banding and gastric bypass. The placement of the adjustable gastric band is performed by creating a small gastric pouch by placing a silastic constricting belt around the upper part of the stomach, with an internal balloon connected to a reservoir placed subcutaneously to allow for adjustments (see figure 1)[14]. The Roux-en-Y gastric bypass is performed by creating a small proximal gastric pouch of about 20 cc, which emptied into a portion of the jejunum in a Roux En Y fashion (see figure 2)[14].

Gastric bypass surgery has multiple weight loss mechanisms. There is a restrictive element from the creation of a small gastric pouch to decrease food intake; there is also a malabsorptive element from the decreased absorption of free fatty acids, vitamins, and minerals. This is particularly relevant in females who wish to get pregnant later in life, as malabsorption is detrimental to fetal growth. Postoperative bariatric patients are at increased risk for malnutrition and require lifelong surveillance for nutritional deficiencies. Current guidelines recommend two chewable vitamins with supplemental calcium and iron for menstruating females.

Outcomes

The mortality rate after placing the gastric band is 0.1%. Gastric perforation is a complication occurring about 0.2%-3.5% in the adult population and the rates are based on a learning curve. Stomach slippage is a common complication as well as stomach obstruction, occurring in about 10%. Erosion and gastric necrosis are also possible complications, but occur in less than 1% [14]. The complications after gastric bypass occur in about 10% of cases.

Anastomotic leak is the most concerning complication; imaging in this situation is difficult and early operative exploration is often the best way to manage this clinical scenario [14].

Limited data exists about the outcomes of bariatric surgery in adolescents. Limited experience suggests that thus far, bariatric surgery is safe and effective. Tsai recently reported complications among adolescent and adult populations as similar in bariatric surgery patients [15]. The most complications included death, wound infection and dehiscence, incisional hernias, abscess, and stomal stenosis. Schilling et al reviewed the KID (Kids Inpatient Database) and found that the most commonly performed procedure among adolescents is the gastric bypass procedure. The adjustable band is second most commonly performed procedure in children; it, however, is currently not approved by the FDA for adolescents under the age of 18 years and insurance carriers do not usually cover this procedure [8].

However there are current debates comparing gastric bypass versus adjustable banding [8]. Favorable arguments for the Lap Band include potential reversibility, potential avoidance of nutritional defects, and low incidence of morbidity and mortality [8]. The concern for placing a laparoscopic adjustable band is the lack of long-term outcomes, the concerns for the longevity of the device, and concerns for high failure and reoperative rate [8]. According to Schilling's study, the average age of adolescent patients undergoing bariatric procedures was 16 years of age, with no one under age 12 years [8]. The majority of patients were female. Most patients report an improved quality of life and a significant psychosocial impact. No studies have indicated an adverse impact on physical or sexual maturation.

Conclusions

The trends in bariatric surgery in the adolescent population appear to have favorable outcomes, although large randomized, prospective trials are nonexistent. The unique features of the adolescent population suggest that bariatric surgery in this population should be performed at centers that specialize in bariatric surgery. As more patients undergo this procedure, more long term data will be available, but at present, bariatric surgery seems to offer the best long term results for weight loss.

References

[1] De Silva NK, Helmrath MA, Klish WJ. Obesity in the adolescent female. J Pediatr Adolesc Gynecol 2007;20(3):207-13.

[2] Flegal KM, Carroll MD, Ogden CL, Johnson CL. Prevalence and trends in obesity among US adults, 1999-2000. JAMA 2002; 288(14):1723-7.

[3] Wang Y. Cross-national comparison of childhood obesity: the epidemic and the relationship between obesity and socioeconomic status. Int J Epidemiol 2001;30(5):1129-36.

[4] Ogden CL, Carroll MD, Curtin LR, McDowell MA, et al. Prevalence of overweight and obesity in the United States, 1999-2004. JAMA 2006;295(13):1549-55.

[5] 5.Dwyer JT, Stone EJ, Yang M, et al. Prevalence of marked overweight and obesity in a multiethnic pediatric population: findings from the Child and Adolescent Trial for Cardiovascular Health (CATCH) study. J Am Diet Assoc 2000; 100(10):1149-56.
[6] Luo J, Hu FB. Time trends of obesity in pre-school children in China from 1989 to 1997. Int J Obes Relat Metab Disord 2002; 26(4):553-8.
[7] 7.Buchwald H, Avidor Y, Braunwald E, et al. Bariatric surgery: a systematic review and meta-analysis. JAMA. 2004; 292(14):1724-37.
[8] Schilling PL, Davis MM, Albanese CT, et al. National trends in adolescent bariatric surgical procedures and implications for surgical centers of excellence. J Am Coll Surg 2008;206(1):1-12.
[9] Xanthakos SA, Daniels SR, Inge TH. Bariatric surgery in adolescents: an update. Adolesc Med Clin 2006;17(3):589-612.
[10] Helmrath MA, Brandt ML, Inge TH. Adolescent obesity and bariatric surgery. Surg Clin North Am 2006;86(2):441-54.
[11] Kane TD, Garcia VF, Inge TH. Bariatric Surgery in Adolescents. In: Schauer PR, Brethauer S, Schirmer BD, eds. Minimally invasive bariatric surgery. New York: Springer, 2007:419-27.
[12] Inge TH, Krebs NF, Garcia VF, et al. Bariatric surgery for severely overweight adolescents: concerns and recommendations. Pediatrics. 2004;114(1):217-23.
[13] Inge TH, Zeller M, Garcia VF, Daniels SR. Surgical approach to adolescent obesity. Adolesc Med Clin 2004;15(3):429-53.
[14] Pories WJ. Bariatric Surgery. In: Fischer JE, Bland KI, Callery MP, et al, eds. Mastery of surgery. Philadelphia, PA: Lippincott Williams Wilkins, 2006.
[15] Tsai WS, Inge TH, Burd RS.Bariatric surgery in adolescents: recent national trends in use and in-hospital outcome.Arch Pediatr Adolesc Med. 2007;161(3):217-21.
[16] Soper RT, Mason EE, Printen KJ, Zellweger H. Gastric bypass for morbid obesity in children and adolescents. J Pediatr Surg 1975; 10(1):51-8.
[17] Anderson AE, Soper RT, Scott DH.Gastric bypass for morbid obesity in children and adolescents.J Pediatr Surg 1980;15(6):876-81.
[18] Rand CS, Macgregor AM. Adolescents having obesity surgery: a 6-year follow-up. South Med J 1994;87(12):1208-13.
[19] Greenstein RJ, Rabner JG.Is Adolescent gastric-restrictive antiobesity surgery warranted? Obes Surg 1995;5(2):138-44.
[20] Strauss RS, Bradley LJ, Brolin RE.Gastric bypass surgery in adolescents with morbid obesity. J Pediatr 2001;138(4):499-504.
[21] Dolan K, Creighton L, Hopkins G, Fielding G.Laparoscopic gastric banding in morbidly obese adolescents. Obes Surg 2003;13(1):101-4.
[22] Sugerman HJ, Sugerman EL, DeMaria EJ, et al. Bariatric surgery for severely obese adolescents. J Gastrointest Surg 2003;7(1):102-8.
[23] Stanford A, Glascock JM, Eid GM, et al. Laparoscopic Roux-en-Y gastric bypass in morbidly obese adolescents. J Pediatr Surg 2003; 38(3):430-3.
[24] Angrisani L, Favretti F, Furbetta F, et al. Obese teenagers treated by Lap-Band System: The Italian experience. Surgery 2005; 138(5):877-81.

[25] Till HK, Muensterer O, Keller A, et al. Laparoscopic sleeve gastrectomy achieves substantial weight loss in an adolescent girl with morbid obesity. Eur J Pediatr Surg 2008;18(1):47-9.

In: Obesity and Adolescence: A Public Health Concern
Editors: H.A. Omar, D.E. Greydanus et al.
ISBN: 978-1-60692-821-9

Chapter XXIV

Obesity and Pharmacotherapy

Donald E. Greydanus**, *Cynthia Feucht and Dilip R. Patel
Pediatrics and Human Development, Michigan State University College of Human Medicine and Ferris State University College of Pharmacy, Michigan State University/Kalamazoo Center for Medical Studies,
Kalamazoo, Michigan, United States of America

Abstract

This chapter reviews various medications currently used and being studied for weight loss induction in adults and adolescents. The search for medication to induce weight loss was stimulated by the US FDA's 1959 approval of phentermine, a sympathomimetic amine, for short-term weight loss despite limited research supporting its claims of causing weight loss. In addition to noradrenergic products like phentermine, other reviewed medications include herbal products (such as Korean herbal formula based on Taeumjowi-tang), sibutramine (mixed noradrenergic-serotonergic chemical), orlistat (lipase inhibitor), metformin (biguanide), rimonabant (CB1-selective cannabinoid receptor antagonist), and others. Only two non-amphetamine-related medications are FDA-approved for adolescents: sibutramine for those 16 years of age and older, and orlistat for those 12 years of age and older. Pharmacotherapy for morbidly obese adolescents should only be used as part of a comprehensive weight loss program that involves diet, exercise, and behavioral modification. The side effects of these products should always be considered as well as the potential for serious adverse events.

* Correspondence: Donald E. Greydanus, MD, Professor, Pediatrics and Human Development, Michigan State University College of Human Medicine, Pediatrics Program Director, Michigan State University/Kalamazoo Center for Medical Studies, Kalamazoo, MI 49008-1284 United States. Tel: 269-337-6450; Fax: 269-337-6474; E-mail: Greydanus@kcms.msu.edu

Introduction

Obesity has become a well-known concern among children, adolescents, and adults throughout the world [1-10]. Pharmacotherapy has been shown to be effective in the treatment of obesity in some adults, however, their use in most youth is often limited at this time to those in research protocols [5,11-21]. The actual safety, effectiveness, and long-term consequences of these medications for obese youth are unknown at this time [2]. The use of anti-obesity medication should be in association with a comprehensive weight reduction program that emphasizes behavioral modification, appropriate diet, and an exercise program [15,22-28].

Pharmacologic management is typically used in obese youth when changes in lifestyle have not worked, medical complications have developed (i.e., hypertension, obstructive sleep apnea, others) and before bariatric surgery is offered [3,7,15,21,28,29]. Weight loss is usually modest, from 2 to 10 kilograms, and usually noted in the first six months of use. Only two non-amphetamine-related antiobesity agents, sibutramine and orlistat, are US Food and Drug Administration (FDA) approved for use under the age of 18: sibutramine for those ≥ 16 years of age and orlistat for those ≥ 12 years of age [5,6]. This article reviews various medications used in the management of adolescent obesity.

Over-the Counter (OTC) Herbal Agents

Various forms of phenylpropanolamine, caffeine, and ephedrine are adrenergic medications which have been used as "weight-loss drugs." They have limited, if any real benefit and with their cardiovascular risk profile, they should be avoided [2,5,30]. Phenylpropanolamine (PPA) is from the phenethylamine family of drugs and has been used as a decongestant and appetite suppressant. On November 6, 2000, the US Food and Drug Administration (FDA) issued a public health advisory against PPA because of increased risk of hemorrhagic cerebrovascular accidents in 18 to 49 year old female users and requested manufacturers to stop marketing products containing PPA [31]. The FDA noted that the risk was low but the event itself was extremely serious.

Yoo and associates from Korea have advocated the short-term effectiveness and safety of a traditional Korean herbal formula (based on Taeumjowi-tang) in children (average age of 11 years)[32]. Korean herbal formula is the most popular herbal weight loss product in Korea advocated for use in obese youth and adults [32]. It consists of a mixture of various seeds, stalks, berries, nuts, and roots as listed in table 1. One of its ingredients is Ephedra sinica (species of ephedra or Ma Huang) that contains alkaloids of ephedrine and pseudoephedrine.

Other herbal or supplement products contained ephedrine (from Ma Huang) and caffeine (from green tea, kola nut or guarana). Ephedrine has been related to reports of sudden death along with some abuse potential. In 1997 the FDA warned against the use of herbal "Phen-Fen" (ephedra and Hypericum perforatum)[33]. More than 800 adverse events related to ephedra had already been reported [33]. In 2001, it was demonstrated that ephedra accounted for 64% of all adverse reactions communicated to poison control centers in relation to herbal products [33]. On April 12, 2004, the FDA banned over-the-counter dietary supplements with ephedrine alkaloids (ephedra)[33]. With the ban on ephedra products, many supplements changed their products to be ephedra-free, utilizing a variety of herbal supplements including caffeine and Citrus aurantium (bitter orange). Other herbal products used without proof of weight loss efficacy and safety include chromium picolinate, chitosan, l-carnitine, Yerba mate, Hoodia, Garcinia cambogia and others [2,5,7,34].

Noradrenergic Products

Amphetamines can lower weight, but lead to severe cardiac and mental health problems, including addiction. They are neither recommended nor approved for use as weight loss products. A number of noradrenergic medications have been tried, and phentermine emerged after receiving FDA approval in 1959 as an appetite suppressing drug. There are limited studies noting the efficacy of this sympathomimetic amine and it has limited use in adolescents because of its Schedule IV DEA classification, its potential for addiction, its structure and side effects being similar to amphetamine, and the lack of evidence for safety and long-tem efficacy. Its link with "Fen-Phen" as noted elsewhere, has led to its reduced use as a weight loss agent, certainly in adolescents.

Table 1. Components of the Korean formula based on taeumjowi-tang

1. Seeds
   a. Coix lacryma-jobi (Job's tears; also found in the US)
   b. Raphanus sativus (Japanese radish also found in the US)
   c. Pinus koraiensis (Korean pine found in parts of Asia)
2. Stalks (Ephedra sinica) (see text)
3. Berries (Schisandra chinensis; woody vine with clusters of red berries found in China, Russia, and Korea)
4. Nuts (Castanea crenata) (Japanese or Chinese chestnut)
5. Roots
   a. Liriope platyphylla (flowering plant in Asia, especially China)
   b. Acorus calamus (plant called "Sweet Flag" found in North America, Europe, and Asia; many medicinal uses claimed)
   c. Pelargonium grandiflorum (Andrews) (large flowery, shrubby plant that is native to South Africa and is a popular house plant)

Several phentermine products are available including Adipex P® and Ionamin®. It is recommended for those individuals with a BMI > 30 kg/m2 or > 27 kg/m2 in the presence of other risk factors such as hypertension, diabetes mellitus, etc. These should only be used for short-term (up to 12 weeks) in those > 16 years of age and in combination with other weight loss measures (such as diet and exercise plans).

Other schedule III noradrenergic drugs approved by the FDA for short-term use to induce weight loss include benzphetamine (Didrex®), and phendimetrazine (Bontril®).2 Diethylpropion (Tenuate®) is a schedule IV noradrenergic agent also FDA-approved for short-term weight loss in adults [17]. Benzphetamine is FDA-approved in adolescents ≥ 12 years of age and diethylpropion in adolescents >16 years of age; both are for short-term use only. These sympathomimetic amines have many side effects including cardiovascular (hypertension, valvular disease), gastrointestinal (diarrhea, constipation, nausea), and sleep dysfunction (insomnia, restlessness).7 Noradrenergic products should be avoided in individuals with cardiovascular disease, moderate to severe hypertension, pulmonary hypertension, hyperthyroidism, and patients with a history of drug abuse.

Serotoninergic Agents

Serotoninergic medications stimulate the release of serotonin from nerve endings, inhibit serotonin reuptake or do both. The result is enhanced serotonin effect at the postsynaptic nerve endings of the brain. Fenfluramine was noted to decrease hunger (and satiety), decrease carbohydrate craving, and decrease binging. Historically, it was marked as Pondimin® (mixed dextro- and levo-fenfluramine) as well as Redux® (dexfenfluramine).

The popular "Phen-Fen" diet (phentermine and fenfluramine) had great success at weight loss with sustained benefit seen up to 3 ½ years with continued use, but discontinuation of the medication was frequently associated with a relapse in weight [2,22]. Therefore, these drugs were used for longer periods of time in the 1990s, and at least in some studies, were associated with cardiac valvulopathy. The FDA withdrew fenfluramine from the market on September 15, 1997 due to findings indicating 30% of patients taking these products had abnormal echocardiograms despite no symptoms [35]. Significantly, fenfluramine and dexfenfluramine have both been associated with pulmonary hypertension, albeit rare. The FDA did not request that phentermine be removed from the market.

Mixed Noradrehergic-Serotonergic Product

The FDA (Food and Drug Administration) has approved the use of sibutramine (Meridia) for the treatment of obesity in adults [17,20,36,37]. Sibutramine (DEA Schedule IV) inhibits the reuptake of norepinephrine, serotonin, and to some degree dopamine, thus, it increases the concentrations of these neurotransmitters in the brain resulting in such effects as reduced appetite. This centrally-acting drug appears to be well-tolerated in most adult patients with a 5% to 10% loss of initial body weight in adults that is sustained in 8 of 10 research studies [5]. However, a dose-related increase in heart rate and blood pressure has been described which can be of clinical significance in some patients [20,37-40]. No valvulopathy has been demonstrated to date. It is given as a dose of 10 mg (5 mg to 15 mg) per day and can be given for up to 2 years.

Research has noted limited weight loss in adolescents (average of 3 kilograms more than controls and reduction of body mass index up to 5.6 kg/m^2) but not beyond six months of use [4,14,20,26-28,38-41]. The FDA has approved sibutramine for weight loss management in patients 16 years of age and older [6]. Research has also noted that sibutramine can be of benefit for children with hypothalamic obesity and exogenous obesity [42]. Side effects and contraindications for use of sibutramine are listed in table 2. There is the potential for drug interactions since sibutramine is metabolized by cytochrome P450 3A4 substrate. Caution should be utilized when combining with agents that can increase the effect of sibutramine (i.e. clarithromycin, nefazadone, verapamil) or decrease the effect of sibutramine (i.e. phenytoin, carbamazepine, rifampin).

Lipase Inhibitor

Orlistat (Xenical) is an inhibitor of lipase (gastric and pancreatic) and has been effective in decreasing weight in clinical trials of adults and adolescents by inducing a dose-dependent fat malabsorption [5,14,17,20,25,43,44]. It blocks about 30% of dietary fat with the 120 mg prescription and 25% with the 60 mg dose [44,45] and can be used in adolescents as well as adults [15,25]. Orlistat can also induce improved lipid levels, glucose levels, insulin sensitivity, and blood pressure [5,15,45]. In a 16 week trial of adults receiving orlistat in combination with a low fat, reduced calorie diet , the orlistat group lost 1.15 kg more than those in the placebo group [46]. In addition, a reduction in BMI up to 4.09 kg/m2 has also been observed [20]. In contrast, some research notes no benefit for this drug in obese adolescents [47]. The FDA has approved its sale as an over-the-counter drug (Alli®) at half the prescription dose for weight loss with the appropriate dieting measures [44].

Orlistat can lead to gastric upset, dyspepsia, abdominal pain, flatulence, steatorrhea, malabsorption, fecal urgency, fecal incontinence, and reduced absorption of fat-soluble vitamins (A, D, E, and K)[7,44,48]. Orlistat (Xenical®) is given in a dosage of 120 mg three times a day with meals. A multivitamin containing fat soluble vitamins should be given daily and at least 2 hours before or after taking orlistat. It was approved by the FDA in 2003 for use in weight management of obese youth ≥12 years of age [6]. However, its side effects have led to its limited acceptance by youth. The effects of orlistat on growing youth is unknown [6]. It is contraindicated in individuals with chronic malabsorption syndrome and cholestasis. It can increase warfarin's anticoagulant effect due to decreased absorption of vitamin K and may interfere with the absorption of various drugs [46].

Another drug, Acarbose (Precose®), inhibits pancreatic alpha-amylase and intestinal alpha-glucoside hydrolase. This results in a delay of ingested carbohydrates leading to reduced postprandial blood glucose concentrations. It can be helpful for obese children and adolescents with evidence of hyperinsulinemia and is used to treat type 2 diabetes mellitus. Side effects include gastrointestinal upset, flatulence, diarrhea, and symptomatic lowering of blood glucose, when used in combination with a sulfonylurea or insulin. It is initiated at an oral dose of 25 mg three times a day with meals and gradually increased as tolerated. Adult maintenance doses are 50 to 100 mg three times daily.

Table 2. Side effects and contraindications for Sibutramine (Meridia)

A. Side effects

1. Dry mouth
2. Headache
3. Dizziness
4. Insomnia
5. Anxiety
6. Depression
7. Suicidality
8. Nausea
9. Constipation
10. Asthenia
11. Increase in pulse (usually minor)
12. Increase in blood pressure (usually minor)

B. Contraindications

1. Avoid in selected heart disease patients
2. Avoid in patients with poorly controlled hypertension
3. Avoid in patients with severe renal or hepatic dysfunction
4. Avoid in patients with a history of substance abuse
5. Avoid in patients with narrow-angle glaucoma
6. Do not use during or within 2 weeks of monoamine oxidase inhibitors (MAOIs)
7. Do not use with serotonergic agents (SSRIs, triptans, tramadol)
8. Do not use in patients with anorexia or bulimia

Metformin

Metformin (Glucophage, Glumetza, Fortamet, Riomet) is a biguanide that is a glucose-sensitizing drug and has been FDA-approved since 1994 to treat type 2 diabetes mellitus. It increases the sensitivity of various tissues (muscle, liver, fat) to the uptake and action of insulin. It reduces hepatic gluconeogenesis as well as improving cell membrane movement of glucose in tissues (adipose tissue and skeletal muscle)[5]. It has also been used to treat polycystic ovary syndrome (PCOS) which is associated with hyperinsulinemia and hyperandrogenism. Metformin acts to improve insulin sensitivity by reducing insulin levels and decreasing symptoms associated with PCOS [49-51]. In PCOS it may lead to better regularity of menstrual cycles, lower levels of androgens, and improved ovulation [49]. Ovulation may also improve because of reduction in weight.

Metformin has been used to treat adults with morbid obesity as well as the metabolic syndrome and can also promote weight loss in non-obese individuals [5,7,52]. In a trial of 9 to 18 year old males in Australia, 1 gram of metformin twice a day resulted in an average weight loss over six months of 4.35 kg [53]. The dose in adolescents (10-16 yrs) is 500 mg twice a day and if treating diabetes mellitus type 2, increase the dose by 500 mg a week to a maximum of 2 grams per day. Side effects (seec table 3), often dose-related, tend to improve with time. One in every 30,000 patients on metformin develops lactic acidosis with a 50% mortality rate and occurrence is more common in patients with renal insufficiency. Though metformin offers some promise for use in overweight adolescents, more research is needed [20,29,52].

Table 3. Side effects and contraindications for metformin (Glucophage, others)

A. Side effects

1. Nausea
2. Emesis
3. Indigestion
4. Abdominal discomfort
5. Flatulence
6. Diarrhea
7. Lactic acidosis
8. Malabsorption of vitamine B12

B. Contraindications

1. Avoid in patients with renal insufficiency (Scr >1.5 mg/dl in men and 1.4 mg/dl in women)
2. Avoid in patients with congestive heart failure requiring pharmacologic management
3. Avoid in patients with liver disease or hypoxia
4. Avoid in patients who are critically ill

Rimonabant

Rimonabant is a new drug that is a CB1-selective cannabinoid receptor antagonist/inverse agonist and is used in Europe as part of a diet and exercise plan for management of obesity in adults [7,21,54,55]. It has also been used and studied in different countries as a smoking cessation product and for management of other addictions [56,57]. It leads to a dose-dependent decrease in appetite, decrease in triglycerides, and an increase in HDL level with no impact on LDL levels [58].

In February, 2006 rimonabant received an approval letter from the FDA for obesity management in adults but not for smoking cessation due to concerns over safety. The endocannabinoids are important modulators during stress conditions as well as in anxiety, phobias, depression, and posttraumatic stress disorder [58]. Concern has been raised over possible worsening for depression and suicidality with a noted relative risk of 1.5-2.5 for psychiatric events in the four Rimonabant in Obesity trials.58 On June 13, 2007, the FDA Endocrinologic and Metabolic Drugs Advisory Committee voted unanimously to not approve rimonabant for obesity due to high risk of serious psychiatric effects, high drop-out rates from the studies, and need for more long-term data [58]. Further research is needed to clarify these ongoing issues.

Other Medications

A number of medications (see table 4) have been studied but not proven to be effective and/or safe for adults or adolescents with obesity. Fluoxetine (Prozac) is an antidepressant medication (selective serotonin reuptake inhibitor) with apparently limited weight loss results [59]. Other antidepessants that have been used because of their anorexic effects include sertraline (Zoloft) and bupropion (Wellbutrin) (see table 4). However, SSRIs and bupropion are approved for use in the treatment of depression and other mental health disorders in adults but not for obesity [2,60]. A number of anticonvulsants (i.e., topiramate, zonisamide) have been studied in research protocols and used off-label for obesity in adults due to their appetite-suppressing effects [17]. Octreotide is a somatostatin receptor analog that has been shown to cause weight loss in pediatric patients with hypothalamic obesity [7].

Table 4. Medications or chemicals studied but not proven benefical or safe in obesity treatment

1. Bupropion (antidepressant)
2. Cholecystokinin
3. Ciliary neurotrophic factor
4. Glucagon-like peptide-1 (exenatide)
5. Leptin (neuropeptide produced by adipose tissue)
6. Neuropeptide Y
7. Selective Serotonin Reuptake Inhibitors (SSRIs: fluoxetine, sertraline)
8. Somatostatin receptor analog: octreotide (for hypothalamic obesity)
9. Synthetic ß-3 agonists
10. Topiramate (anticonvulsant)
11. Zonisamide (anticonvulsant)

Conclusions

Pharmacologic therapy of obesity is recommended only in conjunction with a comprehensive weight loss program that involves diet, exercise, and behavioral modification. The sympathomimetic amine, phentermine, was the first FDA approved product for short-term weight loss in adults in 1959. Since then, other amines with FDA-approval for short-term use in adults include benzphetamine, phendimetrazine, and diethylpropion. The only products that are FDA-approved for long-term use in obese adults are sibutramine (mixed noradrenergic-serotonergic product) and orlistat (lipase inhibitor). Sibutramine is FDA approved for adolescents as young as 16 years of age and orlistat is FDA approved down to 12 years of age.

Other drugs under research for use in obese adults include metformin (a biguanide used to treat diabetes mellitus type 2 and the metabolic syndrome in adolescents as well as adults), rimonabant (a CB1-selective cannabinoid receptor antagonist), and select antidepressants as well as select anticonvulsants with appetite-suppressant effects (see table 3). Attention to the potential side effects of these products is important to consider. Long-term safety of these drugs remains unknown and awaits future research to elucidate. Herbal products have long been popular for weight loss and while ephedra is no longer available, many products now contain caffeine, Citrus aurantium, and a variety of other supplements and herbs. A lack of standardization, supportive research, and the potential for side effects make these products less than desirable as a treatment alternative.

References

[1] Reddy V. Eating disorders in Children and Adolescents. In: Greydanus DE, Patel DE, Pratt HD, eds. Behavioral pediatrics, 3rd ed. New York: Novo Sci, 2009, in press.

[2] Yanovski SZ, Yanovski JA. Obesity. N Engl J Med 2002;346(8): 591-602.

[3] Kirk S, Scott BJ, Daniels SR. Pediatric obesity epidemic: treatment options. J Am Diet Assoc 2005;105(5 Suppl 1):S44-S51.

[4] Godoy-Matos A, Carraro L, Vieira A, et al. Treatment of obese adolescents with sibutramine: a randomized, double-blind, controlled study. J Clin Endocrinol Metab 2005;90:1460-5.

[5] Rowlett JR. Obesity in the adolescent. In: Greydanus DE, Patel DE, Pratt HD, eds. Essential adolescent medicine. New York: McGraw-Hill Med Publ, 2006:651-65.

[6] Barlow SE, et al. Expert committee recommendations regarding prevention, assessment, and treatment of child and adolescent overweight and obesity: Summary report. Pediatrics 2007;120 (Suppl 4): S164-92.

[7] Skelton JA, Rudolph CD. Overweight and obesity. In: Kliegman RM, Behrman RE, Jenson HB, Stanton BF, eds. Nelson textbook of Pediatrics, 18th ed. Philadelphia, PA: Saunders/Elsevier, 2007:232-42.

[8] Eneli I, Davies HD. Epidemiology of childhood obesity. In: Davies HD, ed. Obesity in childhood and adolescence. Westport, CT: Praeger Publishers, 2008:3-23.

[9] Jones KL, Role of obesity in complicating and confusing the diagnosis and treatment of diabetes in children. Pediatrics 2008;121 (2): 361-8.

[10] Kiess W, Boettner A. Obesity in the adolescent. Adolesc Med 2002;13:181-90.

[11] Atkinson RL, Hubbard VS. Report on the NIH workshop on pharmacologic treatment of obesity. Am J Clin Nutr 1994;60 (2):153.

[12] Bray GA, Tartaglia L. Medicinal strategies in the treatment of obesity. Nature 2000;404:672-7.

[13] Jensen MD. Medical management of obesity. Sem Gastrointest Dis 1998;9:156-62.

[14] Freemark M, Kiess W. Anti-obesity medication use in adolescents: risks and benefits. Pediatr Endocrinol Rev 2004;2(Suppl 1):168-70.

[15] McDuffie JR, Calis KA, Uwaifo GI, et al. Efficacy of orlistat as an adjunct to behavioral treatment in overweight African American and Caucasian adolescents with obesity-related co-morbid conditions. J Pediatr Endocrinol Metab 2004;17:307-19.

[16] Molnar D. New drug policy in childhood obesity. Int J Obes (Lond). 2005;29(Suppl 2):S62-5.

[17] Snow V, Barry P, Fitterman N, et al. Pharmacologic and surgical management of obesity in primary care: A clinical practice guideline from the American College of Physicians. Ann Intern Med 2005; 142:525-31.

[18] Joffe A. Pharmacotherapy for adolescent obesity: a weighty issue. JAMA 2005; 293:2932-4.

[19] Lean M, Finer N: ABC of obesity. Management: part II—drugs. BMJ 2006;333:794-7.

[20] Dunican KC, Desilets AR, Montalbano JK: Pharmacotherapeutic options for overweight adolescents. Ann Pharmacother 2007;41: 1445-55.

[21] Eneli I, Mantinan KD: "Managing the overweight child" In: Obesity in Childhood and Adolescence. Volume 2. Eds: HE Fitzgerald and V Mousouli. Westport, CT: Praeger Publishers, 2008:191-225.

[22] Hofmann AD. Obesity. In: Hofmann AD, Graydanus DE, eds. Adolescent medicine, 3rd ed. Stamford, CT: Appleton Lange, 1997:663-82.

[23] Greydanus DE, Bricker LA, Patel DR. The benefits of sports participation in childhood and adolescence to prevent obesity in adolescents and adults. Asian J Paediatr Pract 2006;9(4):1-7.

[24] Greydanus DE, Bhave S. Obesity in the adolescent. Indian Pediatrics 2004;41(6):545-50.

[25] Chanoine JP, Hampl S, Jensen C, et al. Effect of orlistat on weight and body composition in obese adolescents: a randomized controlled trial. JAMA 2005;293:2873-83.

[26] Berkowitz RI, Wadden TA, Tershakovec, et al. Behavioral therapy and sibutramine for the treatment of adolescent obesity. A randomized controlled trial. JAMA 2003;289:1805-12.

[27] Berkowitz RI, Fujioka K, Daniels SR, et al. Effects of sibutramine treatment in obese adolescents: A randomized trial. Ann Intern Med 2006;145:81-90.

[28] Reisler G, Tauber T, Afriat R, et al. Sibutramine as an adjuvant therapy in adolescents suffering from morbid obesity. Isr Med Assoc J 2006;8:30-2.

[29] Webb E, Viner R. Should metformin be prescribed to overweight adolescents in whom dietary/behavioural modifications have not helped? Arch Dis Child 2006;91:793-4.

[30] Silverstone T. Appetite suppressants. A review. Drugs 1992;43(6):820.

[31] US Food and Drug Administration. Food and drug administration science background safety of phenylpropanolamine. Available from: http://www.fda.gov.cder/drug/infopage/ppa/science.htm

[32] Yoo JH, Lee EJ, Kwak CK, et al. Clinical trial of herbal formula on weight loss in obese Korean children. Am J Chin Med 2005;33:713-22.

[33] Seamon M, Clauson K. Ephedra: yesterday, DSHEA, and tomorrow-a ten year perspective on the dietary supplement health and education act of 1994. J Herbal Pharmacother 2005;5:67-86.

[34] Greydanus DE, Patel DR. Sports doping in the adolescent athlete: The hope, hype, and hyperbole. Pediatric Clin North Am 2002;49: 829-55.

[35] US Food and Drug Administration. FDA announces withdrawal of fenfluramine and dexfenfluramine (Fen-Phen). Available from: http://www.fda.gov/cder/news/phen/fenphenpr81597.htm.

[36] Sibutramine for obesity. Med Lett Dr Ther 1998;40:32.
[37] Early JL, Apovian CM, Aronne LJ, et al. Sibutramine plus meal replacement therapy for body weight loss and maintenance in obese patients. Obesity 2007;15:1464-72.
[38] Violante-Ortiz R, Rel-Rio-Navarro BE, Lara-Esqueda A, et al. Use of sibutramine in obese Hispanic adolescents. Adv Ther 2005;22: 642-9.
[39] Garcia-Morales LM, Berber A, Macias-Lara CC, et al. Use of sibutramine in obese Mexican adolescents: Aa 6 month, randomized, double-blind, placebo-controlled, parallel-group trial. Clin Ther 2006;28:770-82.
[40] Daniels SR, Long B, Crow S, et al. Cardiovascular effects of sibutramine in the treatment of obese adolescents: results of a randomized, double-blind, placebo-controlled study. Pediatrics 2007;120:147-57.
[41] Doggrell SA. Sibutramine for obesity in adolescents. Expert Opin Pharmacother 2006;7:2435-8.
[42] Danielsson P, Janson A, Norgren S, Marcus C. Impact sibutramine therapy in children with hypothalamic obesity or obesity with aggravating syndromes. J Clin Endocrinol Metabol 2007;92:4101-6.
[43] Davidson MH, et al. Weight control and risk factor reduction in obese subjects treated for 2 years with orlistat: A randomized trial. JAMA 1999;281:235-42.
[44] Orlistat OTC for weight loss. Med Lett Drugs Ther 2007;49(1263):49.
[45] Orlistat for obesity. Med Lett Drugs Ther 1999;41(1055):55-6.
[46] Anderson JW. Low-dose orlistat effects on body weight of mildly to moderately overweight individuals: a 16 week, double-blind, placebo-controlled trial. Ann Pharmacother 2006;40:1717.
[47] Maahs D, de Serna DG, Kolotkin RL, et al. Randomized, double-blind, placebo-controlled trial of orlistat for weight loss in adolescents. Endocr Pract 2006;12:18-28.
[48] Ozkan B, Bereket A, Turan S, Keskin S. Addition of orlistat to conventional treatment in adolescents with severe obesity. European J Pediatr 2004;163(12):738-41.
[49] Nestler JE. Metformin for the treatment of polycystic ovary syndrome. N Engl J Med 2008;358(1):47-54.
[50] Hoppin AG, Katz ES, Kaplan LM, Lauwers GY. Case 31-2006: A 15-year-old girl with severe obesity. N Engl J Med 2006;355(15): 1593-1602.
[51] Harborne L, Fleming R, Lyall H, et al. Metformin or antiandrogen in the treatment of hirsutism in polycystic ovary syndrome. J Clin Endocrinol Metabol 2003;88:4116-23.
[52] Freemark M. Pharmacotherapy of childhood obesity: an evidence-based, conceptual approach. Diabetes Care 2007;30:395-402.
[53] Srinivasan S, Ambler GR, Baur LA, et al: Randomized, controlled trial of metformin for obesity and insulin resistance in children and adolescents: Improvement in body composition and fasting insulin. J Clin Endocrinol Metabol 2006;91(6):2074-80.
[54] Pagotto U, Pasquali R: Fighting obesity and associated risk factors by antagonizing cannabinoid type 1 receptors. Lancet 2005;365: 1363-4.
[55] Pi-Sunyer FX, Arrone LJ, Heshmati HM, et al. Effect of rimonabant, a cannabinoid-1-receptor blocker on weight and cardiometabolic risk factors in overweight or obese patients. JAMA 2006;295:761-75.

[56] Huestis MA, Gorelick DA, Heishman SJ, et al. Blockage of effects of smoked marijuana by the CB1-selective cannabinoid receptor antagonist SR141716. Arch Gen Psychiatr 2001;58(4):322-8.

[57] Maldonado R, Valverde O, Berrendero F. Involvement of the endocannabinoid system in drug addiction. Trends Neurosci 2006; 29(4):225-32.

[58] US Food and Drug Administration. FDA Briefing Document; NDA 21-888 (rimonobant). Available from: http://www.fda.gov/ohrms/dockets/ac/07/briefing/2007-4306b1-fda-backgrounder.pdf

[59] Fluoxetine (Prozac) and other drugs for treatment of obesity. Med Lett Drugs Ther 1994;36(936):107.

[60] Greydanus DE, Calles J, Patel DR. Pediatric and adolescent psychopharmacology : A primer for the pediatrician. Cambridge: Cambridge Univ Press, 2008.

IX. Acknowledgments

Chapter XXV

About the Editors

Hatim A Omar, MD, FAAP, Professor of Pediatrics and Obstetrics and Gynecology and Director of the Section of Adolescent Medicine, Department of Pediatrics, University of Kentucky, Lexington. Dr. Omar has completed residency training in obstetrics and gynecology as well as Pediatrics. He has also completed fellowships in vascular physiology and adolescent medicine. He is the recipient of the Commonwealth of Kentucky Governor's Award for Community Service and Volunteerism He is the recipient of the Commonwealth of Kentucky Governer's Award for community service and volunteerism in 2000, KY teen Pregnancy Coalition Award for outstanding service 2002, Awards for suicide prevention from the Ohio Valley Society for Adolescent Medicine and Kentucky Pediatric Society in 2005 and 2007, Sexual Abuse Awareness Month Award for his work with sexual abuse victims from the KY association of sexual assault professionals in 2007, Special Achievement Award from the American Academy of Pediatrics 2007 and the Founders of Adolescent Medicine Award from the AAP in 2007. He is well known internationally with numerous publications in child health, pediatrics, adolescent medicine, pediatric and adolescent gynecology. Email: haomar2@uky.edu
Website: https://weblink.ukhealthcare.uky.edu/weblink/phyPro.do?poid=161106&ofid

Donald E. Greydanus, MD, FAAP, FSAM, FIAP (H) is Professor of Pediatrics and Human Development at Michigan State University College of Human Medicine (East Lansing, Michigan, USA) and Director of the Pediatrics Residency Program at Michigan State University/ Kalamazoo Center for Medical Studies (Kalamazoo, Michigan, USA). Received the 1995 American Academy of Pediatrics' Adele D. Hofmann Award for "Distinquished Contributions in Adolescent Health", the 2000 Mayo Clinic Pediatrics Honored Alumnus Award for "National Contributions to the field of Pediatrics," and the 2003 William B. Weil, Jr., M.D. Endowed Distinguished Pediatric Faculty Award from Michigan State University College of Medicine for "National & International Recognition as well as Exemplary Scholarship in Pediatrics." Received the 2004 Charles R. Drew School of Medicine (Los Angeles, CA) Stellar Award for Contributions to Pediatric Resident Education and awarded an honorary membership in the Indian Academy of Pediatrics—an honor granted to only a few pediatricians outside of India. Was the 2007 Visiting Professor of Pediatrics at Athens

University, Athens, Greece and received the Michigan State University College of Human Medicine Outstanding Community Faculty Award in 2008. Past Chair of the National Conference and Exhibition Planning Group (Committee on Scientific Meetings) of the American Academy of Pediatrics and member of the Pediatric Academic Societies' (SPR/PAS) Planning Committee (1998 to Present). Member of the Appeals Committee for the Pediatrics' Residency Review Committee (RRC) of the Accreditation Council for Graduate Medical Education (Chicago, IL) in both Adolescent Medicine and General Pediatrics. Numerous publications in adolescent health and lectureships in many countries on adolescent health. E-mail: Greydanus@kcms.msu.edu

Dilip R Patel, MD, FAAP, FSAM, FAACPDM, FACSM, is professor in the Department of Pediatrics and Human Development at the Michigan State University College of Human Medicine, East Lansing, Michigan, USA. He is a full time teaching faculty member in the Pediatric Residency Program at the Michigan State University Kalamazoo Center for Medical Studies, Kalamazoo, Michigan, USA. Dr Patel has subspecialty training and interests in neurodevelopmental disabilities, developmental-behavioral pediatrics, adolescent medicine and sports medicine. He has published numerous papers on a wide ranging topics in these areas and has edited several special symposia and books. E-mail: patel@kcms.msu.edu

Joav Merrick, MD, MMedSci, DMSc, is professor of pediatrics, child health and human development affiliated with Kentucky Children's Hospital, University of Kentucky, Lexington, United States and the Zusman Child Development Center, Division of Pediatrics, Soroka University Medical Center, Ben Gurion University, Beer-Sheva, Israel, the medical director of the Division for Mental Retardation, Ministry of Social Affairs, Jerusalem, the founder and director of the National Institute of Child Health and Human Development. Numerous publications in the field of pediatrics, child health and human development, rehabilitation, intellectual disability, disability, health, welfare, abuse, advocacy, quality of life and prevention. Received the Peter Sabroe Child Award for outstanding work on behalf of Danish Children in 1985 and the International LEGO-Prize ("The Children's Nobel Prize") for an extraordinary contribution towards improvement in child welfare and well-being in 1987. E-Mail: jmerrick@internet-zahav.net; Website: www.nichd-israel.com; Home-page: http://jmerrick50.googlepages.com/home

In: Obesity and Adolescence: A Public Health Concern
Editors: H.A. Omar, D.E. Greydanus et al.
ISBN: 978-1-60692-821-9

Chapter XXVI

About the Division of Adolescent Medicine at the University of Kentucky in Lexington, Kentucky, United States

The Division of adolescent medicine was founded in 1998 to provide state of the art care for adolescent patients from all areas of the commonwealth of kentucky, to serve as a state wide resource for education and training for local providers on adolescent issues, to study specisifc factors on the local level affecting youth in the state, to help teach medical students and residents and to provide community service to help improve teen future in the commonwealth.

The division provides comprehensive, holistic team approach to adolescents, where teans receive all aspects for care from mental health to routine care from a team of professionals including physicians, mental health providers, social workers, nutritionists and nursing staff. One unique program within the division is the Young Parent Program, where pregnant teens are cared for throughout pregnancy then they and their babies are cared for together in the program.

The division is active in research with more than 10 peer reviewed articles published each year as well as several books and special journal editions.

In the community, the program has founded several grass route programs to help prevent youth suicide, teen pregnancy, accidental death and substance abuse among adolescents in Kentucky.

The division has provided more than 300 lectures, worshops, media events and teaching for community providers, parents, teachers and school counselors. It also provides adovocacy work on behalf of teens with active work at the state legislative and executive government as well as local governments to help improve the lives of teens.

Collaborations

The division collaborates locally with school boards, youth service centers, state and local goverments, other universities and child advocacy centers as well as with regional adolescent medicine programs.

Internationally with the Institute for Child Health and Human Development in Israel, the Division of Adolescent Medicine at Santa Casa University, Brazil, Quality of Life Research Center and Nordic School of Holistic Health, Copenhagen, Denmark, School of Social Work, Chinese University, Hong Kong.

The Vision

The vision of the Division of Adolescent Medicine is to improve the health and long term wellbeing of Kentucky Youth to grow into productive adults. We also invision global work to help positive youth development world wide.

Target Areas of Interests

The interest areas of the division are all aspects of youth development and adolescent health with focus on prevention and community involvement in colloboration on the local, national and global level with programs having the same goal.

Contact

Hatim Omar, MD, FAAP
Professor of Pediatrics and Obstetrics/Gynecology
Director of Adolescent Medicine & Young Parent programs
J422, Kentucky Clinic
Department of Pediatrics, Kentucky Children's Hospital
University of Kentucky College of Medicine
Lexington, KY 40536
Tel. 859-323-6426 ext. 311
Fax. 859-257-7706
E-mail: haomar2@uky.edu
Website://www.mc.uky.edu/

In: Obesity and Adolescence: A Public Health Concern ISBN: 978-1-60692-821-9
Editors: H.A. Omar, D.E. Greydanus et al.

Chapter XXVII

About the Department of Pediatrics and Human Development, Michigan State University College of Human Medicine, MSU/Kalamazoo Center for Medical Studies, Kalamazoo, Michigan, United States

The Department of Pediatrics and Human Development (PHD) at Michigan State University College of Human Medicine (MSUCHM) was developed in 1968 with the formation of the College of Human Medicine (CHM) at Michigan State University (MSU) in East Lansing, Michigan. It is a nationally-recognized Department of PHD that involves four Michigan State University (MSU) campuses including East Lansing and Kalamazoo, Michigan. Michigan State University/Kalamazoo Center for Medical Studies (MSU/KCMS) is a nationally recognized university/community based residency program with over 170 residents in over 12 disciplines including Pediatrics that is located in Kalamazoo, Michigan, USA.

Mission and Service

The MSUCHM PHD has a unique balance between behavioral science, basic biological research, and clinical pediatrics. The Department has a commitment to a comprehensive approach to the health and development of the child, adolescent, and the family. PHD has a unique blend of community integrated medical training centers with a unified educational mission that serves medical students, pediatric residents, and four communities in Michigan, USA.

The mission is to "advance the healthy development and well being of children and adolescents through innovative medical education, research, clinical care, and advocacy, emphasizing community-based partnerships." To this end, the department offers a broad range of clinical and laboratory services to the children and adolescents of Michigan. PHD draws on the talents of over 100 faculty members and over 500 volunteer teaching faculty members. The mission of the Kalamazoo, Michigan program (MSU/KCMS Pediatrics Program) is to train both medical students in their 3rd and 4th year as well as many residents in the field of Pediatrics. MSU/KCMS Pediatrics is a fully accredited, three year program preparing physicians for board-certification in Pediatrics.

Values of MSU/KCMS include compassionate service, leadership training, commitment to lifelong learning, emphasis on teamwork, and commitment to excellence in health care. Trainees at MSU/KCMS become skilled at providing patient care that is compassionate, appropriate, and effective for the treatment of health problems and the promotion of health. They learn to demonstrate interpersonal and communication skills that result in the effective exchange of information and collaboration with patients, their families, and health professionals. They are taught to develop a commitment to carrying out professional responsibilities and an adherence to ethical principles throughout their training with a goal of these values becoming a lifelong habit that reveals professional compassion, integrity, and respect for others. Kalamazoo is the home of the Kalamazoo Promise, a truly unique program that guarantees college education for students who graduate from the Kalamazoo public schools.

Research Activities

MSU/KCMS has a variety of research projects in adolescent medicine, neurobehavioral pediatrics, adolescent gynecology, pediatric diabetes mellitus, asthma, cystic fibrosis, and pediatric oncology. MSU/KCMS Pediatrics is involved with a number of studies with the Children's Oncology Group in the United States.

MSU/KCMS Pediatrics has recently published a number of medical textbooks: Essential adolescent medicine (McGraw-Hill Medical Publishers), The pediatric diagnostic examination (McGraw-Hill), Pediatric and adolescent psychopharmacology (Cambridge University Press), Behavioral pediatrics, 2nd Edition (iUniverse Publishers in New York and Lincoln, Nebraska), and Pediatric practice: Sports medicine (McGraw-Hill).

MSU/KCMS Pediatrics has edited a number of journal issues published by Elsevier Publishers covering Pulmonology (State of the Art Reviews: Adolescent Medicine—AM:STARS), Genetic disorders in adolescents (AM:STARS), Neurologic/ neurodevelopmental disorders (AM:STARS), Behavioral pediatrics (Pediatric Clinics of North America), Nephrologic disorders in adolescents (AM:STARS), College health (Pediatric Clinics of North America), Adolescent medicine (Primary Care: Clinics in Office Practice), Behavioral pediatrics in children and adolescents (Primary Care: Clinics in Office Practice), and Developmental disabilities (Pediatric Clinics of North America). The Department has also edited a journal issue on musculoskeletal disorders in children and adolescents for the American Academy of Pediatrics' AM:STARS.

The department has developed academic ties with a variety of international medical centers and organizations, including the Queen Elizabeth Hospital in Hong Kong, National Taiwan University Hospital (Taipei, Taiwan), Indian Academy of Pediatrics (New Delhi,

India), and the University of Athens Aghia Sophia Children's Hospital (First and Second Departments of Paediatrics) in Athens, Greece.

Contact

Professor Donald E Greydanus, MD and professor Dilip R. Patel, MD
Pediatrics and Human Development
Michigan State University College of Human Medicine PHD Department
Michigan State University/Kalamazoo Center for Medical Studies
1000 Oakland Drive, Kalamazoo, MI 49008-1284 United States
E-mail: Greydanus@kcms.msu.edu and Patel@kcms.msu.edu
Website: http://www.kcms.msu.edu/ and http://phd.msu.edu/

In: Obesity and Adolescence: A Public Health Concern ISBN: 978-1-60692-821-9
Editors: H.A. Omar, D.E. Greydanus et al.

Chapter XXVIII

About the National Institute of Child Health and Human Development in Israel

The National Institute of Child Health and Human Development (NICHD) in Israel was established in 1998 as a virtual institute under the auspicies of the Medical Director, Ministry of Social Affairs and Social Services in order to function as the research arm for the Office of the Medical Director. In 1998 the National Council for Child Health and Pediatrics, Ministry of Health and in 1999 the Director General and Deputy Director General of the Ministry of Health endorsed the establishment of the NICHD.

Mission

The mission of a National Institute for Child Health and Human Development in Israel is to provide an academic focal point for the scholarly interdisciplinary study of child life, health, public health, welfare, disability, rehabilitation, intellectual disability and related aspects of human development. This mission includes research, teaching, clinical work, information and public service activities in the field of child health and human development.

Service and Academic Activities

Over the years many activities became focused in the south of Israel due to collaboration with various professionals at the Faculty of Health Sciences (FOHS) at the Ben Gurion University of the Negev (BGU). Since 2000 an affiliation with the Zusman Child Development Center at the Pediatric Division of Soroka University Medical Center has resulted in collaboration around the establishment of the Down Syndrome Clinic at that center. In 2002 a full course on "Disability" was established at the Recanati School for Allied Professions in the Community, FOHS, BGU and twice a year seminars for specialists in family medicine. In

2005 collaboration was started with the Primary Care Unit of the faculty and disability became part of the master of public health course on "Children and society". In the academic year 2005-2006 a one semester course on "Aging with disability" was started as part of the master of science program in gerontology in our collaboration with the Center for Multidisciplinary Research in Aging.

Research Activities

The affiliated staff has over the years published work from projects and research activities in this national and international collaboration. In the year 2000 the International Journal of Adolescent Medicine and Health and in 2005 the International Journal on Disability and Human development of Freund Publishing House (London and Tel Aviv), in the year 2003 the TSW-Child Health and Human Development and in 2006 the TSW-Holistic Health and Medicine of the Scientific World Journal (New York and Kirkkonummi, Finland), all peer-reviewed international journals were affiliated with the National Institute of Child Health and Human Development. From 2008 also the International Journal of Child Health and Human Development (Nova Science, New York), the International Journal of Child and Adolescent Health (Nova Science) and the Journal of Pain Management (Nova Science) affiliated.

National Collaboration

Nationally the NICHD works in collaboration with the Faculty of Health Sciences, Ben Gurion University of the Negev; Department of Physical Therapy, Sackler School of Medicine, Tel Aviv University; Autism Center, Assaf HaRofeh Medical Center; National Rett and PKU Centers at Chaim Sheba Medical Center, Tel HaShomer; Department of Physiotherapy, Haifa University; Department of Education, Bar Ilan University, Ramat Gan, Faculty of Social Sciences and Health Sciences; College of Judea and Samaria in Ariel and recently also collaborations has been established with the Division of Pediatrics at Hadassah, Center for Pediatric Chronic Illness, Har HaZofim in Jerusalem.

International Collaboration

Internationally with the Department of Disability and Human Development, College of Applied Health Sciences, University of Illinois at Chicago; Strong Center for Developmental Disabilities, Golisano Children's Hospital at Strong, University of Rochester School of Medicine and Dentistry, New York; Centre on Intellectual Disabilities, University of Albany, New York; Centre for Chronic Disease Prevention and Control, Health Canada, Ottawa; Chandler Medical Center and Children's Hospital, Kentucky Children's Hospital, Section of Adolescent Medicine, University of Kentucky, Lexington; Chronic Disease Prevention and Control Research Center, Baylor College of Medicine, Houston, Texas; Division of

Neuroscience, Department of Psychiatry, Columbia University, New York; Institute for the Study of Disadvantage and Disability, Atlanta; Center for Autism and Related Disorders, Department Psychiatry, Children's Hospital Boston, Boston; Department of Paediatrics, Child Health and Adolescent Medicine, Children's Hospital at Westmead, Westmead, Australia; International Centre for the Study of Occupational and Mental Health, Düsseldorf, Germany; Centre for Advanced Studies in Nursing, Department of General Practice and Primary Care, University of Aberdeen, Aberdeen, United Kingdom; Quality of Life Research Center, Copenhagen, Denmark; Nordic School of Public Health, Gottenburg, Sweden, Scandinavian Institute of Quality of Working Life, Oslo, Norway; Centre for Quality of Life of the Hong Kong Institute of Asia-Pacific Studies and School of Social Work, Chinese University, Hong Kong.

Targets

Our focus is on research, international collaborations, clinical work, teaching and policy in health, disability and human development and to establish the NICHD as a permanent institute at one of the residential care centers for persons with intellectual disability in Israel in order to conduct model research and together with the four university schools of public health/medicine in Israel establish a national master and doctoral program in disability and human development at the institute to secure the next generation of professionals working in this often non-prestigious/low-status field of work. For this project we need your support. We are looking for all kinds of support and eventually an endowment.

Contact

Professor Joav Merrick, MD, MMedSci, DMSc
Medical Director, Division for Mental Retardation
Ministry of Social Affairs, POBox 1260
IL-91012 Jerusalem, Israel
E-mail: jmerrick@zahav.net.il
Website: www.nichd-israel.com;

Index

A

B

C

D

F

G

H

M

N

O

P

Q

R

S

T

U

V